The AIDS Pandemic

D0209934

The collision of epidemiology with political correctness

James Chin MD MPH
Clinical Professor of Epidemiology
School of Public Health, University of California at Berkeley
Formerly, Chief of the Surveillance, Forecasting and Impact Assessment (SFI)
Unit of the Global Programme on AIDS (GPA) of the World Health
Organization (WHO), Geneva, Switzerland

Foreword by

Jeffrey Koplan MD MPH

Radcliffe Publishing
Oxford • Seattle

Radcliffe Publishing Ltd
18 Marcham Road
Abingdon
Oxon OX14 1AA
United Kingdom

www.radcliffe-oxford.com
Electronic catalogue and worldwide online ordering facility.

British Library Cataloguing in Publication Data

A catalogue record for this book is available from the British Library.

ISBN-10 1 84619 118 1
ISBN-13 978 1 84619 118 3

Typeset by Lapiz Digital Services, Chennai, India
Printed and bound by Alden (Malaysia)

Contents

Foreword

The AIDS Pandemic is the story of AIDS, with an emphasis on its epidemiology and approaches to preventing and controlling it, from a unique perspective. That perspective is one of a renowned, well-respected epidemiologist whose approach in domestic and global public health discussions is thoughtful, direct, passionate, rational and willing to challenge conventional wisdom. These same characteristics permeate this book, which has elements of autobiography, history, epidemiology, public health politics and a status report on the AIDS pandemic.

The author, Dr. James Chin, has been a mentor, colleague and friend for over 30 years, since I worked in his Infectious Diseases Section at the California Health Department in Berkeley and later when we shared responsibilities for CDC's Advisory Committee on Immunization Practices (ACIP). Whilst, in this book, he challenges "mainstream" thinking and conclusions, by any standard he is a pillar of the public health mainstream. As a distinguished state epidemiologist, WHO consultant, editor of The American Public Health Association's *Control of Communicable Diseases Manual,*[1] and section editor for infectious diseases of the classic text, *Maxcy-Rosenau Public Health and Preventive Medicine,*[2] his careful analyses and views carry the weight of long experience and considerable expertise.

Some readers may find some of the discussion and conclusions provocative and even disagree with them. I certainly disagree with some (tobacco control and reductions in motor vehicle deaths have been public health triumphs, not failures). But challenging the reader to reassess how AIDS is viewed and addressed is part of the author's objective. A case has been made by many public health authorities and organizations that AIDS must be seen as a risk for whole populations globally, that projected future rates will be high, and that poverty, discrimination, and poor access to health care are the most important determinants. Chin disputes all of these conclusions. The issue of targeting interventions toward those at highest risk vs. a broader population has been well considered by the late Professor Geoffrey Rose in *The Strategy of Preventive Medicine.*[3] Rose argues that population strategies are the most effective. Chin offers another perspective particular to AIDS; the reader will have to reconcile these two compelling alternative approaches.

Chin argues that: (1) AIDS has a different pattern in different countries based on behaviors and for some countries it is better to target high risk groups than dilute resources in interventions aimed at the general population; (2) rates of disease projected by public health agencies are often higher than the epidemiology would support and (3) social determinants while playing an important role in all health outcomes are less relevant for AIDS transmission than patterns of sexual behavior and opportunities for parenteral exposure. On the whole, there is probably more agreement than conflict between the author and the "mainstream" authorities but this book is making a case for a particular perspective, which urges the reader to reassess the alternatives using data and the scientific literature.

Controversy and differing opinions have been hallmarks of the AIDS epidemic since its onset. The scope of the problem, how to identify high risk groups without increasing the burden of stigma, the safety of blood products, the best balance between prevention and treatment, have all been hot issues sometimes dividing the public health community. The passion and conflicts about how to consider and address the AIDS pandemic reflect the huge impact this disease has had globally and its interplay with macro economic, legal, social, political, national security and ethical domains.

Chapter 6 and 7 on how AIDS data are collected and analyzed and the validity of conclusions then drawn should find their way into the reading lists for graduate epidemiology courses. After such discussions of AIDS epidemiology and projections of occurrence, the author offers his perspective on public health politics and personalities in the closing chapters of the book. His insights, when considered with those of others involved in the early days of the global AIDS crisis, will be vital for future historians of this major public health challenge. The vignettes of conversations, personnel conflicts and personal opinions that are interspersed throughout the book are further concentrated in these closing pages.

The AIDS Pandemic is filled with information, rational arguments and opinions, often intermingled. It is a rare book on epidemiology that puts so much of the author's personality and viewpoints, along with his knowledge and experience, before the reader. The result is a thought-provoking, likely-to-be-controversial, contribution to the AIDS literature that should engage and stimulate the reader. As Dr. Chin advises students who consider signing up for his course on AIDS at the University of California (Berkeley) School of Public Health: a prerequisite is having "an open mind regarding the past, present and probable future of the HIV/AIDS pandemic." I suspect he would make the same request of readers of this book.

Jeffrey Koplan, MD, MPH
Vice President for Academic Health Affairs
Robert W. Woodruff Health Sciences Center
Atlanta, Georgia, USA
September **2006**

References

1 Chin J (2000) *Control of Communicable Diseases Manual* (17e). American Public Health Association, Washington DC.
2 Last JM and Wallace RB (1992) *Maxcy-Rosenau Public Health and Preventive Medicine* (13e). Appleton-Century-Croft, New York.
3 Rose G (1992) *The Strategy of Preventive Medicine*. Oxford University Press, Oxford.

Preface

For close to a half century, my work as a public health epidemiologist has involved field research, program management, and teaching, mostly on public health surveillance and prevention and control of communicable diseases. Since 1981, I have been involved virtually full time with the international response to the AIDS pandemic which is without question one of the most severe infectious disease pandemics in modern times. During my public health career that began in the early 1960s, I have always been considered a part of conventional or mainstream medical science. However, since the mid-1990s, I have found myself swimming upstream against mainstream AIDS organizations. I have, during this period, gradually come to the realization that AIDS programs developed by international agencies and faith–based organizations have been and continue to be more socially, politically, and moralistically correct than epidemiologically accurate.

I therefore felt obligated to write this book to present an objective assessment of the AIDS pandemic that is at marked variance with the prevailing position of UNAIDS and AIDS program activists. The unique natural history of HIV and its basic epidemiology is complex but not difficult to understand. However, to understand HIV transmission dynamics one must have an open mind, since UNAIDS and other AIDS advocacy organizations have distorted HIV epidemiology in order to perpetuate the myth of the great potential for HIV epidemics to spread into "general" populations. This has been done either unintentionally out of honest ignorance or misunderstanding, or intentionally by deliberate exaggeration.

HIV is transmitted from person to person primarily via blood and sexual fluids such as semen and any other body fluid that may contain some blood. The probability or risk of HIV transmission for any single exposure is related to the amount of infected blood or semen that is exchanged. All published sex partner studies have shown that the risk of HIV transmission via sexual intercourse is a minuscule fraction of the risk associated with most other sexually transmitted diseases (STD). As a result, extensive epidemic sexual HIV transmission can occur only in those populations where there are large numbers of persons who have unprotected sex with *multiple* and *concurrent* sex partners. How high HIV prevalence may reach in these populations depends on: the prevalence of *facilitating factors* such as ulcerative STD (chancroid and genital herpes) that can greatly increase the amount of blood and sexual fluids exchanged during intercourse; and the prevalence of *protective factors* such as male circumcision and consistent condom use.

HIV prevalence is low in most populations throughout the world and can be expected to remain low, not because of effective HIV prevention programs but simply because HIV infection rates can rise only to the level(s) permitted by the prevailing patterns and prevalence of HIV risk behaviors and the prevalence of facilitating and protective factors. The vast majority of the world's populations do not have sufficient HIV risk behaviors to sustain significant epidemic HIV transmission. This epidemiologically sound conclusion is sufficient to explain past, current, and future HIV patterns and prevalence, but has been minimized and ignored by UNAIDS and AIDS program activists. UNAIDS' more politically and socially acceptable public health message is to say that HIV risk behaviors are present in all populations and therefore all populations are at risk of HIV epidemics.

A survey by the Kaiser Foundation in 2003 found that over 70 percent of those surveyed obtained their information about AIDS from the news media. Most journalists and reporters who cover the AIDS pandemic are more socially and politically correct than epidemiologically accurate. Furthermore, most uncritically accept and use information distributed by UNAIDS, an organization that doesn't deny it is primarily an AIDS advocacy agency – not a scientific or technical agency. As a result, there continues to be inadequate understanding of basic HIV epidemiology – especially its transmission dynamics – along with gross ignorance of how current HIV/AIDS estimates and projections are "cooked" or made up. Most of the public, policy makers, and the news media have uncritically accepted high HIV prevalence estimates and refuse even to consider the possibility that lower prevalence estimates may be more accurate.

In reviewing textbooks and other books about HIV/AIDS, I have not run across any that present a clear and objective assessment of the major determinants of epidemic HIV transmission. Furthermore, none presented a critical analysis and evaluation of the reliability or validity of HIV prevalence estimates and projections. Michael Fumento in his book *The Myth of Heterosexual AIDS*, first published in the late 1980s, accurately analyzed the very low potential for epidemic heterosexual HIV transmission in the "general" US population. However, he completely missed the boat when he cast doubt on the epidemic spread of HIV in heterosexual populations in Africa and a few Asian countries.

I had some problems deciding what type of book I should write and who would be the target audience. In briefing new GPA/WHO staff members on the status of the AIDS pandemic during the late 1980s, it became apparent to me that a major difficulty new staff faced was their inadequate understanding of basic infectious disease epidemiology. Thus, in order to adequately comprehend the natural history of HIV infection, its epidemiology and transmission dynamics, they needed to know the basics of epidemiology; the epidemiology of different types of infectious disease agents; and the basics of HIV epidemiology. They also required information about differences between all the HIV/AIDS numbers and how all these numbers are obtained. I also had to decide whether this book should be written as a textbook on AIDS, i.e., HIV/AIDS 101, or as a description of my personal and professional experience in studying this pandemic from its initial recognition in California in 1981 up to 2006. I finally decided that I would write a book anyone interested or involved with AIDS programs can easily understand yet provide sufficient technical details to be credible to HIV/AIDS experts.

As an accredited infectious disease epidemiologist for close to a half century, it has been difficult for me to understand how, over the past decade, mainstream AIDS scientists, including most infectious disease epidemiologists, have virtually all uncritically accepted the many "glorious" myths and misconceptions UNAIDS and AIDS activists continue to perpetuate. Up to mid-2006, there has been no significant criticism of UNAIDS' prevailing paradigm which states that – in the absence of effective HIV prevention programs, directed primarily at the general public, especially youth – epidemic HIV transmission will inevitably occur in populations where HIV prevalence is very low. Any criticism of UNAIDS' HIV prevalence estimates and projections as being too high is immediately labeled as a blatant attack on AIDS programs and an irresponsible denial of the potential infectiousness and severity of the AIDS pandemic.

I hope that this book will, at a minimum, lead to further dialog and a reappraisal of the validity of the prevailing UNAIDS paradigm and to a better understanding of the most probable past, present and future of the AIDS pandemic.

James (Jim) Chin
Stockton, California
August 2006

Acknowledgement

I want to thank Florence Morrison for her editorial assistance over the past four decades and especially for her hard work helping me to get this book ready for publication.

Dedication

I dedicate this book to my wife Anne who has been more than supportive and understanding of my sudden career decisions to take early retirement in 1987 to join Jon Mann at WHO in Geneva, and my abrupt resignation from GPA/WHO in early 1992 to return to an unemployed status in California.

About the author

James (Jim) Chin has been a public health epidemiologist for close to a half century. His work has entailed field research, program management, and teaching, mostly in public health surveillance and prevention of communicable diseases. He has had the unique opportunity to study the AIDS pandemic from the early 1980s in California – where he was responsible for surveillance and control of communicable diseases – to the late 1980s at WHO, where he was responsible for developing the methods and guidelines for global and regional HIV/AIDS surveillance. During his public health career, he has held leadership positions at State, National, and International organizations and received recognition for his work as an infectious disease epidemiologist. Since his resignation from GPA/WHO in 1992, he has worked as an independent consultant for different international agencies to evaluate the patterns and prevalence of HIV in developing countries – primarily in Africa and Asia.

Glossary

ABC	**A**bstinence, **B**e faithful, and **C**ondom use
ACIP	Advisory Committee on Immunization Practices
ADB	Asian Development Bank
AES	American Epidemiological Society
AFEB	Armed Forces Epidemiological Board
AIDS	Acquired Immune Deficiency Syndrome
AMRO	Regional Office for the Americas [of WHO]
ANC	Antenatal clinic
APHA	American Public Health Association
ART	Anti-Retroviral Treatment
ATM	AIDS, TB, and Malaria
AZT	Azidothymidine [Zidovudine]
BAIS	Botswana AIDS Impact Study
BOVD	Board of Vaccine Development
CCCD	Combating Childhood Communicable Diseases
CCDM	Control of Communicable Diseases Manual, formerly Control of Communicable Diseases in Man
CD_4	An antigen of a sub-type of T-lymphocytes – these CD molecules (or Clusters of Differentiation) are markers for identifying these cells
CDC	Centers for Disease Control and Prevention
CIA	Central Intelligence Agency
CMV	Cytomegalovirus
CNS	Central nervous system
CSTE	Conference of State and Territorial Epidemiologists
DCPP	Disease Control Priorities in Developing Countries
DFID	Department for International Development [UK]
DG	Director General
DHS+	Demographic Health Survey (HIV testing)
DHS	Department of Health Services
DOS	Disk Operating System
DOTS	Directly observed treatment strategy [for TB]
DSHS	Division of Special Health Services [USPHS]
EIS	Epidemic Intelligence Service
EMRO	Eastern Mediterranean Regional Office [of WHO]
EPP	Estimation and Projection Package
EURO	European Regional Office [of WHO]
FHI	Family Health International
FIC	Fogarty International Center
FSW	Female sex worker
G6PD	Glucose 6-phosphate dehyrogenase
G-8	Group of 8 [richest countries]
GBD	Global Burden of Disease

GF	Global Fund
GFATM	Global Fund for AIDS, Tuberculosis, and Malaria
GPA	Global Programme on AIDS
GRID	Gay-related immune deficiencies
GTZ	Gesellschaft für Technische Zusammenarbeit [German international aid agency]
HAART	Highly active anti-retroviral therapy
HIV	Human immunodeficiency virus
HS	High school
HSS	HIV sentinel surveillance
HSV-2	Herpes simplex virus − 2
ICD-10	International statistical classification of diseases and related health problems − 10
ICMRT	International Center for Medical Research and Training
IDS	Infectious Disease Section
IDU	Injecting drug user
IHRA	International Harm Reduction Association
IMR	Institute for Medical Research
IOM	Institute of Medicine
ITM	Institute of Tropical Medicine
IQ	Intelligence Quotient
KABP	Knowledge, Attitudes, Behavior, and Practices [sexual surveys]
KL	Kuala Lumpur
LAN	Local area network
MC	Male circumcision
MMWR	Morbidity, Mortality, Weekly Report
MPH	Master in Public Health
MSM	Men who have sex with men
Mtbc	*Mycobacterium tuberculosis*
MTCT	Mother to child [HIV] transmission
NAS	National Academy of Science
NASA	National Aeronautics and Space Administration
NCI	National Cancer Institute
NGO	Non-governmental organization
NIAID	National Institute of Allergy and Infectious Diseases
NIC	National Institute of Cancer
NIH	National Institute of Health
NYC	New York City
PAHO	Pan American Health Organization
PCP	Pneumocystis pneumonia
PCR	Polymerase chain reaction
PJ	Petaling Jaya
PNG	Papua New Guinea
PPP	Purchasing Power Parity
PS	Public school
P&S	Primary and secondary [syphilis]
RAF	Royal Air Force
RAM	Random Access Memory
RBG	Risk behavior group

RD	Regional Director
R_0	Reproduction number of an infectious disease agent
RSV	Respiratory syncytial virus
SARS	Severe acute respiratory syndrome
SCID	Severe combined immune deficiency
SEARO	South East Asia Regional Office [of WHO]
SF	San Francisco
SFI	Surveillance, Forecasting, and Impact Assessment Unit of GPA/WHO
SIDA	French acronym for AIDS
SIV	Simian immunodeficiency virus
SPA	Special Programme on AIDS [before GPA]
SSA	Sub-Saharan Africa
STC	Short-term consultant
SW	Sex workers
TA	Temporary assignment
TB	Tuberculosis
T cells	A subset of lymphocytes that play a large role in the immune response. "T" stands for thymus, where their final stage of development occurs.
TOR	Terms of reference
UC	University of California
UCSF	University of California San Francisco
UK	United Kingdom
UNAIDS	United Nations Joint Programme on AIDS
USBOC	US Bureau of the Census
UNDP	United Nations Development Programme
UNICEF	United Nations Children's Fund
UNPOP	United Nations Population Division
USA	United States of America
USAID	US Agency for International Development
USPHS	US Public Health Service
VRDL	Viral and Rickettsial Diseases Laboratory
VTC	Voluntary [HIV] testing and counseling
WB	World Bank
WER	Weekly Epidemiological Report
WHO	World Health Organization
WPRO	Western Pacific Regional Office [of WHO]

Chapter 1

Introduction and Book Overview

Cases of **A**cquired **I**mmune **D**eficiency **S**yndrome[*] (AIDS) were probably present in low numbers in sub-Saharan Africa (SSA) for decades or centuries before this disease syndrome was recognized as a distinct clinical entity in 1981 in several young homosexual males[†] in southern California. At the time, I was the State Epidemiologist responsible for the prevention and control of communicable diseases in California. Since then, I have been involved virtually full-time with the international response to the AIDS pandemic, which is without question one of the most severe infectious disease pandemics in modern times. During my public health career that began in the early 1960s, I have always been considered a part of conventional or mainstream medical science. However, since the mid-1990s, I have found myself swimming upstream against mainstream AIDS organizations. I have, during this period, gradually come to the realization that AIDS programs developed by international agencies and faith-based organizations have been and continue to be more socially, politically, and moralistically correct than epidemiologically accurate.

My understanding of how human immunodeficiency virus (HIV) infections are spread (HIV transmission dynamics) and of the very low potential for epidemic transmission in populations with current low HIV prevalence "fits" exactly with what has occurred. However, my conclusions are at marked variance with the beliefs of many AIDS "experts" and with the prevailing Joint United Nations Programme on HIV/AIDS (UNAIDS) paradigm. According to UNAIDS, if effective HIV/AIDS prevention programs are not directed to the general public, especially all youth, epidemic heterosexual HIV transmission will inevitably break out in most populations where HIV epidemics have not yet occurred. My HIV/AIDS paradigm is that *epidemic* HIV transmission requires human behaviors that involve having unprotected sex with *multiple* and *concurrent* sex partners[‡] and/or routinely sharing needles and syringes with other injecting drug users (IDU). According to my understanding of HIV transmission dynamics, HIV epidemics cannot occur in populations where high risk patterns and the highest prevalence of such risk behaviors are not present.

Exaggeration of the potential for HIV to spread into the "general" population is a "glorious"[§] myth perpetuated by UNAIDS, AIDS program advocates, and activists, partly to avoid further stigmatization of persons with the highest levels of HIV risk behaviors (MSM, IDU, and sex workers (SW)[**] and their clients). UNAIDS also wants the public and policy makers to be fearful about HIV infections "jumping out" from these foci of infection to spread into the "general population." Yet no such spread into any general population has occurred! In well

---

[*] AIDS is not a simple infectious disease. It is a disease syndrome because it is a group of illnesses that collectively indicate or characterize a specific disease syndrome.
[†] As of the mid-1980s usually referred to as men who have sex with men (MSM).
[‡] Traditionally defined as sexual promiscuity.
[§] An example of *splendide mendax* – gloriously or nobly false for a good cause.
[**] Formerly referred to as prostitutes.

over 100 IDU and/or MSM epidemics documented worldwide, no significant spread to the general population has occurred except to the regular sex partners of infected IDU or bisexual MSM. This myth of a high potential for "generalized" HIV epidemics has resulted in a large and unnecessary amount of effort and funds being used for programs directed to the general population and especially youth. Yet these groups, outside of SSA, are at minimal to no risk of acquiring HIV from risky sexual behaviors. This major focus on preventing "generalized" HIV epidemics means that there is usually insufficient effort given to preventing infections in persons with the highest HIV risk behaviors. UNAIDS, AIDS program advocates, and activists have used this myth effectively in their aggressive struggle for an increasing share of the limited international health budget at the expense of other equally urgent public health needs. I'll detail these fundamental disagreements and problems in this book and let readers decide whether I'm more on target than UNAIDS and many other AIDS "experts."

Book Overview

AIDS was recognized as a newly emerging disease just over a quarter of a century ago. From the outset, there were many uncertainties about this invariably fatal disease syndrome that seemed to have appeared out of nowhere. These initial uncertainties and questions about what AIDS was, what caused it, and why at that time AIDS primarily affected MSM and IDU populations spawned many misconceptions and myths about this emerging pandemic. Most of the extreme, "far out" myths have been dismissed by mainstream* science, but some persist, including some that are defended with a cult-like faith and fervor by UNAIDS and many AIDS "experts." These latter myths are "glorious" myths like the one mentioned earlier – since they are for a good cause, but they have no epidemiologic basis or support.

For close to a half century, my work as a public health epidemiologist has involved field research, program management, and teaching, mostly on public health surveillance and prevention and control of communicable diseases. In these positions, I have had a unique opportunity to study the epidemiology of HIV from the initial investigations in the early 1980s in California to the Global Programme on AIDS (GPA) at the World Health Organization (WHO). There I was responsible for developing the methodology and guidelines for global and regional HIV/AIDS surveillance. One of my responsibilities at GPA/WHO was to "brief" new staff members on the epidemiology of HIV. In addition I provided them with updates on global patterns and prevalence of HIV/AIDS. I found that most of the new staff (also probably the older staff) had an inadequate understanding of HIV epidemiology and a poor understanding of HIV/AIDS numbers. Now, close to two decades later, in thinking about what is needed to provide anyone involved or interested in AIDS with a better understanding of the most probable past, present and future of the pandemic, I felt obligated to write this book.

I had problems in deciding what type of book I should write and who would be the target audience. Should this book be written as a textbook or primer on AIDS, i.e., HIV/AIDS 101, or should I write it to describe my personal and professional

---

* In this book, "mainstream" will refer to the conclusions about HIV/AIDS by WHO, UNAIDS, CDC, and NIH. I'll try to alert readers when I may stray or depart from "mainstream" conclusions and positions.

experience in studying this pandemic from its recognition in California in 1981 up to late-2006. I finally decided that I would include:

1 primers on the basic epidemiology especially the transmission dynamics of HIV related to different patterns and prevalence of risk behaviors
2 descriptions of the methods and data used for estimating and projecting HIV infections and AIDS deaths, along with a detailed discussion of the limitations and problems of current UNAIDS estimates and projections
3 my response to the many myths and misconceptions about the AIDS pandemic, and
4 my personal and professional views of the international response to the AIDS pandemic.

Prevailing Beliefs About the AIDS Pandemic

Several hundred theories about what AIDS is and its possible origin have probably been developed. I will not address most of these theories but will comment on a few of the most persistent in this book.

As of late-2006 two extreme views about this pandemic persist.

- *The position of Duesberg and other AIDS "dissidents"*: Human immunodeficiency virus (HIV) is *not* the cause of AIDS! The driving force of the AIDS pandemic is poverty, not sexual promiscuity.
- *The prevailing UNAIDS paradigm:* HIV is the cause of AIDS: without effective prevention programs, it is only a matter of time before heterosexual HIV epidemics will erupt in almost all populations where HIV infection rates are currently low.

The reality of the HIV/AIDS pandemic lies between these extremes.

HIV is the cause of AIDS, but epidemic HIV transmission requires the highest level of risk behaviors: HIV transmission in any population is determined by the pattern and prevalence of HIV risk behaviors present in that population, as well as the prevalence of facilitating and protective factors. *Heterosexual risk behaviors in most populations outside of SSA are insufficient to sustain significant epidemic HIV transmission.*

There is no question that HIV is the cause of AIDS, as all evidence collected over the past couple of decades by thousands of medical scientists supports this conclusion. Since the first report of AIDS, epidemic HIV transmission has been found only in populations with the highest levels of risk behaviors. With the exception of transmission from infected MSM and IDU to their regular sex partner(s), no significant HIV spread to surrounding heterosexual populations has been documented following hundreds of MSM and IDU epidemics. Nevertheless, UNAIDS and many AIDS "experts" are still sounding alarms that epidemic HIV transmission is "on the brink" of occurring if education and prevention programs are not aggressively directed to the general population, especially all youth! Peter Piot, the head of UNAIDS, in one of his speeches about AIDS in Asia said: "Let's stop the nonsense of trying to determine a 'natural limit' to the [HIV/AIDS] epidemic in Asia and the Pacific..." My response is that it is epidemiologic nonsense to deny that there are no natural limits to epidemic HIV transmission based on the patterns and prevalence of HIV risk behaviors!

In addition to my contrary conclusions about HIV transmission dynamics, I also consider most of the HIV/AIDS estimates and projections made or accepted by UNAIDS to be grossly overestimated. Several years ago I received a telephone call from Laurie Garrett who was, as usual, calling from an airport and was in a great rush. She told me that some of my former colleagues in Geneva were accusing me of "low-balling" the AIDS pandemic and she asked me to comment or defend myself. I told Laurie that those persons who were accusing me of "low-balling" were themselves "high-balling" the pandemic. Laurie had to hang up to catch her plane and she never to my knowledge followed up on this subject.* As will be described in detail in this book, UNAIDS in late 2003 significantly reduced HIV prevalence estimates in many SSA countries as a result of improved surveillance data and the increasing use of population-based HIV serosurveys.

Aside from grossly overestimating prevalence in those populations where epidemic HIV transmission has occurred, UNAIDS in its December 2005 update on the AIDS pandemic included statements such as "…the pandemic is ever increasing and expanding and the numbers of persons living with HIV continues to reach all time record highs." I have been saying that annual global HIV incidence peaked almost a decade ago. UNAIDS in its mid-2006 report on the AIDS pandemic finally acknowledged that "Overall, globally, the HIV incidence rate (the annual number of new HIV infections as a proportion of previously uninfected persons) is believed to have peaked in the late 1990s and to have stabilized subsequently, notwithstanding increasing incidence in a number of countries …" In this book, I'll provide data reported by UNAIDS that supports my conclusion that global HIV incidence and prevalence are not ever-increasing and expanding.

In all my contacts with journalists and reporters about the accuracy of reported or estimated HIV/AIDS numbers I try to convey the message that, because of the major limitations of HIV data, estimation of HIV/AIDS numbers cannot be very precise or accurate. However, even with limited data, HIV prevalence in populations can be confidently classified as low (less than 1 per thousand in the 15–49 year age group), moderate (more than 1 per 1000 and less than 1 per 100), high (more than 1 per 100 and less than 1 per 10), or very high (more than 1 per 10). Even if HIV prevalence estimates in many or most SSA countries were reduced by 50 percent or more, HIV prevalence will still be high or very high in most SSA countries. I caution journalists not to throw out the *baby* (high and very high HIV infection rates in Africa and to a lesser extent in several Caribbean countries and a few SE Asian countries, as well as in MSM and IDU populations throughout the world) with the *bathwater* (the general overestimation of HIV in Africa, the Caribbean and Asia and the exaggerated potential for "generalized" HIV epidemics).

I also have significantly different views and conclusions regarding the UNAIDS litany of poverty, discrimination, and lack of access to healthcare as major factors for the high HIV prevalence rates in SSA. In my opinion, a double standard is used by "mainstream" AIDS organizations which attribute high HIV and other STD rates in black populations in the USA and in SSA primarily to poverty,

---

* I suspect that Laurie believes that I have been too conservative or low with my HIV estimates and projections, but most of my conservative estimates and projections are probably still a bit high! In February 2005 she was quoted in a news release supporting Susan Hunter's new book *AIDS in Asia: A Continent in Peril*, that claims that figures for HIV prevalence in Asia are vastly underestimated, whereas I believe they are overestimated.

discrimination and lack of access to healthcare while clearly pointing out that the major reason for high HIV and other STD rates in MSM populations is high sexual risk behaviors. This double standard is clearly shown in the editorial comments made by CDC following two reports of syphilis in the same issue of MMWR in 2001.

Primary and Secondary Syphilis – USA, 1999

...Syphilis continues to disproportionately affect minority populations – the 1999 reported rate of P&S [primary and secondary] syphilis in blacks was 30 times the rate reported in whites (0.5). [This] is, in part, attributable to differences between blacks and whites regarding *poverty* and in *access to and use of health-care services*, especially in the rural South...

Outbreak of Syphilis Among Men Who Have Sex With Men – Southern California, 2000

...The results of this investigation and other similar outbreaks suggest that an increasing number of MSM are participating in *high-risk sexual behavior* that places them at risk for syphilis and HIV infection.

(2001) MMWR. February 23, 50(07)

Since my resignation from GPA/WHO in early 1992,[*] I have been an independent consultant to evaluate the patterns and prevalence of HIV in developing countries – primarily in Africa and Asia for different international agencies. I have prepared dozens of country reports and a few regional reports for USAID, the Asian Development Bank, the World Bank, and the WHO Regional Offices in Manila (WPRO) and New Delhi (SEARO). Much of what is presented in this book was prepared for these reports. In addition, some of the text and graphics are from material I have prepared for the classes and seminars I teach at the School of Public Health, University of California at Berkeley.

Chapter Previews

Chapter 2: Personal and Professional Background

This chapter is not essential for understanding the AIDS pandemic. It provides readers with details of my personal and professional background up to the time I joined Jon Mann at WHO in Geneva, Switzerland in early 1987. I was born in China[†] and I arrived in Brooklyn, NY, when I was about 5 years old. My formal education started in PS 99 in Flatbush and ended with my receiving an MPH in Epidemiology from the School of Public Health, UC Berkeley in 1961. My professional training and experience as an infectious disease epidemiologist began in 1961 with my appointment as an International Research Fellow first with the Hooper Foundation at the UCSF Medical Center and subsequently at the Institute for Medical Research (IMR), in Kuala Lumpur, Malaysia. I became chief of the Infectious Disease Section, California State Department of Health Services in Berkeley, California from the early 1970s until 1987. My experience with the

---

[*] Details as to why I resigned from GPA/WHO are provided in Chapter 11.
[†] My older brother, Bill, and I had derived US citizenship from our father who was a naturalized US citizen.

Global Programme on AIDS (GPA) and my work on HIV/AIDS since my GPA tenure are described in the last chapter – Chapter 11.

Chapter 3: The Most Probable Origin and Initial Global Spread of HIV

This chapter provides "documentation" for what most mainstream scientists and public health workers believe to be the origin of HIV: it includes a description of the origin of most human infectious disease agents and a brief review of emerging infectious diseases since 1950. An interesting note is that since starting my classes on the AIDS pandemic at the UC School of Public Health in Berkeley, I have had very few students who know anything about Jon Mann. None of them had any idea of why and when he went to Kinshasa, Zaire.[*] This chapter provides details taken from several oral histories that can be accessed via the internet about how and why Project SIDA[†] was established in 1983 in Kinshasa by NIH, CDC, and the Belgium Institute of Tropical Medicine. What amazes me is how few people who are currently interested in or working in AIDS programs are aware of Jon Mann and the Haiti to Zaire connection in the 1960s and 1970s.

Chapter 4: A Basic Primer on HIV Infections and AIDS Cases (HIV/AIDS)

When I was responsible for briefing GPA staff on HIV epidemiology and global trends, I was surprised at their general lack of knowledge about epidemiology and infectious diseases. Some hardly knew the difference between a bacterium and a virus. Thus, I decided to include a chapter that would bring all readers up to speed on the basics of epidemiology, especially infectious disease epidemiology. Readers who do not have a biology or science background will find here basic information on the epidemiology of infectious diseases so that they can understand that HIV is not a simple or "classical" infectious disease agent. I believe that even those who consider themselves to be very knowledgeable about infectious diseases should at least skim this chapter to see if we are in general agreement on the natural history and epidemiology of HIV infection.

Chapter 5: HIV Epidemiology and Transmission Dynamics

This chapter is the most detailed, technical section in the book and is the only one in which I have included detailed references as endnotes. Of special importance is that this chapter explains why *HIV is not and cannot become a "generalized" infectious disease agent*. The information here is essential for understanding HIV epidemiology and transmission dynamics; such an understanding is needed to identify populations in whom epidemic HIV transmission may be expected. Key epidemiologic and infectious disease concepts include:

1 the definition of an infectious disease epidemic, including when an epidemic can be considered a "generalized" epidemic
2 the basic reproductive number (R_0) of an infectious disease agent
3 the generally low infectivity of HIV via sexual intercourse

---

[*] Zaire is now the Democratic Republic of the Congo.
[†] SIDA is the French acronym for AIDS.

4 the paramount importance of patterns, prevalence, and frequency of sex partner exchanges for sexual transmission, including the size and extent of overlapping sex networks

5 the importance of major facilitating factors (not cofactors) and protective factors such as male circumcision and condoms for epidemic sexual HIV transmission, and

6 the fact that there are major differences in the patterns and prevalence of sexual risk behaviors as well as facilitating and protective factors within and between countries and regions.

These concepts are described in this chapter along with a detailed description of HIV epidemiology and transmission dynamics.

Chapter 6: Understanding HIV/AIDS Numbers

There has been and continues to be tremendous misunderstanding and confusion about HIV/AIDS numbers. HIV is not a simple infectious disease agent because the disease syndrome it causes (AIDS) does not usually develop until years, perhaps up to a decade or longer, after infection. Thus, in measuring and monitoring HIV infections and AIDS cases and deaths, these different stages of HIV infection need to be kept in mind constantly. HIV/AIDS programs need to know how many persons may have acquired an HIV infection in a year (annual HIV incidence); how many persons are living with an HIV infection at the end of a year (HIV prevalence); and how many AIDS deaths occur in a year. Specific definitions for each of these numbers and rates are given here as well as description of the methods and data used to estimate these numbers and rates. It's fair to say that in 2005, both the heads of UNAIDS and the Global Fund revealed that they do not fully understand how annual incidence numbers in India are estimated. They would do well to read this chapter through carefully.

Chapter 7: How Credible are HIV/AIDS Estimates?

This chapter describes HIV/AIDS patterns, prevalence levels, and trends in all the major global regions. It also reviews and evaluates the problem of overestimation and projection of HIV prevalence in SSA and in selected Asian countries. In mid-2005 UNAIDS issued a press release on the status of the AIDS pandemic that declared that there was a "quantum worsening in the [HIV] epidemic's trajectory." However, since the late 1990s, there has been a clear trend of leveling or slightly decreasing HIV prevalence rates in SSA and most other global regions. There is no marked increase in HIV prevalence – except for a few countries where HIV epidemics in IDU populations have continued almost unabated. Many countries in SSA and the Caribbean region have, in recent years, carried out population-based HIV surveys. These indicate HIV prevalence has been overestimated on average by about 50 percent. HIV prevalence estimates probably remain too high in those SSA countries where population-based surveys have not been carried out and so are likely too high in many Caribbean, eastern European and Asian countries. UNAIDS finally acknowledged in mid-2006 that epidemic HIV transmission peaked in SSA almost a decade ago. UNAIDS will now need to modify their previous standard press releases to expunge the words "ever-increasing" or "expanding" to describe the current status of the AIDS pandemic.

Chapter 8: HIV/AIDS Prevention

HIV prevention programs have been implemented throughout the world over the past two decades with only limited success. Explosive HIV epidemics in IDU populations continue to occur. Explosive sexual HIV transmission has been more successfully controlled by the 100 percent condom program for commercial sex encounters. However, little progress has been made in preventing transmission from HIV-infected persons (regardless of how the infection was acquired) to their regular sex partners. This latter pattern may now be the predominant mode of HIV transmission throughout the world. This chapter describes: primary HIV preventive measures along with the major issues associated with these public health interventions; and problems of measuring and evaluating the success of HIV/AIDS programs in reducing HIV incidence and prevalence. HIV prevention programs need to re-evaluate their prevention strategies to respond more effectively to current patterns of HIV transmission. This means directing attention primarily to HIV-discordant couples and regular sex partners of HIV-infected persons. All HIV prevention programs now need to identify HIV-infected persons systematically and nominally (by name) to: provide them with secondary and tertiary prevention services (i.e., ART) as needed; and routinely follow-up on all of their regular sex partners to provide them with primary, secondary, or tertiary prevention services, as needed.

Chapter 9: Dispelling "Glorious" HIV/AIDS Myths and Misconceptions

Most of the far out "flat earth" type theories of the origin of AIDS and what AIDS is or isn't, were dismissed by mainstream science by the mid-1980s. However, several glorious myths and/or misconceptions about HIV epidemiology continue to be accepted and used by UNAIDS as well as other mainstream AIDS agencies and activists. These myths are needed to support the UNAIDS paradigm that without aggressive HIV/AIDS prevention programs – especially directed to adolescents and young adults – it is just a matter of time before heterosexual HIV epidemics erupt in current low HIV prevalence populations. The studies and observations of HIV epidemiology and transmission dynamics have led me to far different conclusions about the potential for epidemic HIV transmission in most heterosexual populations. My conclusions are:

1 HIV prevalence can rise only to those levels permitted by the prevailing patterns and prevalence of HIV risk behaviors and the prevalence of facilitating and protective factors, and
2 in most heterosexual populations, the patterns and frequency of sex partner exchange* are not sufficient to sustain epidemic sexual HIV transmission.

The "glorious" myths and misconceptions of UNAIDS cannot be dispelled until there is a willingness among current "believers" to at least accept the possibility that the UNAIDS paradigm has little or no clothes! UNAIDS and all AIDS activists should be happy to hear that global HIV incidence probably peaked about a decade ago, but they have been reluctant even to consider this possibility because it undermines their paradigm. UNAIDS has finally accepted the fact, or at least

---

* Also referred to as sexual promiscuity.

the possibility, that the AIDS pandemic has peaked. UNAIDS will now have to prepare the public and policy makers to accept the reality that, even though HIV incidence has peaked, the pandemic is not over. I totally agree with mainstream AIDS experts who declare that this is not a time to be complacent about HIV prevention, since annual global HIV incidence will still be at least 2 to 3 million.

Chapter 10: The Most Probable Past, Present, and Future of the AIDS Pandemic

This chapter compares the AIDS pandemic with other major infectious disease pandemics to put AIDS in historical perspective. It also compares AIDS deaths with other leading causes of death to provide a global perspective on the current impact of the pandemic. The AIDS pandemic is without question one of the most severe infectious disease pandemics in modern times. Yet compared to the estimated **billion** or more TB deaths in the 18th and 19th Centuries alone, AIDS has a long way to go to catch up to the death tolls of old human diseases like TB and malaria. In addition, the global impact of AIDS has been and will continue to be very uneven. AIDS deaths in SSA will continue to be the leading cause of death in this region for at least the next several decades. In many or most MSM and IDU populations throughout the world, AIDS has been, is, and will continue to be the leading cause of death in these populations for decades to come. However, the demographic impact of AIDS deaths in countries outside of SSA will be minimal to non-measurable. In most of the world's heterosexual populations, epidemic sexual HIV transmission has not occurred. Furthermore, there are no valid epidemiologic reasons to expect epidemic HIV transmission in populations without high risk patterns and the highest prevalence of HIV risk behaviors.

Chapter 11: The International Response to the AIDS Pandemic

This chapter presents my observations and biases regarding the international response to the AIDS pandemic from WHO's initial efforts in the early 1980s to the past decade of effort by UNAIDS and more recently the Global Fund for AIDS, Tuberculosis, and Malaria (ATM). The personal jealousies and politics that I believe prompted Jon Mann to resign his position as Director of GPA in 1990 are described. In addition, I describe how GPA was converted into a "typical" WHO program after Jon's departure by his successor – Mike Merson. This chapter also includes a brief overview of the international response to the AIDS pandemic after UNAIDS replaced GPA/WHO in the mid-1990s.

The AIDS pandemic has exposed the major problems and inequity of international health programs. Prior to the AIDS pandemic, no international agency or donor provided support for routine treatment for any disease as part of its international health commitment. Effective, but expensive, anti-retroviral drugs needed on a daily to weekly schedule have significantly extended the lifespan of HIV-infected persons. These drugs are now provided to virtually all HIV-infected persons who need them in most developed countries. The WHO's 3 by 5 program established an international health precedent by setting a target for the provision of anti-retroviral treatment (ART) for HIV-infected persons in resource-poor countries. The responsibility for further development of international support for ART in developing countries has been assumed by the Global Fund. As of late-2006, it is not clear if the moral commitment made in late-2005 by the richest (G-8) countries to assure universal access to ART in developing countries by 2010 will or will not be met.

In concluding this introduction and overview, I'm copying the first couple of sections from the flyer posted for my course at UC Berkeley, since it succinctly describes what I'll be presenting in this book and what the prerequisites are for reading it.

PH 295: The Epidemiology and Transmission Dynamics of the AIDS Pandemic

Overview: This course provides a detailed review of the past, present, and probable future of the HIV/AIDS pandemic based on the basic epidemiology and natural history of HIV, especially HIV transmission dynamics and the paramount importance of the patterns and prevalence of HIV risk behaviors. A major focus will be to evaluate official HIV/AIDS estimates and projections. Readings and discussions will focus on the primary determinants of epidemic HIV transmission. Most of the papers and reports used are available via the Internet.

Prerequisites: Good access to the Internet and an open mind regarding the past, present and probable future of the HIV/AIDS pandemic.

Chapter 2

Personal and Professional Background

This chapter can be skimmed or skipped since it is not essential for the understanding of the AIDS pandemic: it provides my personal background and my professional training and experience as a public health epidemiologist. This chapter covers my arrival in the USA from China in the late 1930s to early 1987 when I took early retirement from the California State Department of Health Services, where I was responsible for the prevention and control of communicable diseases, to join Jon Mann at the World Health Organization in Geneva, Switzerland. My experience with WHO and my involvement and observations of the international response to the AIDS pandemic is included in the last chapter – Chapter 11.

From Southern China to Flatbush, Brooklyn

I was born in 1933 in the small village of Fausik, near Taishan City in the Pearl River Delta region of Guangdong province, China close to the city of Macau. This is a region in southern China from where the largest proportion of the Chinese in the USA came during the latter part of the 19th Century up to close to the mid-20th Century. In this region the rural/village dialect spoken was Sei Yap (4 counties). The predominate Chinese dialect spoken in the majority of Chinatowns throughout the United States up to the latter part of the 20th Century was Sei Yap. My father had immigrated to the USA via Cuba and Mexico during the 1920s as a young man seeking his fortune. He worked as a laborer in Chinese laundries in New York City and State and returned to China to marry in the mid-1920s. My older brother, Bill was born in 1928 and I was born in 1933. I have almost no recollections of my childhood in China. As the Japanese invasion of China became more intense during the late 1930s, my father sent for us to join him in Brooklyn, New York where he had established his own hand laundry in a middle-class Jewish area of Flatbush.

I arrived in Flatbush when I was about five years old and almost immediately entered public school. I have no recollection of learning English, but at that age I guess that I was a fast learner. I have a vague recollection that Brother Bill was in my kindergarten class for a short time before he was quickly advanced to his age/grade level. I attended Public School (PS) 99 that was about six long blocks from the hand laundry near the corner of Avenue J at 1010 East 14th Street. My parents worked in the front of the laundry and we lived in the back. In those days, each neighborhood in Flatbush had at least one Movie Theater, one Chinese restaurant, and one Chinese hand laundry. We were essentially the only Chinese family in this quiet neighborhood of mostly middle-income Jewish families. I recall that during the Jewish holidays only the Italian kid and I would be in class and we spent those holidays reading comic books and visiting with each other. In this environment, I quickly began to lose whatever Chinese language I still had: I rarely had a chance to use it since both my parents worked about 16 hours a day and we had little time to talk together except at our evening meal. At one point, I think I may have been able to spout more Yiddish than Chinese.

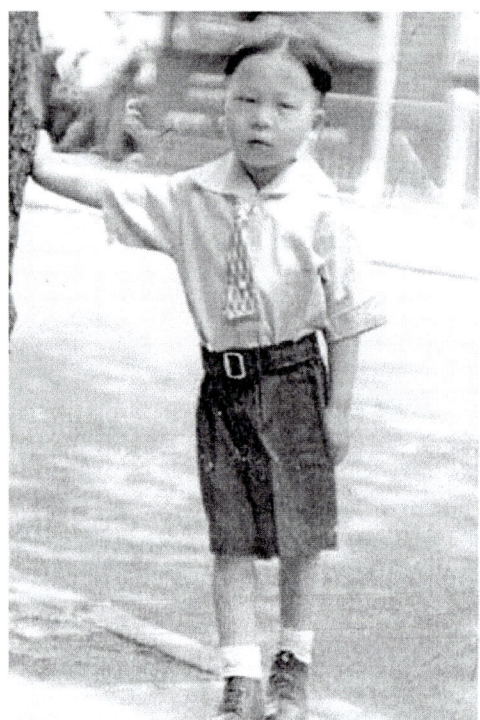 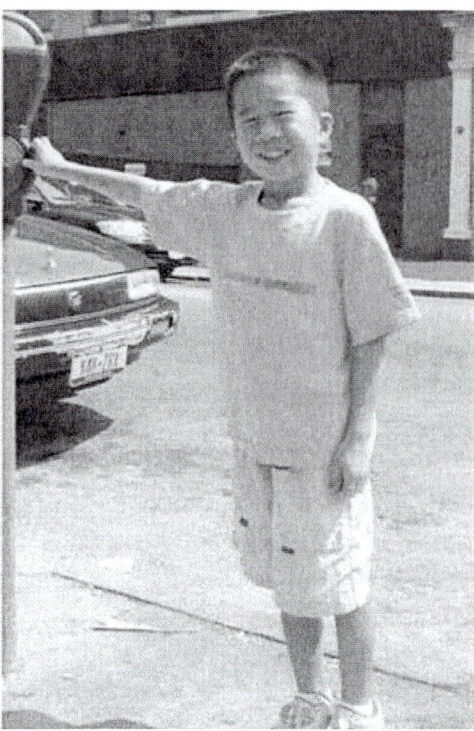

The photograph above (left) shows me leaning against a tree in front of my father's hand laundry in 1940 when I was about seven years old. The photograph on the right shows my grandson, Garrett, leaning on a parking meter (the tree had been cut down) in about the same spot in 2002 when he was about seven years old – my daughter (Elise) was taking my grandchildren to visit grandpa's Brooklyn "roots."

I adapted to school and my schoolmates well. I was very small for my age and still am but I was able to make friends with all of the really bigger boys who shielded me from any physical or racial abuse. At some point at PS 99 I was given an IQ test and was selected to attend a special rapid advancement class at Seth Low Junior High School that was a fairly long bus ride from my neighborhood. My memories of Seth Low Jr. HS are mixed. I was well received by my classmates, most of who were from the Seth Low neighborhood, but they were all super bright and really advanced in both written and spoken English whereas I was always struggling with English classes. I was able to get a respectable overall B minus grade, but my classmates were mostly all A's or A pluses. I was thought of as a very bright kid at PS, but I was near the bottom of my rapid advancement class at Seth Low Jr. High. I nevertheless was able to "skip" a year of school because I was in the rapid advancement class.

When I went to Midwood high school,* I found myself to be one of the youngest in all my classes and also at the top of all my classes except for English

---

* Midwood High is located in the heart of Flatbush next to Brooklyn College. It is in a middle-to-upper income area of Brooklyn. Midwood High was distinguished by having a football team that had never won a game and an alumnus by the name of Woody Allen. He apparently was a couple of years behind me!

class. While I really struggled at Seth Low because all my classmates there were super bright, I found myself at the top in classes with average students. Thus, during high school I was an A student and had no problems in getting accepted to the University of Michigan (Ann Arbor) after graduating from Midwood in June 1949 when I was 16 years old. My parents would not let me attend any university out of NYC, but allowed me to go to Ann Arbor because Brother Bill was a junior at the University of Michigan.

As a product of the NYC school system and a resident of a Jewish neighborhood, I became a "pre-med" almost from the start at Seth Low and I declared myself officially a pre-med when I got to Ann Arbor. The academic momentum I acquired at Midwood High where I competed with "average" students carried over to my freshman and sophomore years at Ann Arbor and I was able to get a 3.5 point average (maximum 4 point) during these years. My study habits were terrible because I found that I did not have to study hard to get good grades. As a result I slacked off considerably during my junior and senior years at Ann Arbor and this was reflected in my average that fell to just a tad over 3 point for my last two years. Fortunately, my grades at the time of my applications to medical schools were good enough to get acceptance from Northwestern and from State University of New York, Downstate Medical College. I elected to return home to Brooklyn to attend medical school in 1954.

As a "professional pre-med," I never really thought much about why I wanted to be a doctor. I was a pre-med because my parents wanted and expected me to be a doctor: one either chose the vocational or academic tracks and most of the boys in the academic track were "pre-meds." When I actually got to medical school, I had to begin thinking hard about why I wanted to be a doctor. Despite my poor study habits, I was near the top of my classes in High School and at Michigan, but I soon found out that most of my medical school class was super bright and it was like Seth Low Jr. High all over again. I was never in danger of not passing any class, but since I couldn't hit the books hard and long, I found myself generally at the top of the lower half of the class. I began smoking in order to extend my attention span for studying to up to one hour. I recall not being able to study for my freshman finals and I must have gone to a dozen movies in downtown Brooklyn during finals week. I graduated from medical school in 1958 and was totally undecided as to what medical specialty I wanted to go into. During my clinical clerkship years I was unable to get interested in any of the medical or surgical specialties. I also knew that I did not want to go into any general type of medical practice. I was leaning towards some laboratory or technical medical specialty such as pathology or radiology but I put off making any decision until my internship year. I elected an internship in San Francisco because this hospital required interns to be on call only one night per week and I wanted to get as far away from Brooklyn as possible.

Public Health Training

My career in public health started when during my internship year in San Francisco a fellow intern told me that the US Public Health Service (USPHS) was recruiting physicians for a career development program in public health. Apparently, the new Division of Special Health Services (DSHS) needed public health physicians and was offering a three-year training program in public health or preventive medicine. This was a very attractive offer because the physician draft was still on in 1959 and I had received deferments from the draft to attend college and then medical school. I could still seek a deferment from the draft for a medical or surgical residency program or I could enroll in the USPHS career development program and fulfill my military draft obligation as a commissioned officer in the USPHS. It was and continues to be confusing, but the USPHS is a uniformed service but not a military service. The USPHS provides staff positions for the National Institute of Health (NIH), the Centers for Disease Control (CDC), and is the medical service for the US Coast Guard. Thus, since I didn't know what I really wanted to do with my MD degree, I had an opportunity to fulfill my draft obligations as a commissioned officer with the USPHS and to explore career opportunities in public health/preventive medicine.

The career development program of the DSHS consisted of a three-year package that would fulfill the requirements for the new Specialty Boards in Public Health or Preventive Medicine. The program included a first year as a public health resident at a local health department, followed by an academic year at a school of public health to get a masters degree in public health (MPH), and a final year as a public health resident at a state health department or in some public health research project. Since I was recruited into the USPHS from San Francisco, I selected the Berkeley City Health Department as the local health department to begin my residency program. I selected the Berkeley City Health Department because this allowed me to stay in the general Bay Area and because I knew that the main staff of this health department also had teaching appointments at the University of California's School of Public Health at Berkeley. I had a marvelous experience with the Berkeley City Health Department. One of my responsibilities was to lecture high school students about the health hazards of smoking. Suddenly, after one of these sessions I made a decision to quit smoking and I have not smoked cigarettes since!* I enjoyed the interaction with local health department staff and the public at vaccine clinics or well baby clinics. Al Leonard, the Health Officer, and Alberta Parker, the Assistant Health Officer, gave me guidance and enough time to develop some research projects such as a program for kindergarten teachers to test for color blindness. However, although it was invaluable to learn how a good local health department works, it was also clear to me that I did not want to spend my career in public health working at a local health department.

For my second year I had to select a school of public health to attend and my mentors in the DSHS wanted me to consider the Johns Hopkins School of Public Health in Baltimore. Since I had married just before starting my residency at Berkeley and my wife, Anne, was pregnant near the end of my first year of residency, I requested permission to get my MPH at Berkeley to avoid moving cross country. Although my mentors did not want me to stay too attached to any one location, they consented to let me attend the School of Public Health in Berkeley.

My year as an MPH student majoring in epidemiology in Berkeley was the turning point of my career in public health because the faculty consisted of Bill Reeves, a most distinguished epidemiologist who was a great teacher and

---

* I was smoking about 1 pack per day, but my wife Anne was a nonsmoker and with her encouragement and support I was able to quit smoking – after I finished the new pack of cigarettes that I had just bought that day!

researcher; Reuel (Stony) Stallones, who was also a superb teacher and who became the first dean of the School of Public Health in Houston, Texas; and Warren Winkelstein, who is now considered one of the "deans" of public health epidemiologists. These teachers introduced me to the fundamentals of epidemiology and it was because of them that I made my decision to pursue a career as an infectious disease epidemiologist.

Why I Left the DSHS Career Development Program

Midway through my MPH year, the DSHS was reorganized and the career development program was discontinued. Thus, my third and last year as a public health resident was withdrawn. I was asked to go to Washington DC during the spring break to interview with several of the special programs of the former DSHS and other USPHS offices to arrange an assignment in the USPHS after my MPH year. I had interviews with: Dr. George Comstock who was the chief epidemiologist in the Tuberculosis Program; staff of the Heart Disease Control Program to explore an assignment with a streptococcal disease prevention study in Bismarck, North Dakota; and with Dr. Robert Coatney, who was head of malaria research at NIH to explore an overseas assignment on monkey malaria. Dr. Comstock wanted me to go to Battey State hospital in Rome, Georgia to do a three-year residency in chest diseases but I told him that I was more interested in field epidemiology and did not want to commit myself to a three-year hospital residency in chest diseases.

I arranged to stop in Bismarck, North Dakota on my way back to Berkeley to have a look at the Heart Disease Prevention Program's field study underway there. I arrived in Bismarck with the temperature near freezing and was told by my hosts that this was one of the warmest days of the season. When we were driving to the study office I asked when we would get into Bismarck and was told that central Bismarck was at the crossroad with the gas station and post office that we passed a few miles back! My hosts also informed me that the State Governor would not be able to meet with me because he was out of town for the day. Bismarck certainly had a nice small town feel and I was excited about working and living in a small town atmosphere after growing up in Brooklyn. The field study was also actually quite interesting, but the resident study microbiologist introduced himself to me and told me that as the senior study staff he would be taking over the responsibilities of the field epidemiologist and I would be assigned to take over his position in the laboratory. I did not want to get into a turf war with him and I decided not to accept this assignment even though I think that Anne and I would have really enjoyed working and living in Bismarck.

When I got back to Berkeley, I called Bob Coatney to let him know that I hadn't accepted any of the assignments I was offered and I was still looking for an assignment within the USPHS. He offered me a dream assignment to join a senior scientist (Dr. Don Eyles) whom he had just sent to the Institute for Medical Research (IMR) in Kuala Lumpur, Malaysia to set up a field study on monkey malaria. Don Eyles would do the laboratory work and I would assist with the fieldwork. I was ecstatic and jumped at this offer. However, a week later, Bob Coatney called to let me know that he had just received a cable from Don Eyles informing him that there was no government housing available for families in Kuala Lumpur and asked that he not send anyone with a family. He told me that he would not be able to send me and my wife and infant son to join Don Eyles in Malaysia but he had another assignment for a physician to go to the Atlanta Penitentiary to carry out studies of monkey malaria with prison volunteers. I told Bob Coatney that I was more interested in field studies and did not want the Atlanta assignment which was clinical research. As it turned out, Bob Coatney had my brother, Bill, and me mixed up.

My brother Bill, who is five years older than I am, was drafted after he graduated from Michigan in 1955. He did not go to medical school until after his discharge from the army and getting his MPH degree from the University of Michigan, School of Public Health. After his internship at the USPHS hospital in San Francisco, he volunteered to go to Ghana as the first Peace Corps medical officer in the field. In 1961, as he was getting ready to return to the States after his Peace Corps assignment, he was looking for a position within the USPHS and he had been in contact with Bob Coatney at NIH about the same time that I contacted him. I remember Dr. Coatney calling me to double check if I was the same Dr. Chin he had talked to a few weeks before. He asked me if: I had graduated from the University of Michigan (I did get my bachelor's degree from UM, and Bill also graduated from UM with a bachelor's degree in addition to his MPH and MD degrees); was I already a commissioned officer in the USPHS (I was in the USPHS because of the DSHS career development program as was Bill because he interned at a USPHS hospital and he was a medical officer in the Peace Corps); was I married (we were both married); and did I have an infant son (my first son was born a couple of weeks before Bill's son, David was born). It took a while for Bob Coatney to realize that there were two Dr. Chins with somewhat similar backgrounds. Bill eventually did accept the malaria research assignment at the Atlanta Penitentiary!

Just when I thought that I would wind up with no assignment, I got a call from Reuel "Stony" Stallones who had just learned that the Hooper Foundation at the San Francisco Medical Center had just been designated one of the five new International Centers for Medical Research and Training (ICMRT).[*] He knew that Ralph Audy, the new director of the Hooper Foundation, was looking for postdoc types interested in an international research fellowship. I made an appointment to see Dr Audy and I talked briefly with him about my background. He passed me onto Fred Dunn who was the designated team leader for the first contingent of Hooper Foundation staff and research fellows who would work out of the IMR in Kuala Lumpur (KL), Malaysia. I told Fred about my exchanges with Bob Coatney about no government housing available in KL. Fred just laughed and said that government housing was very scarce in KL but there was a great abundance of good housing available in the private market and I should not worry about housing in KL.

I was accepted as an ICMRT fellow and the program I was offered included an initial fellowship year at the Hooper Foundation in San Francisco to prepare myself for research studies that I would carry out in Malaysia. Then the second

---

[*] In the late 1950s, NIH was aware that the capacity of the American medical establishment to deal with tropical diseases was atrophying. In 1960 NIH began funding several training centers in the United States. The International Centers for Medical Research and Training (ICMRT) program was designed to increase the number of US scientists competent in biomedical research and knowledgeable about health problems in other countries.

and third years of the fellowship would be devoted to implementing the studies in Malaysia with the IMR as home base. Essentially, I was given a blank check to design epidemiologic studies to be carried out at the IMR. The first year at the Hooper Foundation would be used to prepare what I might need in laboratory equipment and supplies. I resigned from active duty in the USPHS after completion of my MPH from Berkeley and since I did not remain on active duty, I was required to pay back the USPHS for my books and tuition/fees.

Hooper Foundation, ICMRT

The Hooper Foundation (The George W Hooper Foundation for Medical Research, San Francisco) established its preeminence early in the field of infectious diseases and diseases transmitted to man by animals (zoonotic diseases). Dr. Karl F Meyer, or "KF" as he was familiarly known, was one of the last scientific giants of infectious disease epidemiology and research during the 20th Century: he was the head of the Hooper Foundation from 1924 to 1954. During the early 1960s, the Hooper Foundation was housed in one of the oldest "Victorian" type buildings on the campus of the University of California Medical Center in San Francisco. I shared a small office in the basement of the Hooper Foundation with KF's last doctoral student who was studying a newly recognized infectious disease agent (Chlamydia). I remember when we introduced ourselves that I didn't hear his name distinctly and I thought he said "I'm a Jewish actor" when he was saying in his full Bronx accent "I'm Julie Schachter." To this day, I remember Julie fondly as the "Jewish actor." Julie and I had our desks pushed together because it was a very small office and late at night we often reminisced about growing up in the Bronx versus growing up in Brooklyn and now finding ourselves thrown together in a small basement office in San Francisco! Julie told me very seriously that he was going to ride to fame and glory on the back of Chlamydia because, at that time, it was a newly recognized infectious agent and the search and race was on to discover the specific diseases that this new agent might be causing both in animals and humans. Julie has indeed gone on to achieve his fame and glory as the pre-eminent chlamydiologist of our times.

During my last year in medical school and during my MPH year, I became interested in the interaction of infectious diseases with genetic polymorphism.[*] I began to plan a study to look into genetic polymorphism and leprosy. This required that I learn how to perform all of the blood typing and other laboratory tests needed for my studies. To learn how to perform the G6PD enzyme test, I arranged to travel to Seattle to spend a few days at Dr. Arno Motulsky's laboratory at the University of Washington. In addition, I was intrigued with the general problem of atypical mycobacteriae and the question of their prevalence and significance in a tropical area like Malaysia. I contacted Dr. Phyllis Edwards at the TB program formerly in the DSHS and discussed my interest in carrying out a field survey by skin testing schoolchildren: she promised to send me a supply of skin testing antigens for several atypical mycobacteriae. The preparatory year

---

[*] The search for evolutionary advantages of some genes – the classic example is the persistence of the gene for sickle cell trait because it confers some protection against Falciparum malaria.

went by fast and in February 1962 our daughter Elise was born and we prepared to leave for Malaysia when she was about six months old.

Institute for Medical Research (IMR)

In July 1962, when Elise was five months old we traveled first class on Pan-Am 1 to Malaysia via Tokyo and Hong Kong. We were sent first class because the arrangements made with the IMR required that Malaysian scientists travel first class to San Francisco. Thus, the University of California was also obligated to send us peons by first class. It was with some trepidation that Anne's family were reconciled to my taking her and our two young children to the wilds of SE Asia, but little did we or they realize how developed Malaysia was. Our trip to Malaysia was memorable aside from flying first class! I remember making reservations at the old Imperial Hotel in Tokyo and was offered a room instead in the new tower. I refused because I wanted to stay at the old Imperial and I was thankful that I was able to enjoy the last days of this section of a truly grand hotel. In Hong Kong, we stayed for a few days so that I could meet with Bob Worth who was also a first year Hooper International Research Fellow, studying the epidemiology of leprosy in Hong Kong.

When we got to Kuala Lumpur, we were housed in temporary government housing. Anne and I both had to get accustomed to British English and to a military type mess/dining hall. Children ate at about 5 to 6 pm with their nannies or parents: adults had an early seating around 7 pm or a later seating for dinner. Children were not permitted at the adult dinner hours. When we tried to get a baby sitter for the evening meals, we were told that we needed to hire a child amah or nanny to take care of our children and there were no readily available baby sitters for hire for a few hours. We quickly settled into a British colonial system of temporary government housing and regimented dining with a full-time child amah while we looked for more permanent housing. We soon found a new house that was just being finished in Petaling Jaya (PJ), a university suburb that was about 20 miles outside of KL. We found out that the British term "fortnight" means a constant two weeks because when we concluded our negotiations to rent the house we were told that it would be ready for occupancy in a fortnight. For the next couple of months, every time we asked when we could move in the answer was consistently "in a fortnight!"

We were very comfortable in the three-bedroom house we rented (with maids quarters). It was very near a Methodist church that was the Church that Anne grew up in. In retrospect, our all-too-short two years in Malaysia spoiled us because with the annual stipend I received from the University of California – about US $10 000 – we were on a par with most of the government Malaysian doctors. So we "had to" hire in addition to our child amah, a full-time house/cook amah and an almost full-time gardener. The total population of Chinese in Malaysia was about 40 percent compared with about 45 percent for Malays, about 10 percent Tamils from India and 5 percent Europeans and others: in the large cities the Chinese usually comprised 70 to 80 percent. The food in KL was and is among the best in the world particularly if you enjoy hot peppers mixed with traditional Chinese dishes and hot spicy Indian curries!

A couple of the other Hooper staff and fellows also found housing in PJ so we were able to car pool from PJ – a new community – across the new federal highway that cut through 25 miles of virgin jungle to deposit us at the IMR in KL. I have been back to PJ and KL on a couple of occasions since we left in 1964 and now the whole expanse from PJ to KL is all built up and the jungle has disappeared.

I was quite busy during my 2 years at the IMR in KL. Early on I made contact with Don Eyles who had by this time contracted with a Malay physician to help him with his field studies. We both had a good laugh about how I was able to get to KL and the IMR in spite of the miscommunications about government housing. I made contact with the leprosy expert (Dr. John Petit) assigned by the British Medical Research Council at Sungai Buloh Leprosarium that was about 25 km outside of KL to begin my genetic studies with the thousands of leprosy patients who were still living there. He welcomed my study and he provided me with the specific leprosy diagnosis/classification for each patient. There are two main types of leprosy and I was trying to find out if genetic factors might play a role in determining whether a leprosy patient developed lepromatous (multibacillary, the more infectious) or tuberculoid (paucibacillary, the less infectious) type of leprosy. I won't go into details about my studies except to say that my genetic fishing expedition among several thousand leprosy patients did not find anything of significance. However, I was able to coauthor a paper with John Petit to document that G6PD deficiency did not significantly modify the course of leprosy or its treatment with sulfa drugs. I was also able to get my study of comparative tuberculin testing of schoolchildren published in the British TB journal *Tubercle* as well as several brief papers/notes on some of my genetic studies in Malayan aborigines.

Towards the end of my two years at the IMR, my Berkeley mentor, "Stony" Stallones came on an official inspection tour of the Hooper's ICMRT assignments and I had a chance to show him what I had been doing in Malaysia. He also was looking for a field epidemiologist to replace him in the evaluation of several viral vaccines at Fort Ord, California and he urged me to consider accepting this assignment at the end of my fellowship in Malaysia. Again, it seems that my career path was being made for me by the epidemiologic gods because when Stony described the assignment to me, it was like a dream come true. I would be taking a Research Epidemiologist position with the California State Viral and Rickettsial Diseases Laboratory, one of the most pre-eminent public health laboratories in the world, and was renowned for its pioneering work in developing viral diagnostic tests.

One of the most interesting and exciting field studies I was involved with during my time at the IMR was the investigation of the cholera outbreak in Malacca in 1963. Anne and I had just returned from an all day Saturday trip to Malacca when the director of the IMR telephoned and informed me that he had just received word that there might be a cholera outbreak in Malacca. Anne and I had not eaten any food other than afternoon English tea and biscuits in Malacca so I was not worried that we might have been exposed to cholera. Since I was the only resident field epidemiologist at the IMR who did not have daily responsibilities, I was considered dispensable and the director asked me to go back down to Malacca to see what was going on. I asked him if I would have laboratory support and he asked me to contact the head of microbiology to find out. I immediately opened my epidemiology 101 notes to refresh myself on the 10 essential steps for investigating a disease outbreak. Step one was to get to the library and get as much information about the suspect disease as possible. It was Sunday morning and the library was closed so I went on to step two which was to arrange whatever laboratory support might be needed. I tracked down the head of the microbiology department at his country club where he was having his Sunday brunch. When asked what laboratory support he could provide me his answer was a simple: *none*! I then threw away my epi-101 investigation notes and headed back down to Malacca to carry out my first infectious disease outbreak investigation by "winging it."

Cholera in Malacca

The facts and complete story about this epidemic have never really been made public but I wrote a detailed report that should be in the files of the IMR. The initial cases of cholera were most likely from barter traders (smugglers) from the straits of Malacca to Malaysia. These cases led to secondary cases in the community and gradually to increasing admissions of enteric disease patients to the General Hospital. The septic tank of the hospital was not functioning and the overflow from the hospital sewage system (with increasing numbers of *Cholera vibrios*) flowed into the Malacca River a few hundred yards downstream from one of the main water intake pipes for the Malacca municipal water supply. During this season, there was regular salt water intrusion up the Malacca River that resulted in occasional salt water in the municipal water supply. The final cap to all these epidemiologic links to the cholera epidemic was the absence of chlorination in the city water supply for a full weekend. The supervisor of the water system went off on a vacation and took the keys to the lime shed. The worker responsible for chlorination did not want to break the lock to get to the lime supplies. The major city cholera outbreak started within a couple of days of the recorded zero chlorine levels in the city's water supply! I recall that I had a letter asking about the *Cholera vibrio* isolates from this outbreak from a Dr. (Major) "Bud" Benenson who was with a US Army research laboratory in Bangkok. More about "Bud" later! I did finally manage to get some basic laboratory support for my field investigation by telling the news media to ask the IMR about the status of the laboratory investigation. Shortly after this interview, the IMR sent an RAF plane to Malacca to deliver laboratory supplies in order to obtain a more definitive isolation and identification of the strains of *Cholera vibrio* that were involved in this outbreak.

Return to California and Vaccine Field Studies at Fort Ord

The California State Viral and Rickettsial Diseases Laboratory (VRDL) was located in the California State Department of Public Health in Berkeley, across the street from the School of Public Health. Dr. Edwin H Lennette,* a national and international leader in public health viral diagnostic research, was chief of the VRDL. During the 1960s, in contrast to most other state laboratories that provided basic laboratory support for public health programs, VRDL was active in the development of viral

---

* It is impossible to overstate his contribution to clinical virology through his research, the people he trained, and the books he wrote. Stony was my mentor, but Dr. Lennette was always my Chief!

diagnostic tests, training of postdoctoral research fellows, and in laboratory and field research. The VRDL had large study grants for cancer studies from the National Cancer Institute (NCI); support for field studies of viral respiratory vaccines in military recruits from the Influenza Commission of the Armed Forces Epidemiological Board (AFEB); and a grant from the Board of Vaccine Development (BOVD), National Institute of Allergy and Infectious Diseases (NIAID). It was these latter two studies that Stony had helped start: he recruited me to take charge of the field office at Fort Ord, California,* where these field studies would be carried out over the next 3 to 4 years.

I spent about 3 years at Fort Ord heading up a small field unit that tried to evaluate the efficacy of influenza and adenovirus vaccines in military recruits as well as a new respiratory syncytial virus (RSV) vaccine and a new parainfluenza virus vaccine in infants and young children. During my time at Fort Ord, I learned much about the epidemiology of respiratory viruses and the difficulties in field evaluations of these viral vaccines. What was referred to as Lennette's law, but was actually Stony's law, was that the efficacy of an influenza vaccine cannot be evaluated in the absence of an influenza epidemic. In the following years, Stony's first corollary to this law was that the relative efficacy of different influenza vaccines cannot be evaluated in the absence of an influenza epidemic. Thus we were able to administer influenza vaccines to our study populations before the start of the influenza season, but year after year, there was insufficient circulation of influenza viruses within our study populations to evaluate the effectiveness of these vaccines. Similarly, we were able to get some important information on the ability of the RSV and parainfluenza vaccines to elicit specific antibody responses, but the pediatric field study of the RSV was discontinued when it was found at Fort Ord and in other NIH field study sites that the RSV vaccine, a formalin-inactivated, alum-precipitated whole virus vaccine, enhanced rather than prevented RSV disease in vaccine recipients.

Shift to the California State Bureau of Communicable Disease Control

After completion of reports and papers about our vaccine field trials at Fort Ord, I was offered a position as head of the general epidemiology unit in the Bureau of Communicable Disease Control of the California Department of Public Health in Berkeley. This was the type of infectious disease epidemiology I had been preparing for when I first started in the USPHS career development program. Again, it was like a dream come true to be given responsibility for the surveillance, prevention, and control of infectious diseases for the State of California. I was literally handed this position because I was already in the state's civil service system as a medical officer (research epidemiologist) with the VRDL while the incumbent medical epidemiologist, Henry Renteln, was given a two-year leave of absence to work on an international health assignment with USAID in Turkey. I was fortunate because the medical officer positions in the general epidemiology unit were, at the time that I assumed my position, vacant due to recent retirements. I was

---

* Fort Ord is about 120 miles south of the San Francisco Bay area, near the cities of Monterey, Salinas, and Carmel. During the 1960s, Fort Ord was the US Army's primary training facility for basic combat and advanced infantry training.

able to recruit a couple of medical epidemiologists, former EIS officers, who had additional academic public health training and who like me thoroughly enjoyed being a public health infectious disease epidemiologist.

When the chief of the bureau retired a couple of years later, I reluctantly* allowed myself to be kicked upstairs as the chief to assume control and management of all the infectious disease program units within the bureau of CDC. These other units included the TB program unit; the immunization program unit; the sexually transmitted diseases (STD) unit; the veterinary public health unit (for zoonotic diseases); and the statistical unit. I subsequently added a new hospital infection control (nosocomial) unit; and also an infant botulism research unit to what was eventually reorganized as the Infectious Disease Section (IDS) during the mid-to-late 1970s. The total staff of the IDS by the early-to-mid 1980s was close to 200, with a mixture of half state employees and the other half federal employees assigned to work in California by the CDC, Atlanta.

I will not go into much detail about my work during my pre-AIDS years as the California State Epidemiologist responsible for public health surveillance, prevention, and control of infectious diseases except to give a brief overview of my experience working with national and international organizations involved with infectious disease prevention/control. My experience and position in California during the 1960s and 1970s qualified me to participate in many national committees on infectious disease epidemiology and infectious disease prevention/control programs. To serve on these national committees and panels required travel out of state (paid for by the national committee or panel) and I had constantly to justify to my narrow-minded bureaucratic superiors why, as a state employee, I should be permitted to travel out of state several times a month. These committees and panels were convened by organizations such as: American Public Health Association (APHA); National Institute of Health (NIH); Centers for Disease Control (CDC); Institute of Medicine/National Academy of Science (IOM/NAS); Armed Forces Epidemiological Board (AFEB); and Conference of State and Territorial Epidemiologists (CSTE). During the 1970s, I assumed leadership roles in several of these national organizations. I was elected a member of the American Epidemiological Society (AES) in 1973; elected president CSTE in 1978; and appointed as chairman of the National Advisory Committee on Immunization Practices (ACIP) from 1982–1985.

In addition to my work as a state epidemiologist, I also began to teach a course on infectious disease control for UC Berkeley's School of Public Health. Since the School was just across the street from the State Public Health Department building, I had students come to class in our building so that I did not have to spend close to a half hour walking to the campus and back. The California State Department of Public Health started a public health residency program during the 1970s and my senior medical staff and I assumed responsibility for up to two to three full-time public health residents in addition to our

---

* I was content to be head of the general epidemiology unit and did not want to manage other units in the bureau, but I was told that I would not be able to recruit Ben Werner to whom I had already committed a position, since the responsibility for recruitment of new staff would be given to the new bureau chief. Thus, in order not to leave Ben dangling to be approved by the new bureau chief, I reluctantly agreed to assume the responsibility of bureau chief.

assigned EIS office during this period. Most of these residents were assigned by their sponsoring military services. At one time we had a resident from the Army, the Navy, and the Air Force. We also accepted Pan American Health Organization (PAHO), World Health Organization (WHO), and CDC (Atlanta) sponsored fellows* for up to 3 months for public health training in infectious disease epidemiology.

I have never considered my writing skills to be one of my professional strengths and I have always had to struggle to put my thoughts onto paper. Thus, to my surprise, I was asked in the mid-1970s by Bud Benenson, editor of the then entitled *Control of Communicable Diseases in Man* (CCDM) – whom I had corresponded with about a decade earlier about cholera in Malacca – to be the associate editor for the 13th (1981) edition of CCDM. At about the same time John Last called from Canada and asked me to be the section editor (for communicable diseases) for the 11th edition of *Maxcy-Rosenau Public Health and Preventive Medicine*. CCDM was and continues to be considered the "bible" for anyone interested or working on public health prevention and control of infectious diseases: Maxcy–Rosenau was *the* standard public health textbook recommended and used in most of my classes when I was an MPH student in Berkeley in 1961. To become the associate editor for CCDM and a section editor for Maxcy–Rosenau at that stage of my public health career meant that I had made my mark as a public health infectious disease epidemiologist.

Recognition of AIDS: 1981

The CDC's Morbidity and Mortality Weekly Report (MMWR) contains data on specific diseases as reported by state and territorial health departments. It contains reports on infectious and chronic diseases of current interest and is a publication that often makes news headlines. Since MMWR provides reports of new disease outbreaks, CDC began to send an advanced copy of the week's reports to state health departments so that they would be better prepared to respond to news media questions. My management style was to foster open communications between all of the other offices and laboratories with which my bureau of CDC interacted. Thus, we had a regular one hour (maximum) infectious disease meeting every Tuesday afternoon that included senior staff from all of my bureau's units as well as representatives from the VRDL, the Microbial Diseases Laboratory, and the Food and Drug Program. I recall vividly that I handed to Tom Ault, who was the deputy chief of the STD unit, a copy of the fax that contained the prepublication report on a cluster of *Pneumocystis carinii* pneumonia in five young males, all active homosexuals, in three separate hospitals in the Los Angeles area during the period from October 1980 to May 1981. I told Tom that there might or might not be anything of significance in this cluster of cases, but I wanted him to make sure to provide LA County with any help that they might request in the investigation of these cases. Little did I realize at the time that this cluster of cases would turn out to be AIDS and that I would be spending the next couple of decades working almost exclusively on this emerging pandemic.

---

* Jeff Koplan who became Director of CDC (Atlanta) in the 1990s was one of our fellows in the 1970s.

In the ensuing weeks and months, it became apparent that the mysterious illness reported from Los Angeles was also present among MSM in San Francisco. From 1981 to 1984, AIDS cases reported from San Francisco rose almost exponentially – from a handful in mid-1981 to well over 800 towards the end of 1984. The impact that AIDS has had in San Francisco is unequaled on a per capita basis anywhere in the developed world. If the AIDS prevalence rate of about one case per 1000 population that was present in San Francisco at the end of 1984 was applied nationally, then there would have been about a quarter of a million AIDS cases nationwide instead of the 7000 that were actually reported. During the first few years of what was initially referred to as GRID (gay-related immune deficiency), there was general denial of the severity of this newly recognized mystery disease, even in San Francisco. The enormity of the AIDS problem was first fully accepted by the gay community in San Francisco. Physicians and researchers in the city rapidly became the leading experts in the country on the medical management, prevention, and control of AIDS. In contrast to Los Angeles and New York, which also had large concentrations of AIDS cases, the gay community in San Francisco has been more unified and organized in developing political and community support for the treatment and care of AIDS patients.

My Involvement With International Health Prior to GPA/WHO

My first venture into international health as a paid consultant was the result of the minority preference policy that was initiated by the Carter administration. This policy shift gave a small minority-owned "beltway bandit" firm the responsibility for recruitment of public health and other types of consultants for specific USAID projects. I was asked by a mother/son operation to be the leader of a USAID project design team to develop an operational plan for Combating Childhood Communicable Diseases (CCCD) in sub-Saharan Africa (SSA). This was a 6-week mission that involved meetings with WHO units in Geneva, visits to USAID regional offices in west and east Africa, and visits to selected SSA countries. Our small design team was royally received by WHO, especially by Ralph Henderson, director of the immunization program, and Mike Merson, newly assigned head of the Programme for Control of Diarrheal Diseases (CDD). They knew we were drawing up plans for a US$50 million disease control project in SSA and there was the possibility that we might recommend routing some project funds through WHO. The CCCD project was, in my opinion, the cornerstone of international health activities at CDC, Atlanta, during the 1980s. In retrospect, many thousands of HIV-infected persons were most likely present throughout SSA at the time that the CCCD project design team traveled throughout SSA in 1979.

My second venture into international health was in 1983 as a temporary advisor (TA) to the South East Asia Regional Office (SEARO) of WHO. At that time, I was Chairman of the National Advisory Committee on Immunization Practices (ACIP). I had thrown my hat into the ring at CDC, to be considered for a two-month appointment as a TA for international health programs, and I may have been jumped to the head of the line to evaluate the measles situation in Burma, now Myanmar. I was able to complete all of my objectives or terms of reference (TOR) for my Burma mission within 6 weeks. I was able to prepare a paper on my general findings and it was published in the Bulletin of WHO.* One of the highlights of my mission was a lecture that I gave to the Burma Medical Association on AIDS in California. At that time, there was no documented AIDS in Burma and HIV had not yet been isolated and identified. I remember the general speculation and discussion we had about what the specific cause of AIDS might be and whether AIDS would ever become a public health problem in Burma. HIV did get into Burma and epidemics in IDU and FSW were reported during the late 1980s.

My next international health consultancy was related to my being the "Godfather" of the CCCD project in SSA. As part of the CCCD project, USAID was to provide support for operational field research studies by African researchers. David Heymann, whom I would a few years later recruit to work for GPA in Geneva, asked me to participate in a 1985 meeting to review and evaluate the applied research component of CCCD. I recall on the evening before the meeting held in Mbabane, Swaziland, that there was an almost full eclipse of the moon. Equally memorable to me was that I was severely scolded when I tried to discuss AIDS in Africa with all of the best and brightest of African researchers. They all jumped on me to say that AIDS was a "western" disease of homosexuals and drug addicts and was not a problem in Africa! I knew better because I was fully aware of Jon Mann's clinical and epidemiological studies with Project SIDA in Kinshasa. I told my African colleagues, as gently as possible, that they needed to collect data to back up their claim that AIDS was not a problem in Africa rather than to just deny the possibility that AIDS was indeed present. In retrospect, the number of Africans living with an HIV infection in 1985 was probably at least 1 to 2 million!

How I Joined the Global Programme on AIDS

I knew Jon Mann when he was a "junior" state epidemiologist in New Mexico during the 1970s. Jon called me in Berkeley sometime during the early 1980s and asked me how he might get into international health work since he was getting restless in New Mexico and he had heard about my work with USAID in 1979 to design the CCCD project. I remember telling him that there were only three avenues or options for him to get some entry into international work as an infectious disease epidemiologist:

1 he could seek work with a university that had research projects overseas
2 he could try to get a position with NIH or USAID or
3 he could throw his hat into the CDC ring to be considered for an international assignment.

Jon obviously chose the latter option and he was ready, willing, and able when CDC needed an infectious disease epidemiologist who was fluent in French to head up Project SIDA in Kinshasa, Zaire in 1983.

Thus, I was well aware of what Jon was doing when he first went to Kinshasa, then to WHO in 1985 (initially as the responsible medical officer for AIDS) and to his appointment as the Head of a Special Programme on AIDS (SPA) in 1986. It was around this time that I responded to the siren call of international health.

---

* Chin J and U Thaung (1985) The unchanging epidemiology and toll of measles in Burma. *Bull WHO.* **63**(3): 551–8.

Don Francis* had joined my staff in Berkeley in 1985. He pretty much covered most of the needs of my office by coordinating HIV/AIDS surveillance with local health departments and the medical community. He was also very active in his professional liaison with gay leaders and groups regarding HIV prevention and HIV/AIDS legislation. By this time, I had concluded that the epidemiology of HIV in California was fairly well understood: the remaining challenge to public health was the apparent epidemic spread of HIV in Africa that was going to be tackled by Jon Mann at WHO, Geneva. I remember driving to Sacramento sometime in 1986 for a legislative hearing with Don and telling him that I felt that I wasn't needed or essential for the AIDS program in California. Rather I felt that I would be able to contribute more to the global challenge of AIDS at WHO.

About a year later in early 1987, I was recruited for a two-month assignment as a short-term consultant for the World Bank to be the communicable disease advisor on a team that was carrying out an evaluation of different health and healthcare programs in Indonesia. Near the end of this mission, I received an invitation from WHO to attend a meeting in Geneva to review the global AIDS situation and its possible significance for international travel. I was able to leave the World Bank team for a few days to fly from Jakarta to Geneva for this meeting where Jon asked me if I would be able to be a short-term consultant (STC) to what was then the Special Programme on AIDS (SPA). He told me that he really needed experienced public health staff to help in developing a global response to the AIDS pandemic. I told Jon that I would be more than willing to join WHO, initially as a STC, and that I was ready to take early retirement from my position in California so I would then be eligible to assume a full-time position with SPA.

---

* Depending on the informant, Don either jumped out or was kicked out of his position in the HIV/AIDS laboratory at CDC, Atlanta. I tend to believe that it was a little of both. Don wanted to come to work "in the trenches" in California, and I fully supported his assignment to my office.

Chapter 3

The Most Probable Origin and Initial Global Spread of HIV

The origin of the human immunodeficiency virus (HIV) remains a controversial and sensitive issue. Whatever "mainstream"* science or public health may have to say about the origin of HIV will be dismissed out of hand by those who refuse to accept HIV as the cause of AIDS. These persons likely comprise a significant percent of the US population and they may comprise an even larger group outside the US, especially in developing countries. In this chapter I'll present all of the available medical and epidemiologic findings that have convinced me that HIV was a natural infectious disease agent in African primates that jumped the species barrier into humans at some as yet undetermined time – decades or centuries ago – and that during the 1960s and 1970s HIV began to spread rapidly within sub-Saharan Africa (SSA) and then to other areas such as Haiti and major cities in North America and Western Europe.

International Sensitivity About the Origin of HIV

It is clear to me that I cannot prove my conclusions about the origin of HIV "beyond any reasonable doubt." However, to readers with an open mind, I believe that I can make a very strong case that the Central African origin of HIV is consistent with all available medical and epidemiologic observations. I believe that "mainstream" AIDS organizations generally accept Africa as the most likely origin of HIV, but they are all acutely aware of the international sensitivity this issue causes, especially among Africans. When and if asked about the origin of HIV, these organizations state that the origin of HIV is irrelevant to the problems at hand: These problems are the prevention and control of HIV transmission and the provision of treatment and care to the millions of HIV-infected persons throughout the world. While I agree with this latter position, I will not duck the question since most of the earliest medical and laboratory documentation of HIV/AIDS point to Africa as the origin of HIV.

I recall that during an AIDS briefing session of delegates to the World Health Assembly in the late 1980s, I made an announcement at the beginning of my presentation on the current status of the AIDS pandemic – that WHO had determined the specific origin of HIV/AIDS. Furthermore, I said that there was near-universal agreement among the AIDS experts we had conferred with about the origin of HIV, and I would divulge the answer at the end of my presentation. Needless to say, there was a bit of a stir in the audience and I particularly noted the frown on Jon Mann's face when I made this bold announcement. At the end of my presentation, I told the assembled delegates and WHO staff that there was

---

* In this book, "mainstream" will refer to the conclusions and positions regarding HIV/AIDS by WHO/UNAIDS, CDC, and NIH. I'll try to alert readers when I may stray or depart from "mainstream" conclusions and positions.

clear consensus that HIV/AIDS originated in *someone else's country*! There was a great sigh of relief from Jon and some of the high ranking WHO staff. I'm convinced that if I had said that without a doubt HIV originated in Africa, I would have had to leave WHO before Jon's resignation about a year after this meeting.

Recognition of AIDS and Initial Theories About its Origin

AIDS was first reported as a distinct clinical entity in 1981 in California. At that time there were many questions as to what the disease was and how it got into the homosexual population. The origin of HIV became one of many contentious and sensitive questions related to the HIV/AIDS pandemic and it is one where the parallel pandemic of AIDS "experts" (actually mostly AIDS activists masquerading as AIDS experts) have been instrumental in fueling and continuing the public's misunderstanding and uncertainties surrounding the AIDS pandemic.

I remember vividly the initial general alarm and panic within the gay communities in the San Francisco Bay Area and Los Angeles shortly after the MMWR reported that a mysterious and unknown disease was killing young gay males. During the latter half of 1981, cases of this invariably fatal disease kept increasing, with a doubling time of reported cases within weeks and months. Then when a few reports indicated this new disease was occurring outside of homosexual males – in injecting drug users and persons who had received blood transfusions or some human blood factors – the alarm and panic spread through the public at large. Theories abounded about the possible cause(s) of this new disease that appeared to be ravaging the immune system: they included several possible and reasonable causes such as a new infectious disease agent or a variety of drugs/poisons/toxins; some rather far-out theories that ranged from an extraterrestrial source (i.e., it came from aliens who had landed on earth); some fundamental evangelical pronouncements that this disease was "God's curse on homosexuals!"; and a host of conspiracy theories that still have staunch believers – that "HIV/AIDS was made by evil-minded scientists" in the developed world as a means of controlling the nonwhite population of the world.

A study report released in early 2005 indicated that a significant proportion of the US black population believes that HIV was made in a laboratory. The study, which was supported by the National Institute of Child Health and Human Development, polled 500 African Americans. Nearly half said HIV is man-made; more than one-quarter said they believed AIDS was created in a government laboratory; and 12 percent said the Central Intelligence Agency created and spread HIV. Kenyan ecologist Dr. Wangari Maathai, the first African woman to win the Nobel Peace Prize, received intense media coverage in late 2004 when she proclaimed that some "evil minded" scientists from the developed world deliberately researched and developed the virus in order to "punish the Blacks." Under pressure from the Norwegian Nobel committee and "mainstream" AIDS organizations she tried to squirm out of her clearly stated and held belief by claiming that she was quoted out of context and released the following statement – "It is therefore critical for me to state that I neither say nor believe that the virus was developed by white people or white powers in order to destroy the African people. Such views are wicked and destructive. I am sure the scientists will continue their search for concluding evidence so that the view, which continues to be quite widespread, that the tragedy could have been caused by biological experiments that failed terribly in a laboratory somewhere, can be put to rest." Unfortunately, Dr. Wangari's assertions appear to have wide resonance within Africa and within a large proportion of blacks in the USA. I don't believe that "mainstream" science will be able to provide her and others like her who believes in such theories with conclusive evidence to dispel their dark suspicions.

President Mbeki of South Africa and probably the majority of Africans are skeptical and just don't want to believe in the African origin of HIV/AIDS and are all too willing to listen to dissident theories such as these conspiracy theories and the theories of dissident scientists who do not believe that HIV is the causative agent of AIDS. Among other dissenting theories on the origin of HIV – rejected by the vast majority of scientists – is one by British journalist Edward Hooper suggesting that HIV emerged from a well-intentioned project by US and Belgian researchers to develop a polio vaccine in what was then the Belgian Congo in the 1950s. However, this theory does not cast doubt on the African origin of HIV, but speculates that instead of a natural jump into humans possibly via hunters skinning monkeys and getting exposed and infected via cuts, etc., that HIV was an inadvertent contaminant of one of the early polio vaccines. His theory has been dismissed by a panel of scientists after their review of all available data.

To understand fully what I believe "mainstream" science has concluded and accepted as the most probable origin of what we now know as the human immunodeficiency virus (HIV) – the etiologic agent of the acquired immunodeficiency syndrome (AIDS) – requires an open mind and some basic understanding of human infectious disease agents and how new or newly recognized infectious disease agents emerge or suddenly appear in human populations.

Zoonotic Infectious Disease Agents

Virtually all human infectious disease agents are or were disease agents of animals – i.e., zoonotic in origin. Over time, many of these agents have adapted to humans and have become *species-specific* or speciated and can no longer easily infect their former host(s). For example human infection and outbreaks due to animal influenza viruses occur constantly. HIV, types 1 & 2 are examples of zoonotic agents that have adapted to humans – i.e., they are now relatively well speciated to humans. The African origin of Simian Immunodeficiency Virus (SIV) is not generally disputed, and there is also almost no dispute that SIV and HIV share a common SIV-like ancestral virus.

The Emergence of New Infectious Disease Agents

During the past 50 years, more than 25 new or newly recognized infectious disease agents have emerged and have been detected (*see* Table 3.1). Included among these emergent infectious disease agents have been about a dozen influenza or influenza-like agents. Influenza A viruses are found in many different animals, including ducks, chickens, pigs, whales, horses, and seals. Wild birds are the primary natural reservoir for all subtypes of influenza A viruses and are thought to be the source of influenza A viruses for other animals. Pigs can be infected with both human and avian influenza viruses in addition to swine influenza viruses. Because pigs are susceptible to avian, human and swine influenza viruses, they potentially may be infected with influenza viruses from different species (e.g., ducks and humans) at the same time. If this happens, it is theoretically possible for the genes of these viruses to mix and create a new virus. While it is unusual for humans to get influenza virus infection directly from animals, sporadic human infection and outbreaks caused by avian and swine influenza A viruses have occurred. However, the emergence of a new influenza virus that "jumps" from animals to humans does not guarantee that a human disease pandemic will occur. The prime example of emergence of a non-pandemic influenza type A virus was the 1976 Swine flu outbreak! The emergence of SARS Corona virus apparently from civet cats to persons in close contact with them in southern China is another example of emergence of a non-pandemic infectious disease agent.

Table 3.1 Newly recognized infectious agents/diseases since 1950

1957 – Asian flu (A/H2N2)	1988 – USA Swine flu (A/H1N1)
1967 – Marburg virus	1988 – Hepatitis E
1968 – Hong Kong flu (A/H2N3)	1989 – Hepatitis C
1969 – Lassa fever	1992 – *Vibrio cholerae* O139
1976 – Ebola	1993 – Hantavirus (pulmonary syndrome)
1976 – Swine flu (A/H1N1)	1993 – Netherlands reassortant flu – human H3N2 and avian H1N1
1976 – Legionnaires' Disease	1995 – UK duck virus (A/H7N7)
1976 – Infant botulism	1996 – New variant of Creutzfeldt-Jakob disease – nvCJD – (Mad cow disease)
1978 – Toxic shock syndrome (TSS)	1997 – Russian flu (A/H1N1)
1981 – HIV (identified in 1984)	1997 – Hong Kong – "Chicken flu"(A/H5N1)
1982 – *Escherichia coli* O157:H7	1999 – Hong Kong – "Bird flu" (A/H9N2)
1982 – *Borrelia burgdorferi* (agent of Lyme disease)	2003 – Netherlands – Avian flu (A/H7N7)
1983 – *Helicobacter pylori* (peptic ulcer agent)	2003 – China – Severe acute respiratory syndrome – Corona virus (SARS-CoV)
1986 – Netherlands swine flu (A/H1N1)	2004/05/06 – SE Asia – "bird flu" (A/H5N1)

It is quite likely that over the past 50 years many more infectious agents have emerged, infected a few or even many persons, and then vanished undetected because human to human transmission of these agents was not high enough to sustain transmission in human populations. The increasing documentation of new flu-like agents over the past decade may not reflect an increasing rate of emergence of these agents but may be the result of increased public health attention and surveillance (or both). The "bird flu" situation in SE Asia that started in 2004 and continued into 2005 and 2006 may be an example of an emerging infectious disease agent that cannot sustain itself in human populations, but is receiving higher visibility because of the intensive surveillance instituted for "bird flu" cases. I believe that we will not need intensive surveillance to detect the next influenza pandemic virus because when it emerges, it will be very efficiently transmitted from person to person so there will be no need to ponder whether this is the next pandemic flu virus. This does not mean I'm against the intensified surveillance for emerging disease agents, including new flu agents, but such efforts need to be placed in proper perspective. Such surveillance should be looked upon as increased research on new emerging infectious disease agents and dire alarms should not be automatically sounded for each human case and death due to chicken or bird flu as the beginning of the next major flu pandemic.

Severe viral infections of primates in Central Africa that have "jumped" into humans include the Marburg virus* (identified in 1967), Lassa fever virus (1969), and Ebola virus (1976). During the 1960s and 1970s, there was significant public health concern that one of these viruses could be introduced or imported into populations outside Central Africa. Accordingly, CDC along with state and territorial epidemiologists developed guidelines and plans for responding to the potential introduction of any of these viral agents. In retrospect, although novels have been written about the potential introduction of agents such as Lassa fever and Ebola, HIV was the agent that sporadically and silently traveled "under the radar" out of Africa during the 1960s and 1970s. However, HIV was not isolated during the 1970s because the laboratory capabilities for isolating and identifying HIV were not available until the early 1980s. In addition, the number of HIV-infected persons in Africa during the 1970s was relatively small and those AIDS cases that may have occurred during this time period were not recognized as a new infectious disease. This clinical aspect of AIDS (i.e., resembling many other prevalent diseases) will be described in detail in the next chapter, which will explain exactly what AIDS is and why it has been so difficult to accept and diagnose AIDS in Africa. AIDS, as a new and invariable fatal clinical entity, was not recognized until HIV was introduced into MSM sex networks in the USA. Epidemic HIV spread in MSM populations in the USA probably began sometime during the mid-to-late 1970s. This resulted in the first wave or cluster of AIDS cases that were recognized and reported as a distinct clinical entity in California in mid-1981.

The Haitian Connection to Africa: How Jon Mann Became Director of Project SIDA

During the early 1980s, in addition to homosexual males and injecting drug users, hemophilia patients and Haitians were added to the national list of populations or subgroups in which AIDS cases were identified. These subpopulations were referred to as the four Hs – hemophilia patients, homosexuals, Haitians, and heroin addicts. While two-thirds of AIDS cases in Florida in 1982 were in recent Haitian immigrants, there were no AIDS cases reported in Haitians who had immigrated to Florida prior to 1975. It was therefore concluded that AIDS was a recent problem in Haiti and this was confirmed by an NIH and CDC team visit to Haiti in 1983. In addition to finding relatively large numbers of apparent AIDS cases equally in males and females during the Haitian visit, the NIH/CDC team also learned about a probable Haiti to Africa connection. It was common knowledge that when the Belgians were thrown out of Zaire in 1960 they contracted for Black, French-speaking teachers and professionals to teach and to work in government positions. From 1960 to 1975, Zaire reportedly imported nearly 10 000 Haitians annually for short-term labor; many of these contract workers returned to Haiti during the late 1960s and early 1970s. To follow-up this African connection, an NIH/CDC team visited Kinshasa, Zaire and they found that since

---

* In March-April 2005, an outbreak of Marburg virus occurred in Angola and resulted in over 300 deaths.

the mid-1970s, AIDS was a new and increasing phenomenon. All of this led to the creation of Project SIDA* in Kinshasa in 1983 and Dr. Jonathan Mann was selected by CDC (Atlanta) as its first director.

There are plenty of anecdotal stories of Haitian workers in Zaire during the 1960s and 1970s, but scant hard documentation of this. I recall a very interesting chat that I had with a Zairian doctor (Dr. MF Nwanatambwe) at an International Public Health Conference in Taipei in 2002. He was working at the National Institute of Infectious Diseases in Tokyo, Japan and we started to talk about AIDS in Zaire and I asked him about the "Haitian HIV/AIDS connection." He told me when he was growing up during the 1960s and 1970s that almost all of his teachers were Haitians and that most of them left sometime during the 1970s. When the official "ambassador" to Taiwan from the Democratic Republic of the Congo (formerly Zaire) joined us after dinner, he vehemently denied that there was such a thing as the "Haitian connection." This has been and continues to be a very sensitive issue.

I recall mentioning the Haitian connection to Laurie Garrett sometime during the early 1990s: she chided me for believing such anecdotal reports since she was not aware of any documentation of this – even though it might be "common" knowledge. I told her that I was confident that documents existed in Belgium that would provide hard proof of the Haitian connection because apparently the Belgian government funded the annual contracting of the thousands of Haitian workers during the 1960s and early 1970s. I told her to look up such documents if she needed "hard" proof. Apparently she did not follow up on this connection or if she did, she may have concluded that it was not newsworthy enough to write about.

In my discussions with Tom Quinn (NIH) in April 2005, he corroborated the Haitian connection, but when asked for "documentation" he said that he must have mentioned this in some of his early publications on AIDS in Africa. However, in the *Science* article AIDS in Africa (1986) for which he was the first author, Haiti was mentioned only as an area where some of the initial AIDS cases were studied – there was no mention of the Haitian connection with Zaire. I suspect that the tremendous sensitivity of Haitians to being labeled as a high-risk area and population for AIDS by CDC in the early 1980s prompted the Haitians to deny any possible HIV/AIDS connection with Zaire. Thus, NIH was very careful in their publications during this time period to avoid any mention of a Haitian HIV/AIDS connection with Zaire – they were content to have the Haitians "blame" CDC for this "insult"!

The following is "documentation" of the Haitian connection to Zaire abstracted from http://aidshistory.nih.gov/home.html – the oral history of AIDS website where NIH and CDC researchers recalled "in their own words" the early investigations of AIDS.

> ...We knew there was a "Haitian connection." Early on we had the four Hs – hemophiliacs, homosexuals, Haitians, and heroin addicts. We could not get into Haiti because they were so damned mad that we called AIDS the Haitian disease...The Haitians were incredibly angry with us, but we had a good discussion, and they extended an invitation for us [NIH] to go to Haiti. It was in the spring of 1983. I took Dr. Tom [Thomas] Quinn, an epidemiologist, and Dr. Clifford

---

* SIDA is the French acronym for AIDS.

Lane, a clinical investigator, with me. Also somebody from the CDC [Dr. Harry Haverkos]...large numbers of them [Haitians] in the 1960s had gone to Zaire as engineers, accountants, etc. When they were kicked out, some of them came back to Haiti, some of them came here [US] and to Canada, and a few went to Europe. AIDS traveled with them from Africa. My own view is that AIDS started in Africa, because of societal changes and urbanization. It had probably been confined and transmitted very sporadically in the rural communities, not spreading very far because people did not travel very far...

http://aidshistory.nih.gov/transcripts/bios/Richard_Krause.html[*]

There were reports coming out of Europe of this syndrome, and we knew the Haitians were getting it. It was pretty obvious to me that if Haitians were getting it, they had to be getting it in Haiti as well as in New York and other places in the US...The Haitians came [to NIH] and they basically said, "We do not want the CDC. They are the ones who have labeled us. But we will allow a team of investigators from the NIH to come down and invite them to find out what is going on." However, the CDC said, "We have to have at least one person on the team."...The first thing that we saw [when we went to Haiti] were these women, who were just wasted away, coughing, probably having Pneumocystis or tuberculosis or whatever, and we were told that they had tuberculosis. They showed us the X-rays. I never actually saw definitive proof of that, but it was suspected...After being in Haiti, we thought it [heterosexual transmission] was very possible, so we were calling it a heterosexual disease and maybe one that went both ways, because we saw equal numbers of men and women. Eventually, the longer we stayed down there, the more equally divided were the numbers of patients, male and female...Then there was a report in Europe of Africans with the same disease who had come from Zaire and other places to Belgium, and France, and the patients were both men and women. That was all I needed to see. It was, I think, just one report, but that was enough for me. I felt this was not just a gay disease, and I doubted that this was [due to] dirty needles. But the only way we were ever going to find out was to go to Africa or go back to Haiti and set up good prospective long-term epidemiologic studies...

http://aidshistory.nih.gov/transcripts/transcripts/Quinn96.pdf[†]

...AIDS was first diagnosed among Haitians migrants by pathologists in Florida in the form of CNS [central nervous system] toxoplasmosis. Two-thirds of the cases of AIDS in Florida in 1982 were among Haitians who were recent Haitian migrants, illegal migrants who came in the boatlift following the Duvalier debacle. As a matter of fact, there were a half a million or more Haitian-Americans who had been migrating into

---

[*] Richard Krause was head of the National Institute of Allergies and Infectious Diseases (NIAID) during the 1980s.
[†] Thomas Quinn was a young clinical research scientist who worked with the earliest AIDS cases in the Baltimore area before he was asked to join NIAID to work on HIV/AIDS.

the country legally since the 1960s, at the rate of about 8000 to 10 000 per year. Most of them lived in the Northeast, the New York and New Jersey area. Almost all the Haitians were in that area. Very few were in Florida, actually. And there were no cases of AIDS in those Haitians who had legally migrated. So, whatever it was, this was something that was a recent problem in Haiti...it was a horrible thing to implicate the Haitian migrants as having AIDS. But the truth was, they had AIDS, we did not know the cause yet, and we had no choice. So Haitians were reported with AIDS. In our studies of Haitians, we learned they were heterosexual...Then, the story in Africa came along...One of the men, who was on our staff at the CDC, was a guy named [Dr. Joseph] Joe McCormick, who was a hemorrhagic fever virus expert, and who is now at the Pasteur Institute. He had worked extensively in Africa. As a matter of fact, when he got out of college, he entered the Peace Corps as a high school teacher in Zaire. That experience was in the late 1960s, before he went to medical school. When the Belgians were removed from power in Zaire, there were very few educated Zairians. They brought in many expatriates, including Haitians, to teach in Zaire. When Joe was over there teaching in the Peace Corps, he was teaching with many Haitians, many of whom, like Joe, subsequently returned to their own country...[Joe] believed that the most plausible idea was that this problem comes from Central Africa, is transmitted to Haiti, and then gets transmitted to the North American continent somehow through a combination of factors. Now that kind of speculation back in the 1980s would be enough to get you severely criticized, but it was the most plausible hypothesis. Then Americans transmitted it through sexual contact to injecting drug users. But the pattern in Haiti looked very much like the pattern in Central Africa...

...Joe McCormick from the CDC; Sheila Mitchell, who was a technician who worked on AIDS, and [Dr.] Peter Piot, who was with the Institute of Tropical Medicine [ITM], visited Zaire with these NIH colleagues. The initiation of that visit had been a combination of Dick Krause talking to the head of ITM at the time and Joe McCormick talking to some of his colleagues in Zaire...During that visit...They were able to determine, with a man named Dr. Kapita, who was the head of medicine at Mama Yemo Hospital, that there were a lot of cases of this illness and wasting syndrome occurring. It was a fairly new phenomenon that he had been seeing with increasing frequency since the late 1970s. They were able to get quite a few blood specimens, interview a few people, and they came back and published a summary article in the *Lancet*. After they came back, the CDC and the NIH were absolutely convinced that there was an epidemic in that city, Kinshasa, and that there should be some additional scientific commitment to a project there. And we agreed to do it together...Jonathan Mann was our first project director [Project SIDA in Kinshasa, Zaire]...he was an enormously productive physician and scientist who spoke fluent French. His wife was French, and he had studied in France. He had been a state epidemiologist in New Mexico. I met him and was very captivated with his abilities and his fluency in French. And his desire to do something like this was very important. So he went over to initiate the project...Jonathan left after two years, and became the founding director of the AIDS program at the World Health Organization.

http://aidshistory.nih.gov/transcripts/transcripts/Curran98.pdf*

The following is the only published paper that I found that provides some additional specific details regarding the Haitian HIV/AIDS connection to Zaire.

In 1960, the new nation of Zaire recruited French-speaking managers to work in this country. To replace the Belgian managers who had abruptly left the country without training local Zairians managers and executives, a significant number of Haitian intellectuals fleeing the Duvalier regime had gone into exile to work in Zaire. These French-speaking managers (administration, health service, and teaching staff) gave Zaire an extraordinary opportunity to avoid failure at the beginning of its independence. These Haitian immigrants made the country function, in particular, in the economically strong provinces of eastern and southern Zaire (Shaba province). After 1968, Zaire completed the training of local national managers, and Haitians began to leave central Africa at the beginning of 1970 and were slowly replaced by native Zairians...Between 1970 and 1975, some Haitians exiles in central Africa emigrated either to Europe (France and Belgium), Canada, and the United States, or returned to Haiti (because of less severe political repression in their native country). Medical investigations made in Haiti from 1985 to 1988 and clinical observations (Henrys D, Molez J-F, unpublished data) reported the deaths of retired Haitian managers who had lived and worked in Zaire and then returned to Haiti (and had lived there for a period of 10–15 years) that were suspected to be due to AIDS. Haitians who returned to Haiti from Zaire indicated that some of their fellow emigrants showed the same lethal pathology...

www.ajtmh.org/cgi/reprint/58/3/273

Molez JF (1998) The historical question of acquired immunodeficiency syndrome in the 1960s in the Congo River basin area in relation to cryptococcal meningitis *Am J Trop Med Hyg.* **58**(3): 273–6.

Despite these observations the author of this paper concluded: "Concerning the implication of the Haitian migration in the emergence of the HIV from the Congo River basin area, complementary research would be necessary to confirm or deny the hypothesis given in this report. This historical research belongs to the demographers and anthropologists; they would have the means to have access and exploit the migratory data in the various countries concerned (if these data exist)." This author also said that the Belgians abruptly left the country without training local Zairian managers and executives. What he didn't say was that the Belgians were abruptly thrown out of Zaire – the following is a quote from the oral history of Zaire by a Zairian painter/historian who was describing events in Zaire in 1960.

---

*Jim Curran was working on STDs when he was tapped to be the first head of the AIDS program at CDC.

The initial recognition of what is now known as AIDS was reported in five young homosexual males in Los Angeles, California in June 1981. Subsequent epidemiologic investigations showed that AIDS was occurring in the USA during the early 1980s in the following populations:

1 homosexual populations in several major cities of the USA
2 [heroin-]injecting drug users (IDU), especially on the northeast coast of the USA
3 Haitians in southern USA who migrated to the USA after 1975 and
4 hemophilia patients who received pooled blood products.

NIH and CDC visited Haiti in 1983 to follow up on the relatively high number of Haitians in Florida who had AIDS and who had recently emigrated from Haiti to the US. There they learned of the probable introduction of AIDS into Haiti by Haitian contract workers returning from Zaire. Dr. Jonathan Mann was sent by the Centers for Disease Control (CDC) to Kinshasa, Zaire in 1984 to investigate the HIV/AIDS link between Haiti and Zaire. His studies and others showed that HIV/AIDS was prevalent in SSA and this led to the eventual development of the World Health Organization's Global Programme on AIDS (WHO/GPA) in 1987.

Whether gay men in the 1970s independently introduced HIV to Haiti cannot be proved or disproved, but it is more likely that gay men from NYC or other urban centers acquired HIV in Haiti and then introduced HIV into bathhouses in NY and SF, and perhaps into "shooting galleries" on the east coast. It should be noted that the HIV epidemics in MSM and IDU in major cities in North America and Western Europe had no effect on HIV transmission in SSA. If, for some reason, the MSM and IDU epidemics had not occurred, the HIV situation in SSA would have progressed as it has. The major difference is that it would have delayed recognition of HIV/AIDS for almost a decade and delayed the start of the massive and unprecedented public health and research efforts to identify and isolate the etiologic agent and the development of drugs to treat this newly recognized viral agent!

AIDS would not have been initially labeled as an American disease of homosexuals and injecting drug users if AIDS were first recognized as an African disease like Marburg, Ebola, and Lassa fever viruses. The stigma and discrimination issues that were integral aspects of the "American" disease would not have been so prominent and nominal (i.e., named) reporting of HIV-infected persons and AIDS cases would have been the norm. However, without the social and political pressures brought by the "gay" lobby to focus national and international efforts on research of HIV/AIDS, it is unlikely that billions of dollars would have been allocated to this problem.

Finally, the actual origin and initial global spread of HIV are irrelevant for the current development and implementation of effective prevention programs. Nevertheless, the most likely origin of HIV/AIDS should not be ignored or denied because of social or political correctness!

Chapter 4

A Basic Primer on HIV Infections and AIDS Cases (HIV/AIDS)

This chapter addresses the fundamental questions: What exactly is AIDS? Is HIV the etiologic (causative) agent of AIDS? Why has it been so difficult to convince dissidents that HIV causes AIDS? The best known AIDS dissident, Peter Duesberg, has received undeserved prominence for his unsupported assertion that HIV has not fulfilled all of Koch's original postulates for causation of an infectious disease, and thus cannot be accepted as the cause of AIDS. In this chapter, I will respond to many of the myths, misconceptions and misunderstanding of HIV/AIDS. First I will provide some basic information on infectious disease agents and the diseases they cause, along with some basic concepts of infectious disease epidemiology. What I'll describe in broad strokes about HIV/AIDS will be covered in much more detail in subsequent chapters that focus on: major HIV risk behaviors and patterns of HIV transmission dynamics (*see* Chapter 5); understanding HIV/AIDS numbers and estimation/projection of HIV prevalence (*see* Chapter 6); global and regional HIV/AIDS patterns and prevalence (*see* Chapter 7); and prevention/control of HIV transmission (*see* Chapter 8).

What is AIDS? Is HIV the Cause of AIDS?

Before I answer these basic questions I need to provide those readers who may not know much about epidemiology and infectious diseases with some basic understanding of infectious disease epidemiology. I believe that there has been a general problem in assuming that everyone involved with or interested in AIDS and AIDS programs has a basic knowledge of infectious disease agents and infectious disease epidemiology. In my briefing sessions with new GPA/WHO staff, I encountered many persons who thought that they were knowledgeable about infectious diseases, especially AIDS, when they were not. Professor Peter Duesberg is a prime example of this general problem and he has used his superficial knowledge about infectious diseases to support his theory that AIDS is not an infectious disease and further that HIV is not the cause of AIDS. Those readers who think they know all they need to know about epidemiology and infectious diseases should at least skim the following pages on epidemiology and specifically infectious disease epidemiology to check out whether they agree with what I consider to be the basics of infectious disease epidemiology. Once we are all on the same page with regard to understanding the concepts and methods of epidemiology, more specifically the basics of infectious disease epidemiology, and finally the natural history of HIV infection and AIDS along with AIDS case definitions, I'll address in detail Duesberg's assertions that:

1 HIV does not behave like a classical infectious disease agent
2 HIV is not the cause of AIDS; HIV is merely a harmless passenger virus and
3 AIDS is not a new disease in Africa but merely old diseases that are now redefined by AIDS organizations as a new infectious disease.

Epidemiology

Epidemiology is basically a measurement science: it is often called the science arm of public health because it is usually left to the epidemiologists to measure and evaluate the occurrence and rate of diseases or conditions in different populations. Epidemiologists study a diverse range of health conditions as well as the impact that various exposures or factors may have on the manifestation of disease. There are many definitions of epidemiology but the one I use is:

> Epidemiology is the study of the factors that influence or determine the patterns and prevalence of a disease or condition in populations.

Epidemiologists are concerned with and study populations rather than individuals. It is the responsibility of epidemiologists to:

1 describe and measure different levels or rates of disease or conditions in different populations and
2 evaluate and decide what factors are responsible for different cases and rates of health or disease.

Epidemiologists are trained to combine observational methods with analytic techniques to describe and compare the risk or probability of developing a disease in both qualitative and quantitative terms. Thus the field of epidemiology is comprised of statistical methods and concepts such as the design of prospective and retrospective studies, use of control populations, and a mind-set that is constantly vigilant to *avoid or minimize bias* and to detect and measure confounding variables. With regard to most infectious diseases, but especially HIV/AIDS, a major problem that I see is that virtually everyone who is interested in or who works in any AIDS program, from laboratory specialists to clinicians, considers themselves to be epidemiologists and thus experts on estimating and projecting the current and future course of the AIDS pandemic.

From my perspective, an epidemiologist is similar to a conductor of a symphony orchestra in that he/she must be knowledgeable about all aspects of the music to be played and of the strengths and limitations of his/her musicians as well as their instruments. An infectious disease epidemiologist does not have to be a licensed physician, or a certified laboratory scientist, or an expert statistician, but he/she must utilize the contributions of all of these allied sciences in order to understand all of the factors that influence or determine the patterns and prevalence of HIV infections and AIDS cases (HIV/AIDS) in different populations. I believe I have a good understanding of basic virology, but I do not consider myself to be an "expert" virologist. However, too often, prominent laboratory scientists will pontificate on the potential for epidemic HIV transmission in different populations as if they were true "experts" on the epidemiology of HIV/AIDS. In late 2003 or early 2004, I was watching Dr. David Ho give a televised presentation about HIV/AIDS in China to an audience in Los Angeles. During the question and answer period at the end of his presentation, he deftly fielded questions about anti-HIV treatment programs and laboratory aspects of HIV in China. However, when he was asked a detailed question about current HIV/AIDS cases and trends and asked to speculate on the future of HIV/AIDS in China, he did not pretend to be an expert on HIV/AIDS numbers in China. He said that such questions need to be answered by an epidemiologist knowledgeable about the epidemiology of HIV/AIDS in China. Unlike many other prominent laboratory scientists, he did not consider himself to be an expert epidemiologist.

Basic Epidemiologic Methods

Unraveling the epidemiology of a specific infectious disease is analogous to detective work. There are many similarities in the basic questions asked and the methods used by police trying to solve a crime and those used by public health epidemiologists trying to determine whether a new disease is emerging and if so, what the cause might be. When the first clusters of what we now know as AIDS were reported in 1981, public health epidemiologists from local and state health departments as well as from CDC, Atlanta all began very intensive investigations to answer the following questions.

Who of **whom**, developed **what, when, where**, and **why**?

These questions provide a simple outline of epidemiologic thinking and methods and we will use this outline to describe the basic epidemiology of HIV infections and AIDS cases (HIV/AIDS).

What we now know as AIDS (Acquired Immune Deficiency Syndrome) was first reported in five young homosexual males in Los Angeles, California in June 1981.* Applying the epidemiologic method above, we had five young male homosexuals as the **who**, and the first epidemiologic question is "**of whom**", i.e., from what specific population were these five males drawn? Were they from the general male homosexual population or from a very specific subgroup of the male homosexual population? This simple question – **who of whom** – represents the most important and challenging aspect of the epidemiologic method. We will see in subsequent chapters that failure to answer this question accurately continues to obscure the full understanding of HIV transmission dynamics and contributes to our failure to target specifically persons with the highest levels of HIV risk behaviors in HIV/AIDS prevention programs. The **who of whom** question also enables the calculation of the prevalence rate for HIV-infected persons or AIDS cases. The **who** is the numerator, and the **of whom** is the denominator for the calculation of the prevalence rate. Since the initial report was a clinical description of a few cases of a new disease syndrome and was not part of a specific population-based study, the epidemiologic question **who of whom** could not be answered with the available data. A more detailed description of incidence and prevalence rates and how they are estimated or calculated are presented in Chapter 6.

The answer to the "**developed what**" question applied to the first MMWR report is that the **what** appeared to be a new disease that resulted in immune deficiency. As we will later realize, there are many possible **what**s, since the natural history of HIV infection begins with HIV transmission followed over many years with different clinical stages of the disease syndrome we now refer to as AIDS. AIDS is a complex disease not easily understood by persons without some medical training. The disease follows a dynamic course from HIV infection

---

* CDC (1981) Pneumocystis pneumonia – Los Angeles. *MMWR*. **30**: 250–2.

to the relentless destruction of the host's immune system and to the progressive development of clinical diseases that are the surrogate or indirect markers of the impaired immune system. More details about the epidemiology and natural history of HIV infections as well as the public health surveillance definitions of AIDS will be presented in a later section of this chapter.

The epidemiologic questions of **when** did this condition/disease/syndrome occur, **where** did it occur, and finally **why** or **how** did this happen are all questions that need to be answered in order to understand the epidemiology of HIV infection. An important point to note: there is a major difference in **when** an AIDS case was reported and **when** the patient developed AIDS. Both dates should be collected, since both are important in evaluating AIDS patients' delays in seeking medical attention and/or the delays of healthcare providers in their recognition, diagnosis and reporting of AIDS cases. The **why** or **how** is the biggest challenge to infectious disease epidemiologists and details of how HIV is transmitted from person to person will be described in detail in Chapter 5.

Epidemiology is the study of the factors that influence or determine the pattern and prevalence of disease in populations – specifically how, when and where they occur. Epidemiologists attempt to determine what factors are associated with diseases (risk factors), and what factors may protect people or animals against disease (protective factors). Epidemiologic studies cannot prove causation; that is, they cannot prove that a specific factor actually causes the disease being studied. Epidemiologic studies and data can show only that a risk factor is statistically associated (correlated) with a higher incidence of disease in the population exposed to that risk factor. The higher the correlation the more certain the association, but the association does not prove causation. Koch's postulates were formulated in the late 19th Century to provide a set of rigorous criteria that had to be fulfilled before a causal relationship for a specific microbe and disease could be accepted. Whether HIV has fulfilled all of Koch's postulates and so may be considered the cause of AIDS will be described in detail later in this chapter.

The strength of an epidemiologic study depends on the number of cases and controls included in the study. If more individual cases are included in a study, the more likely it is that a significant association will be found between the disease and a risk factor. Just as important is the determination of what behavioral, environmental, and health factors should be studied as possible risk or protective factors. If inappropriate factors are chosen, and the real factors are missed, the study will not provide any useful information. It is possible that an association may be found between an inappropriate factor and the disease because the inappropriate factor (call it factor 1), is associated with another factor (factor 2), which is actually related to the disease, but which was not studied. In this case, factor 1 is called a confounding variable, because it confounds the interpretation of the study results. Thus, it is very important that an epidemiologist choose the proper factors to study at the outset, and not study too many factors at once, since the possibility of finding confounding factors increases with the addition of more variables.

Such a confounding factor or variable was that of toxic drugs or some poisons identified as the cause of AIDS. Duesberg, along with many other scientists who were studying AIDS in California in the early 1980s, recognized the relatively high rate of "recreational" drug use among some MSM and postulated that AIDS was caused by these drugs or some unknown toxins or chemicals contained in these drugs. When injecting drug users also began to develop AIDS, this reinforced Duesberg's belief that AIDS was not caused by an infectious disease agent but by toxic drugs, a belief to which he continues stubbornly to hold onto. Another example of a confounding factor that obscured a very important protective factor for sexual HIV transmission was that of male circumcision. Comparison of HIV rates showed high HIV prevalence in uncircumcised males compared with low HIV prevalence in circumcised males. Circumcision was not generally accepted as being a specific protective factor because it was also directly correlated with religion and different patterns and prevalence of sexual risk behaviors. Thus, it required additional epidemiologic analyses and studies to show that male circumcision is indeed a major protective factor for sexual HIV transmission, independent of the differences in the patterns and prevalence of sexual risk behaviors!

Infectious Disease Agents

Table 4.1 Infectious disease agents

Type	Description	Diseases
Parasites	Large multi-cellular parasites to single-cell Protozoa	Tapeworm infestation, Amebiasis, Malaria
Fungi	Simple organisms that resemble plants but lack chlorophyll	Athlete's foot to severe systemic Histoplasmosis
Bacteria	Single-cell organisms that lack chlorophyll and have no internal cell membranes. Their taxonomy is complex and some bacteria have been considered as viruses or plants. Antibiotics are effective for treating many bacterial infections	Anthrax, Tuberculosis, Syphilis, Gonorrhea, Whooping cough, Plague, Cholera, Epidemic typhus, Rocky Mountain spotted fever, Q fever
Viruses	Obligate intra-cellular agents that use host cells to reproduce. Antibiotics are ineffective against viruses.	AIDS, Genital herpes, Smallpox, Measles, SARS, Rubella, Chickenpox, Monkeypox, Influenza,
Prions	An infectious protein particle similar to a virus but lacking nucleic acid	BSE ("Mad cow disease"), new variant CJD [nvCJD], Kuru, Scrapie

We live in a world teeming with many other life forms and we can easily recognize the tremendous differences and diversities within the visible animal and plant kingdoms. As with the higher orders of animals and plants, there are also tremendous differences and diversity in what are commonly referred to as germs or microbes. The vast majority of microbes are harmless for humans but many are needed or essential for human life: some (microbial disease agents) are harmful. In Chapter 3, I described the general origin of human infectious disease agents, i.e., they are virtually all derived from animals – zoonotic. There are many major types of infectious disease agents (*see* Table 4.1), ranging in size from microscopic single-cell organisms to parasitic worms that can grow to several feet in length. The most common human infectious disease agents are bacterial and viral agents. In its simplest form, a virus is a minute capsule that contains genetic material. The major mission of a virus is to reproduce. However, unlike bacteria, viruses aren't self-sufficient – they need to gain entry into a suitable host cell to "take over" the cell and to get the cell to manufacture the parts it needs for reproduction. Host cells are eventually destroyed during this process. HIV is a viral agent that "jumped" from nonhuman primates in Central Africa to humans probably sometime during the early-to-mid 20th Century. Unlike bacterial infections for which many drugs and antibiotics have been developed for effective treatment, there is generally no effective drug treatment for most viral infections.

Epidemiology of Infectious Diseases

To understand infectious disease epidemiology one must know the exact meaning of the following words or terms:

1 *Exposure* to an infectious disease agent occurs when there is actual or potential physical contact with an agent that may result in an infection. Not all exposures result in infections.
2 *Infection* occurs when an infectious disease agent enters a host and grows and multiplies.
3 *Clinical spectrum of infection* – from virtually no clinical signs and symptoms to mild or severe disease and death. Not all infections result in any obvious disease in the host.
4 *Disease syndrome* – a recognizable pattern or group of multiple signs, symptoms or malformations that characterize a particular condition; syndromes are thought to arise from a common origin.

Transmission Patterns of Infectious Disease Agents

There are many different types of infectious disease agents. Each agent has specific epidemiologic characteristics such as how it is transmitted and how infectious the agent may be. It is important to know the specific modes or routes of transmission for any infectious disease agent in order to develop appropriate interventions to limit or prevent its transmission. Similarly, it is important to know how infectious the agent may be in order to estimate the probability or risk of infection for any specific exposure to the agent. Some infectious disease agents such as measles virus are extremely infectious: virtually all exposures to this virus in persons who never had measles or never received measles vaccine will result in typical measles disease within a week or so after exposure. In contrast, HIV transmission requires the transfer of HIV-infected blood or of body fluids such as sexual secretions (semen). Furthermore it may require up to a thousand or more unprotected sexual exposures to transmit HIV infection to a susceptible sex partner. Each infectious disease agent has its own unique epidemiologic characteristics or profile as shown in Table 4.2.

Table 4.2 Selected epidemiologic and natural history characteristics of different infectious diseases

Disease	Influenza	Tuberculosis	Genital Herpes	AIDS
Type of agent	Influenza viruses	*Mycobacterium tuberculosis* (bacteria)	Herpes simplex virus, type 2 (HSV-2)	Human immuno-deficiency virus (HIV)
Transmission	Airborne via respiratory tract	Airborne via respiratory tract	Primarily via sexual contact	Primarily via sexual contact and via blood
Infectivity	High	Low to moderate	Moderate to high	Low
Period from exposure to infection/ disease	1–3 days	2–10 days, with variable latent period for TB disease	2–12 days, with variable recurrences	Acute infection (1–3 months) – to AIDS (median of 8 years)
Clinical spectrum of infection	Majority of infections asymptomatic, mild or moderate	Majority of infected persons do not develop clinical TB	Majority of infected persons develop acute genital lesions	Vast majority (>90 percent) will develop severe immune deficiency
At risk population	General population	Close personal and household contact	Sex contacts	Sex and blood sharing contacts
Case fatality	Generally low	Moderate without treatment	Low	Among the highest
Treatment	Limited new drugs	Effective drugs and antibiotics	Limited new drugs	New drugs effective but require lifetime use

The major point this table demonstrates is that an infectious disease agent such as HIV which requires sex or blood contact for transmission from person to person cannot become a "generalized" epidemic agent. By contrast, an agent such as influenza can be very infectious and does not require direct physical contact to spread from person to person. HIV and genital herpes virus (HSV-2) are both viral agents primarily transmitted from person to person via direct physical contact (unprotected sexual intercourse). The general pattern and prevalence of these infections in any population are similar: only persons who have multiple sex partners or who are the regular sex partner of an infected person are at any risk of acquiring or transmitting these viral infections via sexual contact. As we will see in Chapter 5 (on HIV epidemiology and transmission dynamics), epidemic HIV transmission requires a very high level of HIV risk behaviors and public health interventions must be directed to persons with the highest levels of HIV risk behaviors and not to the general public.

HIV is Not a Simple, "Classical" Infectious Disease Agent

It is essential to have some knowledge of the natural history of HIV infection and the clinical and public health definitions of an AIDS case to fully understand HIV/AIDS numbers. The following section presents the current mainstream medical science view of HIV infections and AIDS. We need to understand the marked differences of infectious disease agents and especially the diseases that they cause in order to respond to the assertion that AIDS is not a new disease in Africa and that HIV is not the cause of AIDS.

Immune Deficiencies and Natural History of HIV Infection

Immune deficiency disorders or conditions can be classified as

1 primary or inherent and
2 secondary or acquired.

Primary immune deficiency is caused by genetic defects in the immune system. An example of a primary immune deficiency disease or condition is Severe Combined Immune Deficiency (SCID), commonly referred to as "boy in the bubble disease." David the "bubble boy" was born in 1971 with SCID, but because he had an older brother who died of SCID, his doctors suspected that David would be similarly affected and prepared a germ-free birth and living environment for him. David lived his entire life in "bubbles" – isolation chambers designed by NASA space engineers. However, as he grew older, David longed for a normal life outside his "bubbles" and at the age of 12 he received a bone marrow transplant from his sister who had a normal immune system. Unfortunately, David died as a result of a Cytomegalovirus (CMV) infection that was present in his sister's bone marrow. Without the germ-free environment provided by David's "bubbles", he would have likely succumbed at a very early age to infections that persons with normally functioning immune systems could easily cope with.

Secondary or acquired immune deficiency is caused by toxic drugs or by viral agents such as the Human Immunodeficiency Virus (HIV). HIV attacks the human immune system: the major target cells of HIV are helper T lymphocytes, or T_4 cells that are vital for the functioning of the human immune system. HIV binds to specific receptors (CD_4 antigen) on the surface of T_4 cells and some macrophages, effectively destroying these cells. The decrease in the number of CD_4 T cells is the primary mechanism by which HIV causes severe immunodeficiency. The result is a serious impairment of the immune system that renders the host susceptible to pathogens – such as viruses, fungi, parasites, and many bacteria – that are normally controlled by the T lymphocytes of the host's immune system. The infected person becomes increasingly vulnerable to many opportunistic infections and cancers. These illnesses are surrogate or indirect indicators of the immunodeficiency due to HIV and collectively they constitute the diagnosis of **A**cquired **I**mmune **D**eficiency **S**yndrome (AIDS). Survival after the onset of AIDS is, in the absence of anti-HIV treatment, short, and is usually less than one year in most developing countries.

Figure 4.1 shows the different clinical stages and estimated approximate intervals from acquisition of an HIV infection to development of AIDS (according to different public health surveillance definitions), and from AIDS to death.

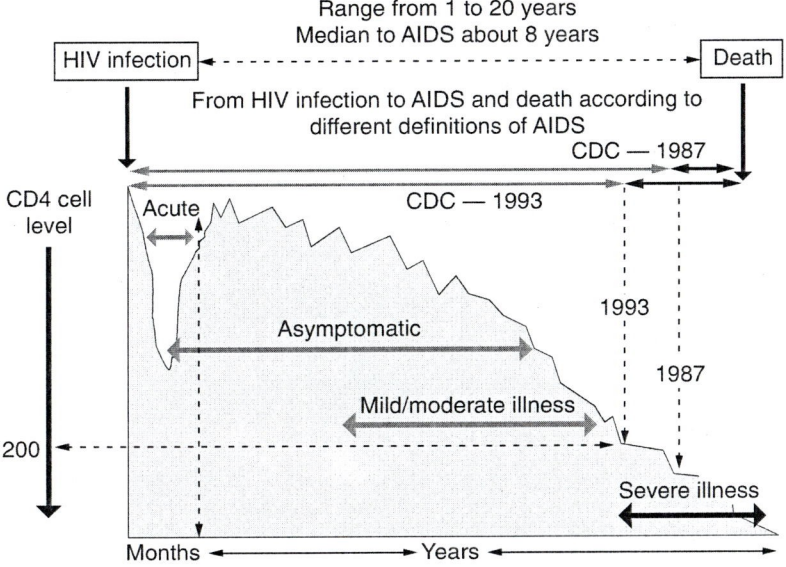

Figure 4.1 Clinical spectrum of HIV infection and CDC definitions of AIDS.

Initial HIV infection is indicated by the presence of antibodies often without any other signs or symptoms but some persons experience a short, mononucleosis-like illness about 2 to 5 weeks after infection. During this acute phase, there may be a significant depression of the cellular immune system. Subsequently, the immune system rebounds to "normal" levels and the infected person becomes asymptomatic for periods ranging from many months to many years. Antibodies to HIV are detectable, but individuals experience no symptoms. Progression to symptomatic disease is highly variable and may rarely occur within a year, or take more than 10 years. Based on the most recent prospective cohort data, it is believed that the median period for the development of severe immune deficiency as measured by a CD_4 cell count of less than $200/mm^3$ is about 8 years. This median period has been shown to be similar in large prospective cohort studies in several developed countries (USA and a few European countries) and in several developing countries (Haiti, Thailand, and Uganda).

Survival after onset of AIDS defining illnesses is also variable, but limited. In most developed countries average survival before the advent of effective anti-HIV drugs in the mid-1990s was about 2 years. In developing countries survival from the development of AIDS to death averaged about 6 months. The shorter survival in developing regions was most likely due to diagnosis at a later stage of disease and limited access to medical care. This very long interval from HIV infection to death (almost a decade) is very, very important to keep in mind when we begin to measure HIV infections and try to determine if they are increasing or decreasing.

Development of Case Definitions for AIDS

The first step in any epidemiologic study of a new disease or condition is to develop a specific case definition in order to define exactly what requirements must be met to classify someone as a "case." When the first few cases of what is now known as AIDS were reported, CDC initiated intense public health surveillance for this new and invariably fatal disease that appeared to attack the immune system. The first priority was to develop a case definition for public health surveillance purposes. This definition needed to be as sensitive and specific as possible, but initially, greater priority was given to sensitivity – i.e., it was important not to miss any possible case. Thus, the definition needed to be as broad as possible even if some diseases or conditions that may not have been AIDS were captured by this broad definition, i.e., for surveillance purposes, the specificity of the definition could be relaxed.

In 1982, the Centers for Disease Control's (CDC) case definition of what was initially named gay-related immune deficiency (GRID) and shortly changed to AIDS was defined as: "a disease at least moderately predictive of a defect in cell-mediated immunity, occurring in a person with no known cause for diminished resistance to that disease" (CDC, *MMWR*, September 1982). More than a dozen opportunistic infections and several cancers were considered to be sufficiently specific indicators of the underlying immunodeficiency for inclusion in the initial case definition of AIDS developed by CDC. As more cases were reported and analyzed, the CDC definition was periodically revised and refined. In 1985 CDC added several additional diseases that would be accepted as indicative of AIDS if the patient were found to be HIV positive. In 1987, the CDC definition was again revised to include additional indicator diseases and to accept as a presumptive diagnosis some of the indicator diseases if laboratory tests showed evidence of HIV infection.

In 1993 CDC again revised its public health surveillance definition of AIDS to include pulmonary tuberculosis, recurrent pneumonia and invasive cervical cancer in HIV-infected individuals. In addition, all HIV-infected persons with a CD_4+ cell count of less than $200/mm^3$ or a total CD_4+ T-lymphocyte percent of less than 14 percent, regardless of clinical status, were considered as having AIDS by this revised definition. The 1993 expanded CDC definition of AIDS resulted in a marked increase of reported AIDS cases in the USA during 1993 and 1994. However, this increase in reported AIDS cases according to the revised definition did not mean that there was any real increase in AIDS cases. This definition change enabled a diagnosis of AIDS to be made at an earlier stage of HIV infection in some persons and the increased number of reported cases in 1993 and 1994 resulted in a relative decrease in diagnosed and reported AIDS cases after the mid-1990s because AIDS cases that were diagnosed earlier (1993–1994) could not be diagnosed later (1995–1996) when they would have met the older (1987) AIDS definition.

Developing countries generally lack adequate laboratory facilities for the histologic or culture diagnosis of the many specified surrogate indicator diseases needed to meet any of the CDC's AIDS definitions. In 1985, WHO developed a clinical case definition of AIDS for public health reporting in Africa (Bangui definition) that relied on specific combinations of major and minor signs/symptoms and diseases for a diagnosis of AIDS. In 1994, an expanded WHO case definition for AIDS surveillance for adults and adolescents in Africa was developed; the 1994 WHO surveillance definition incorporated major features of the initial WHO clinical definition and the 1987 CDC definition. Major features of the 1994 WHO definition included both pulmonary and extra-pulmonary manifestations of tuberculosis associated with features of the wasting syndrome, and HIV serologic testing.

The continuing problem for public health surveillance of AIDS cases in most countries throughout the world is that most physicians and public health workers (including many national and local AIDS program staff) are not familiar with these case definitions and make a diagnosis of AIDS in almost any patient who has some illness and who is found to be HIV positive. In contrast to a "simple" infectious disease such as measles where the measles virus is very infectious and the incubation period from infection to disease is short (1–2 weeks) and the clinical manifestations of high fever and a distinctive skin rash are easy to recognize and diagnose, the epidemiology and natural history of HIV infections are much more complex. Severe damage to the immune system may take up to a decade or more and the clinical manifestations of immunodeficiency can range from common "opportunistic" diseases such as tuberculosis to less common diseases such as *Pneumocystis carinii* pneumonia.[*]

Another important point is that the background or population floras of infectious disease agents differ in different populations. Thus, the surrogate or indirect disease markers of the immune deficiency due to HIV will be different for different populations. In addition, AIDS is not a simple infectious disease because it is a disease syndrome. A disease syndrome is defined as a recognizable pattern or group of multiple signs, symptoms or malformations that characterize a particular condition that all result from a common origin. HIV attacks the immune system and all of the infections and rare cancers that are considered indicative of AIDS result from the immunodeficiency caused by HIV. There are significant problems in the recognition and diagnosis of an AIDS case that were compounded by the changing public health surveillance definitions. As I will repeatedly point out, reported AIDS case data have to be critically evaluated: these data cannot be used without a complete understanding of the inherent deficiencies in the public health reporting of a complex disease syndrome such as AIDS.

The Parallel Epidemics of AIDS and Tuberculosis

Potential interactions between HIV and other infectious disease agents have caused great medical and public health concern. The major interaction identified is with *Mycobacterium tuberculosis* (*Mtbc*), the etiologic agent or cause of pulmonary tuberculosis (TB). Initial infection (i.e., primary infection with *Mtbc*) usually goes undetected. Early lung lesions commonly heal, leaving no residual changes except occasional pulmonary or tracheobronchial lymph node calcifications. About 5 percent of patients initially infected by *Mtbc* will progress to active pulmonary disease (TB) within the first year after primary infection (early progressive disease); and another 5 percent will progress to active infection and disease

---

[*] The organism that causes human PCP is now named *Pneumocystis jiroveci*, Frenkel 1999. Changing the organism's name does not preclude the use of the acronym PCP because it can be read "Pneumocystis pneumonia."

over the remainder of their lives (reactivation disease). Thus, only about 10 percent of persons infected with *Mtbc* are expected to develop clinical TB disease during their lifetimes. Persons with latent *Mtbc* infection and who are also infected with HIV develop clinical tuberculosis (TB) at an increased rate. Clinical studies have shown that dually infected persons develop clinical TB (pulmonary or disseminated) when their CD_4 cell counts are moderately depressed (about $350/mm^3$). This contrasts with *Pneumocystis jiroveci* pneumonia (PCP) that usually occurs in HIV-infected persons with less than 200 CD_4/mm^3. In populations where the prevalence of infection with *Mtbc* and HIV are both very high, such as in sub-Saharan Africa, huge increases in the annual number of TB cases related to HIV infection can be expected.

Is HIV the Cause of AIDS?

Karry Mullis, who won the Nobel prize in 1993 for the discovery of the Polymerase Chain Reaction (PCR), wrote in the introduction to the book *Inventing the AIDS Virus* by Peter H Duesberg (1996) – "We have not been able to discover any good reasons why most of the people on earth believe that AIDS is a disease caused by a virus called HIV. There is simply no scientific evidence demonstrating that this is true." Over the past couple of decades "mainstream" science has compiled an unprecedented amount of evidence to prove that HIV is the cause (etiologic agent) of AIDS and it is somewhat puzzling to see such a blatant denial of all of the clinical, laboratory, and epidemiologic findings by a scientist who should know better.

We are almost ready to respond to misconceptions and misunderstanding of HIV/AIDS perpetuated by scientists who deny that HIV is the cause of AIDS. Before that it would be helpful to review Koch's postulates that were developed as criteria that need to be fulfilled to accept an infectious disease agent as the cause of a specific disease. Virtually everyone who has taken a basic science course on microbiology and the germ theory should be aware of the postulates that were developed by Robert Koch in 1890 to prove the causal association of an infectious agent with a specific disease. The critical elements of Koch's postulates include:

1 a specific association of the agent with the disease state
2 scientific concordance of microbiological, pathological, and clinical evidence
3 isolation of the agent by culture on lifeless media and
4 reproduction of disease by inoculation of the cultured organism into a host.

These postulates were intended to convince skeptics that microbes can cause disease by requiring rigorous criteria before claiming a causal relationship for a specific microbe and a disease. However, even Koch was aware of the shortcomings and limitations of his own postulates. He was convinced that cholera and leprosy were caused by specific visible microbes, but he could not isolate and grow these agents in pure culture and thus fulfill all of his postulates for disease causation. Koch's postulates have frequently been applied to issues of causation with a mathematical rigidity that is not warranted in the biological world. The dogmatic insistence that viruses and newly identified infectious disease agents such as prions, that are difficult if not impossible to culture in a lifeless culture medium, be cultured in a lifeless medium in order to fulfill all of Koch's postulates, has impeded the understanding of these infectious disease agents and have led to revisions of Koch's postulates.

The fundamental limitations of Koch's postulates were brought into sharp focus by scientists who were pioneers in identifying and working with many of the newer classes of microbes such as viruses, Chlamydia, and Rickettsial agents. These agents cannot be propagated in pure culture and require other cells for reproduction. Viruses propagate by usurping the host's cellular machinery, they cannot be propagated in pure (lifeless or cell-free) culture and therefore cannot fulfill all of Koch's postulates. Technological advances in virology during the first half of the 20th Century led to the discovery of hundreds of new viruses. Some of these viruses were found typically to establish chronic or latent infections in humans, and this posed a major challenge to the dogmatic use of Koch's postulates as the gold standard for proof of causality. In his review "Causation and Disease,"[*] Al Evans documented the evolution of thought on causal theory in medicine following the enunciation of Koch's postulates. Evans developed a set of criteria for causation based on modern technology, improved understanding of pathogenesis, and an appreciation of the limitations of the original Koch's postulates. This unified concept of causation was intended to apply to acute and chronic diseases with diverse etiologies. The use of Evans' criteria shows clearly that HIV can be accepted as the causative agent of AIDS. In addition, NIH has compiled all of the available studies of HIV and AIDS and concluded in the late 1990s that according to the most recent studies of HIV and AIDS, HIV has, in fact, fulfilled all of Koch's postulates and has posted all of the detailed facts and supporting studies on a website.[†] A summary of the evidence that HIV fulfills Koch's postulates as the cause of AIDS is copied below.

HIV Fulfills Koch's Basic Postulates as the Cause of AIDS.

With regard **to Koch's postulate #1**, numerous studies from around the world show that virtually all AIDS patients are HIV seropositive; that is, they carry antibodies that indicate HIV infection.

With regard to **Koch's postulate #2**, modern culture techniques have allowed the isolation of HIV in virtually all AIDS patients, as well as in almost all HIV seropositive individuals with both early- and late-stage disease. In addition, the polymerase chain (PCR) and other sophisticated molecular techniques have enabled researchers to document the presence of HIV genes in virtually all patients with AIDS, as well as in individuals in earlier stages of HIV infection.

Koch's postulate #3 has been fulfilled in tragic incidents involving three laboratory workers with no other risk factors who have developed AIDS or severe immunosuppression after accidental exposure to concentrated, cloned HIV in the laboratory. In all three cases, HIV was isolated from the infected individual, sequenced and shown to be the infecting strain of virus. In another tragic incident, transmission of HIV from a Florida dentist to six patients was documented

---

[*]Evans AS (1976) Causation and disease: the Henle-Koch postulates revisited. *Yale J Biol Med.* **49**: 175–95.

[†] www.niaid.nih.gov/Factsheets/evidHIV.htm. This fact sheet provides detailed and documented responses to all of the questions raised by persons who are skeptical about HIV being the causative agent of AIDS.

by genetic analyses of virus isolated from both the dentist and the patients. The dentist and three of the patients developed AIDS and died, and at least one of the other patients has developed AIDS. Five of the patients had no HIV risk factors other than multiple visits to the dentist for invasive procedures.*

In addition, through December 1999, the CDC had received reports of 56 healthcare workers in the United States with documented, occupationally acquired HIV infection, of whom 25 have developed AIDS in the absence of other risk factors. The development of AIDS following known HIV seroconversion also has been repeatedly observed in pediatric and adult blood transfusion cases, in mother-to-child transmission, and in studies of hemophilia, injection drug use and sexual transmission in which seroconversion can be documented using serial blood samples.

Koch's postulates also have been fulfilled in animal models of human AIDS. Chimpanzees experimentally infected with HIV have developed severe immuno-suppression and AIDS. In severe combined immunodeficiency (SCID) mice given a human immune system, HIV produces similar patterns of cell killing and pathogenesis as seen in people. HIV-2, a less virulent variant of HIV which causes AIDS in people, also causes an AIDS-like syndrome in baboons.

Misconceptions, Misunderstanding, and Myths About HIV/AIDS

From the observations and studies described in Chapter 3, and those described in the preceding sections of this chapter, there should not be any major lingering questions or uncertainties about the origin of HIV/AIDS, what AIDS is and that HIV is the cause of AIDS. Yet, in spite of all of these observations and studies that have been accepted by mainstream medical science and public health epidemiologists some staunch supporters of the theory that HIV is not the cause of AIDS persist in their fervently held belief. In the developed world, such AIDS dissidents are summarily dismissed and are viewed as mainstream science views those who continue to believe that the earth is flat. However, such dissident views about AIDS have found receptive believers among many Africans, especially President Mbeki of South Africa, and these dissident views and conclusions about AIDS in Africa have significantly hindered the rapid development of HIV/AIDS prevention programs and more recently seriously questioned the need for anti-HIV treatment programs for AIDS.

The following section presents the many arguments and questions that AIDS dissidents still raise as of the new millennium about AIDS in Africa along with my specific answer or response.

The pattern of AIDS cases in the USA and Africa does not fit that of "classical" infectious disease epidemics such as measles or influenza.

The pattern (i.e. epidemic curve) of AIDS cases in the USA and Africa indeed does not fit that of "classical" infectious disease epidemics such as measles or influenza because HIV is simply not a "classical" infectious disease agent! When "classical" infectious disease agents such as influenza or measles viruses appear in

---

* Some investigators of this incident suspect that the dentist deliberately infected some of his patients.

a virgin (i.e., totally susceptible) population, these agents sweep through and infect virtually everyone in an explosive epidemic and then cases begin to decrease as most of the susceptible persons in the population are infected. As originally described by one of the first recognized epidemiologists in the early 19th Century, and is known as Farr's law: "the curve that represents the incidence of new cases in an [classical infectious disease] epidemic ascends rapidly at first, then gradually levels off to a maximum, and finally descends more rapidly than it ascended, thus approximating a bell-shaped curve." The rise reflects the exponential spread of contagion and the fall reflects the resulting natural vaccination or immunity of survivors. Such epidemic patterns (a bell-shaped curve) are seen for infectious disease agents where there is generalized or almost universal exposure of the population and the infectivity of these agents following exposure is very high. However, such a "classical" epidemic pattern cannot be expected for all infectious diseases, especially not for an agent such as HIV that requires blood or sex contact for transmission.

In addition, as will be repeatedly described in detail in latter chapters, epidemic transmission of HIV requires the highest levels of HIV risk behaviors. The occurrence of HIV epidemics has been and will be restricted to those populations that have extremely high levels of these risk behaviors. Indeed, that is exactly what has been observed over the past couple of decades regarding HIV epidemics. It is naive and incorrect to believe that all infectious disease epidemics must have a random and generalized pattern. Since AIDS cases in the USA are concentrated in MSM and IDU, AIDS dissidents believe this should rule out an infectious cause of AIDS. They totally ignore the different distribution of different infectious disease agents within any population. The patterns of HIV epidemic curves resemble more closely such infectious agents as hepatitis B and genital herpes viruses. HIV and these latter infectious disease agents are concentrated in those persons who have risk behaviors that enable person-to-person transmission of these agents.

"Classical" bacterial/viral diseases are very specific for clinical signs and symptoms. Yet according to CDC's AIDS case definitions over 30 different diseases may be considered diagnostic of an AIDS case.

Again, this argument shows that AIDS dissidents are ignorant of the unique characteristic of HIV as an infectious disease agent. As described earlier in this chapter, HIV attacks the host's immune system and when there is sufficient immune damage, the HIV-infected person is then susceptible to a whole range of infectious agents (both endogenous and exogenous) that a normally functioning immune system would be able to inhibit or destroy. Thus, persons infected with the tubercle bacillus or *Pneumocystis jiroveci* (formerly *carinii*), who subsequently acquire an HIV infection are at very high risk of developing pulmonary tuberculosis (TB) or *Pneumocystis* pneumonia (PCP). These are common AIDS defining diseases in persons whose immune system is severely damaged as a result of HIV infection. AIDS dissidents simply ignore all of the thousands of clinical and laboratory studies that demonstrate progressive damage to the HIV-infected person's immune system. They further refuse to accept that this acquired immune deficiency is the underlying cause of all of the diseases and conditions considered indicative or diagnostic of a case of Acquired Immune Deficiency Syndrome.[*]

---

[*] A syndrome can be defined as a collection of signs, symptoms, and diseases with a common etiology.

AIDS dissidents should review the natural history of syphilis. Syphilis has many diverse signs and symptoms – in its late stages, untreated syphilis can cause serious heart abnormalities, mental disorders, blindness, other neurologic problems, and death.

AIDS in the USA and other developed countries is totally different from what is being labeled as AIDS in SSA.

This argument appears on the surface to be valid because the basic HIV risk behaviors in SSA are markedly different compared to the USA and other developed countries. In addition, the indicator diseases for AIDS in SSA are also markedly different from the major AIDS indicator diseases in developed countries.

In SSA the vast majority of HIV infections are attributed to heterosexual HIV transmission while in the USA epidemic heterosexual HIV transmission is virtually absent. The majority of HIV transmission in the USA is attributed to anal intercourse in male homosexuals and to sharing needles and syringes for injecting drug use. According to AIDS dissidents, the African AIDS diseases are generated by their conventional, widespread causes – malnutrition, parasitic infections and poor sanitation – and have nothing to do with sexual risk behaviors. This hypothesis offers a simple and politically correct explanation for the predominant heterosexual distribution of AIDS in SSA, a view that has apparently been accepted by President Mbeki of South Africa.

The answer of mainstream medical science to the question – why is epidemic heterosexual HIV transmission so rampant in SSA and not in most other regions – should be simple and direct. Epidemic heterosexual HIV transmission requires a high prevalence and frequency of sex partner exchange (i.e., having multiple sex partners on a concurrent basis) and the pattern and prevalence of these heterosexual risk behaviors in most SSA populations are sufficient to sustain epidemic HIV transmission whereas the patterns and prevalence of these risk behaviors in most other populations are not sufficient to fuel epidemic heterosexual HIV transmission. WHO and UNAIDS and all national AIDS programs have avoided giving such a direct answer to this question and have instead tiptoed around the issue by stating that the major determinants of high HIV prevalence are poverty, social and gender discrimination, and lack of access to healthcare. The direct and blunt answer is considered offensive and any official who tries to say this is automatically branded as a racist bigot. In Chapter 5, I'll present the data that show very clearly that sexual risk behaviors, sexually transmitted diseases, and other factors that can facilitate sexual HIV transmission are all collectively at least one order of magnitude greater and possibly up to a hundred-fold greater in many SSA populations compared with most populations outside of SSA.

The answer to the question raised as to why AIDS indicator diseases in SSA are so much different from the major AIDS indicator diseases in the USA and other developed countries is simply because the background flora of infectious disease agents (endogenous and exogenous) are so very much different. Just as the animal and plant flora in Africa are different from those in most developed countries, the background flora of animal and human infectious agents are also markedly different. HIV-related TB cases are found in higher numbers and proportion of AIDS cases in SSA compared to the USA because up to half of the adult population in SSA are infected with *Mycobacterium tuberculosis* whereas in the USA only about 10 percent or less of adults are infected with the tubercle bacillus.

AIDS in the USA is different from AIDS in Africa.

In his presentation to President Mbeki's "scientific" panel on AIDS in South Africa, Duesberg used CDC and WHO reports and statistics to reinforce his belief that AIDS in the USA is totally different from what has been labeled as AIDS in Africa. He used the major differences in patterns and prevalence of reported AIDS cases in the USA compared with Africa and could not understand why they were so different. This led him to conclude that AIDS in Africa is not a new disease and the AIDS industry is merely labeling diseases that were and continue to be prevalent in Africa as AIDS cases.

In his presentation, Duesberg's misuse of HIV/AIDS numbers point out his profound ignorance of the different accuracy of these numbers.* He used the 1999 UNAIDS *estimate* of 23 million prevalent HIV-infected persons in the 15–49 year age group in SSA and the annual number of 75 000 AIDS cases *reported* to WHO and he came up with a ratio using these 75 000 annual *reported* AIDS case divided by the 23 million *estimated* HIV infections for a ratio of *1:300*. For the USA he used CDC's *estimated* annual AIDS cases of about 45 000 and divided this number by the 900 000 *estimated* number of HIV-infected persons to arrive at a ratio of *1/20*. However, he compared apples with oranges! He should have used *estimated* HIV prevalence with *estimated* AIDS cases for SSA because reported AIDS case numbers in developing countries are grossly under-reported and represent at most only about 5–10 percent of the actual number. A better estimate of the actual annual number of AIDS cases during that year would be 1.25 million† assuming that only about 5–10 percent of actual AIDS cases were recognized, diagnosed correctly and reported. Dividing the *estimated* HIV prevalence of 23 million by the *estimated* annual number of AIDS cases of about 1.25 million gave SSA the same *1/20* ratio as estimated for the USA population! However, Duesberg believed that his perceived marked discrepancies between African and USA AIDS/HIV ratios and the marked differences in the indicator diseases for AIDS in Africa compared to those commonly found in the USA can be both readily explained by the hypothesis that AIDS is caused by non-contagious risk factors and that HIV is a harmless passenger virus.

The average annual number of reported AIDS cases in Africa up to the year 2000 was about 75 000. Such small numbers will have minimal impact on population growth in Africa and are inconsistent with some projections that AIDS will result in negative population growth in Africa.

HIV infection rates in Africa only began to increase markedly during the late 1980s, and the resulting increase of AIDS cases and deaths lags close to a decade behind. AIDS cases and deaths in SSA only began to increase markedly during the last half of the 1990s. Using a conservative but reasonable HIV scenario based on the most recent HIV prevalence estimates, the cumulative number of adult AIDS deaths in SSA countries up to the year 1990 was less than 1 million and the total estimated number of adult AIDS deaths during the 1990s was about 10 million or an average of less than a million annually. However, annual adult AIDS deaths in SSA are expected to continue to increase and in 2005 the estimated number of AIDS deaths was from 2 to 3 million. The estimated numbers

---

* Chapter 6 will provide basic information and definitions of all HIV/AIDS numbers.
† Such an estimate is also reached by use of a model such as EPIMODEL.

of AIDS deaths in SSA up to the year 2000 were not sufficiently large to have had any major impact on the overall population growth rate in the region. However, annual AIDS deaths since the new millennium are estimated to be over 2 million (with over 90 percent of these deaths in the 25–49 year old age group) and these deaths will begin to reduce the overall population growth rate from 2 to 3 percent down to 1 to 2 percent during the latter half of this decade. Details of HIV prevalence trends and estimation and projection of AIDS deaths in SSA are presented in Chapters 6 and 7.

HIV antibody tests are grossly inaccurate – in some HIV surveys, over 90 percent of persons who were found positive by these tests were not infected with HIV!

The HIV antibody tests are one of the most accurate biologic tests available. The detractors of these tests are ignorant of the specific characteristics of any biologic test for a specific antibody or antigen. These characteristics are sensitivity and specificity.

Sensitivity is the accuracy of identifying the specific antibody – in this case, HIV antibody. The sensitivity of HIV antibody tests are all very high and can be as high as 99.9 percent, i.e., if this test was performed on 1000 persons who were infected with HIV, this test would identify 999 out of the thousand as HIV positive and because it is not 100 percent accurate, it would fail to detect one of the infected blood samples (false negative). The other major characteristic of biologic tests is the specificity of the test.

Specificity is the accuracy of not identifying the specific antibody or antigen in question when it is in fact not present. The specificity of HIV antibody tests are also all very high and can be as high as 99.9 percent, i.e., if this test was performed on 1000 persons who were not infected with HIV, this test would identify 999 out of the thousand as HIV negative and because it is not 100 percent accurate, it would falsely identify one of the blood samples as HIV positive (false positive).

The problem of "inaccurate" results from using these very accurate HIV antibody tests arises when these tests are used in populations with very low HIV prevalence. For example, let us take a population of 1 million where we "know" there are no HIV infections. In this population, because the specificity of the HIV antibody test is 99.9 percent, 1000 persons will be reported as HIV positive because one of every thousand blood samples tested will be a false positive. In this situation, the predictive value of a positive HIV test in identifying a person infected with HIV is zero! If HIV prevalence in this population was 0.1 percent (1 per 1000), then there would be 1000 HIV-infected persons and when this population is tested, 99.9 percent of the 1000 HIV-infected persons would be identified as HIV positive because the sensitivity of the test is 99.9%. In this latter example, the test would report close to 2000 HIV positive results – close to 1000 would be true positives (HIV-infected persons), and about 1000 false positive because the specificity of the test is 99.9 percent. In the first example, the predictive value of a positive test was zero and in this second situation, the predictive value of a positive test is about 50 percent.

Thus, these tests are very accurate, but because they are not perfect, for clinical purposes and for HIV prevalence surveys in low HIV prevalence populations, there is a need to re-test an initial positive test with a test from a different manufacturer to be more confident that the initial positive test result is a true positive.

Summary/Conclusions

As of late-2006, a significant number of persons throughout the world continue to doubt that AIDS is caused by a retrovirus, the human immunodeficiency virus (HIV), and that this virus originated in Africa. The reasons why some doubt and skepticism about AIDS remains are because most of the general public obtains their information about AIDS primarily from news sources and most news services provide almost equal, if not more, attention to "flat earth" type theories compared with conventional mainstream sources of information. In addition, the severe social stigma that was first associated with the initial recognition of AIDS and the international sensitivity of the origin of HIV makes some of the dissident theories more socially and politically attractive.

AIDS cases were first recognized in male homosexuals and subsequently in injecting drug users (IDU) in the early 1980s. Questions and uncertainty about what AIDS was and what caused it were rampant when this new and invariably fatal disease syndrome emerged seemingly out of nowhere. There were many diverse theories about AIDS but as public health epidemiologists, clinicians, and laboratory scientists focused an almost unprecedented number of studies on this mysterious disease syndrome, the cause of AIDS was narrowed to an infectious agent. By the mid-1980s, there was an overwhelming consensus among "mainstream" scientists and public health professionals that HIV which was first isolated in 1983 was the cause of the acquired immune deficiency syndrome (AIDS). The development of laboratory tests to identify HIV infections enabled clinicians to study the natural history of HIV-infected persons.

Epidemiologic studies rapidly established that HIV was transmitted by anal intercourse in men who have sex with men (MSM) and the sharing of drug injection equipment by IDU – risk behaviors that were and are generally socially unaccepted and/or illegal in most countries. As a result, in addition to AIDS being an invariably fatal disease, HIV-infected persons were subjected to severe social stigma and discrimination. These factors complicated the development of public health surveillance of HIV/AIDS because MSM and IDU did not want to be identified in any registry listing, even if it were in a confidential public health registry. Since no specific treatment was initially available for AIDS, public health programs reluctantly adopted a non-nominal or even anonymous system of surveillance for HIV/AIDS. I'm convinced that if AIDS was first recognized in SSA populations, that routine public health surveillance of HIV/AIDS would have developed as a traditional nominal reporting system such as those developed for Ebola or Lassa fever outbreaks. Epidemic heterosexual HIV transmission requires a high prevalence and frequency of sex partner exchange (i.e., having multiple sex partners on a concurrent basis) and the pattern and prevalence of these heterosexual risk behaviors in most SSA populations are sufficient to sustain epidemic HIV transmission whereas the patterns and prevalence of these risk behaviors in most other populations are not sufficient to fuel epidemic heterosexual HIV transmission.

During the past couple of decades, the natural history and epidemiology of HIV have been almost completely determined but some uncertainties and problems in the full understanding of HIV pathogenesis and transmission dynamics remain. These uncertainties include: why there are such major differences in HIV prevalence levels within SSA; why some HIV-infected persons progress rapidly, within a few years, to develop AIDS and some take more than a decade to progress to AIDS; and are there some who will never develop AIDS? However, with anti-HIV drugs now available for effective treatment, these latter questions may never be fully answered. Similarly, the median interval from HIV infection to the development of severe immune deficiency is now believed to be about 7–8 years in all adult populations, but it is now unethical to develop or continue cohort studies to measure annual progression rates since there are anti-HIV drugs that retard progression to AIDS.

During the early 1980s, AIDS was labeled as an "American disease" of MSM and IDU and the origin of HIV was a very sensitive international issue. In the previous chapter I described the Haiti to Zaire connection that was vehemently denied during the early 1980s and continues to be denied. Denial of AIDS as an indigenous disease in Africa during the early to mid-1980s was also prominent. Because of the social stigma surrounding AIDS in MSM and IDU, many of the alternative theories of dissident scientists that included that HIV was not the cause of AIDS but was the result of poverty or that HIV was developed by Western scientists to reduce African populations have been accepted or at least still being considered as possible or even probable by large numbers of Africans and African Americans. As of late-2006, there should not be any question that AIDS is a very severe infectious disease problem in most SSA countries and will be the leading cause of death in this region for at least several more decades.

Chapter 5

HIV Epidemiology and Transmission Dynamics

The explosive increase in reported cases of AIDS in the early 1980s among men who have sex with men (MSM) and subsequently injecting drug users (IDU) in North America and Western Europe – initially with reported doubling times of a few months – created the false perception that AIDS is caused by a very infectious agent. As a result, during the mid-to-late 1980s, there was significant public health fear that the "next wave" of HIV epidemics would occur in heterosexuals following the hundreds of explosive HIV epidemics in MSM and IDU documented throughout the world. Heterosexual HIV epidemics did not materialize in any developed country and this led to the conclusion that perhaps heterosexual AIDS was a myth.[1] Documentation by the late 1980s and early 1990s of heterosexual HIV epidemics in sub-Saharan Africa (SSA), several Caribbean countries, and a few Asian countries dispelled this myth. However, as of the new millennium, another myth, the myth of the "next waves" of heterosexual HIV epidemics sweeping through low HIV prevalence countries in Asia has been created by UNAIDS and many AIDS "experts." This myth has been fully accepted by AIDS activists, most policy makers as well as most of the general public. Some of the more zealous AIDS "experts" also predict such dire HIV epidemics in many Middle East and central Asian countries.

Some simple common sense reasoning should dispel such myths since:

HIV is primarily a sexually transmitted infection (STI) and there are no credible sexually transmitted disease (STD) experts who are concerned that an STI such as genital herpes virus (HSV-2) that has been present in human populations probably for centuries or longer and that is perhaps a hundred times more infectious than HIV could ever become a "generalized" infection.

To understand the epidemiology and transmission dynamics of HIV, especially to identify populations where epidemic HIV transmission may be expected, requires an awareness of several key epidemiologic and infectious disease concepts that include:

1 the definition of an infectious disease epidemic, including when an epidemic can be considered to be a "generalized" epidemic
2 the basic reproductive number (R_0) of an infectious disease agent
3 epidemic versus nonepidemic sexual HIV transmission patterns
4 the generally low infectivity of HIV via sexual intercourse
5 the paramount importance of patterns, prevalence, and frequency of sex partner exchanges, including the size of and extent of overlapping of sex networks
6 the importance of major facilitating factors (not cofactors) and protective factors for epidemic sexual HIV transmission
7 the reality that there are major differences in the patterns and prevalence of sexual risk behaviors as well as facilitating and protective factors within and between countries and regions and
8 understanding and accepting that the majority of all populations have no measurable risk of acquiring an HIV infection.

These epidemiologic and infectious disease concepts will be described in this chapter along with a detailed description of HIV epidemiology and transmission dynamics.

The Reproductive Number (R_0) of an Infectious Disease Agent[*]

As with any field of science, exact definitions are needed in order to avoid misunderstanding. The general definition of "epidemic" found in most dictionaries – a disease or condition that affects many individuals in an area or a population at the same time – is not helpful in understanding the major differences inherent in different patterns of HIV transmission. The epidemiologic concept of the reproductive number of an infectious disease agent (R_0) is very specific and is more useful to describe HIV transmission dynamics, especially the difference between epidemic and nonepidemic HIV transmission. R_0 describes in a single value, the epidemic potential of an infectious agent. When, *on average*, one infected person infects more than one other person, R_0 is greater than (>) 1 and the result will be epidemic spread of the agent. However, when, *on average*, one infected person does not infect more than one other person, R_0 is less than (<) 1 and epidemic spread does not occur. When R_0 is <1, the infectious agent will slowly disappear and if R_0 stays close to 1 the agent will maintain itself in the population with no or minimal growth (i.e., becomes endemic).

Examples of the spread of an infectious agent where R_0 is much >1 include influenza and measles epidemics in a largely susceptible population. In such situations, one infected person at the start of an epidemic can easily infect scores of persons (R_0 >20), who in turn infect scores more so that epidemic spread is rapid. Persons infected who recover are then immune to re-infection with the same infectious agent. As the epidemic continues, the number of persons who were infected and become immune increases while the number of susceptible persons decreases. Thus, R_0 in these examples decreases over time and eventually becomes <1: then the infectious agent either becomes endemic or dies out depending on how rapidly new susceptible persons may become available. Epidemic (R_0 >1) HIV transmission occurs primarily as a result of those human behaviors that place an individual at some risk of acquiring or transmitting an HIV infection. These behaviors include: (1) having unprotected sexual intercourse with *multiple* and *concurrent* sex partners; and/or (2) routinely *sharing drug injecting equipment* with many other injecting drug users (IDU).

An appreciation of the concept of the reproductive number of an infectious disease agent is not enough to understand HIV transmission dynamics in populations with varying patterns and prevalence of HIV risk behaviors and HIV infections. The ability to calculate the *risk of acquiring an HIV infection* in different epidemiologic situations is also needed. Many countries with pockets of heterosexuals who engage in high-risk sexual behaviors (e.g., FSW and their male clients) have not experienced epidemic HIV transmission because in addition to the very low risk of transmission per single coital act, HIV prevalence is also very

---

[*] Calculation of R_0 for an HIV-infected FSW and calculation of risk of or probability of acquiring an HIV infection from or to a FSW in the Philippines are presented in an appendix to this chapter.

low. In populations where HIV prevalence is very low, a high prevalence of heterosexual risk behaviors can be present yet the risk of acquiring an HIV infection can still be extremely low. However, if HIV prevalence is allowed to rise to a "high" level (arbitrarily over one percent), then, depending on the underlying pattern(s) and prevalence of sex partner exchange rates and the presence of multiple facilitating factors, the risk of acquiring an HIV infection can increase markedly. If HIV prevalence rises above five percent, sustained HIV transmission becomes more likely, especially in the presence of facilitating factors or the relative lack of protective factors. This latter situation is now a prominent factor in the continuing epidemic HIV transmission in many African countries.

HIV Transmission

HIV is transmitted from person to person primarily via blood and sexual fluids such as semen as well as any other body fluid that may contain some blood. The probability or risk of HIV transmission for any single exposure is directly related to the amount of infected blood or semen that is exchanged. This risk ranges from a low of <1 per 1000 coital acts from an HIV-infected female to her male sex partner up to about 90 percent or more from receiving a transfusion of HIV-infected blood. The majority of persons in any "general" population are not at any measurable risk of contracting an HIV infection. However, the following persons or groups may be at varying risk of HIV infection (*see* Figure 5.1):

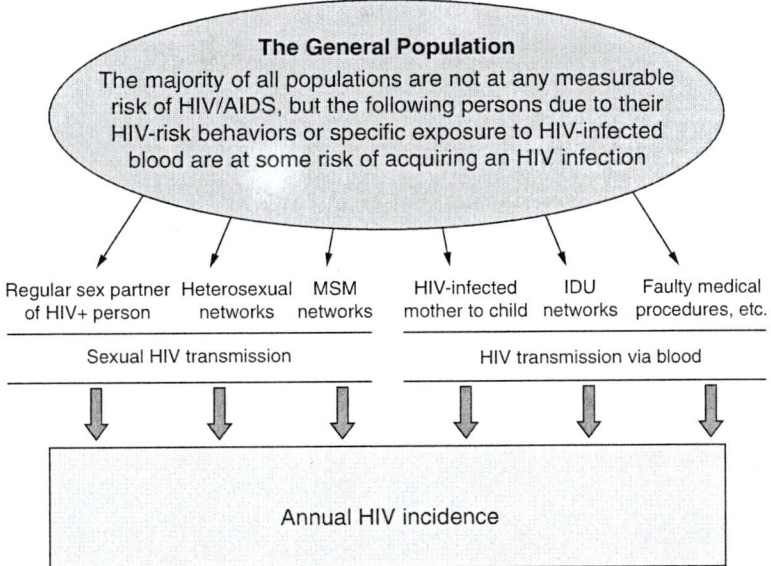

Figure 5.1 Annual HIV incidence.

1 heterosexuals or MSM who have unprotected sex with multiple sex partners, especially within large and overlapping sex networks
2 IDU who share needles/syringes with other IDU, especially within large IDU networks
3 persons who are the regular sex partners of HIV-infected persons

4 infants born to HIV-infected mothers
5 persons who receive HIV-infected blood or blood products and persons in healthcare settings who are accidentally injected with HIV-infected medical equipment (includes persons who are infected by faulty plasma collection methods).

Mother to Child Transmission (MTCT)

Mother to child transmission occurs when an HIV positive woman passes the virus to her baby during pregnancy, labor and delivery, or by breastfeeding. Without treatment, around 15 to 30 percent of babies born to HIV-positive women will become infected during pregnancy and/or delivery. A further 10 to 20 percent will become infected through breastfeeding. During the late 1980s and early 1990s, field studies consistently showed that mother to infant transmission rates in Africa were almost twice as high as in Europe. Even though breastfeeding was known to be a possible factor to explain this marked difference in HIV transmission rates, there was great reluctance by most official agencies to accept this association with breastfeeding without additional and more conclusive data. By the mid-to-late 1990s, increasingly available data confirmed that breastfeeding by HIV-infected mothers did not represent just a small increment of risk, but increased HIV transmission to their infants by up to 50 percent. It is now accepted that about 25 to 30 percent of HIV-infected pregnant females will infect their infants – about 5 percent *in utero* (during gestation), about 15 percent around the delivery period, and about 10 percent in the postnatal period, primarily due to breastfeeding.

HIV Transmission From Infected Blood/Blood Products

1 Wherever injecting drug users (IDU) are infected with HIV, there is a risk of HIV transmission through sharing needles and syringes with other IDU. While the risk associated with a single shared exposure is considered to be relatively low (generally well less than 1 percent), the specific risk depends on the amount of infected blood transferred to a susceptible individual. Worldwide, less than 5 percent of all adult HIV infections are attributed to IDU. Extensive and explosive HIV epidemics in IDU have been documented in more than 100 populations throughout the world. As of late-2006, this is the primary mode of HIV transmission in many countries in Asia and in Eastern and Southern Europe.
2 HIV transmission via blood transfusion occurs rarely in low HIV prevalence countries, even in those with limited HIV testing capabilities: however, it is probably an extensive problem in high HIV prevalence countries in SSA.
3 Many thousands of hemophilia patients in many countries throughout the world received HIV-infected blood products in the early-to-mid 1980s. This mode of transmission has not been a problem since the mid-to-late 1980s, when manufacturing methods were changed to make these products safe.
4 Extensive HIV transmission associated with HIV-contaminated plasma collection equipment was documented in Mexico during the mid-1980s and in China up to about the mid-1990s. It has been estimated that the Chinese problem was widespread and may have infected several hundred thousand persons.
5 Hospital or medically acquired HIV infections due to reuse of injection equipment or to administration of small amounts of blood or serum for treatment

have been documented in Russia, Romania and more recently possibly in Libya. HIV transmission via accidental needle sticks in a medical setting is always a potential problem, but the probability of such transmission from HIV-infected needles and syringes is relatively low (about 3 of 1000 HIV contaminated needle sticks).[2]

HIV Transmission Via Sexual Intercourse

A major factor that makes the epidemiology and transmission dynamics of HIV different from most other STI is the generally very low infectivity of HIV via sexual intercourse. In the absence of facilitating factors,[*] the risk of HIV transmission via vaginal or anal intercourse can be several hundred times lower than most other STI. The transmission probability per episode of vaginal intercourse has been estimated from studies of HIV-discordant sex partners: transmission probabilities per act in such couples vary from 1 per 7000 to 1 per 700 in the USA, Europe and Uganda[3,4,5,6,7] and to 1 per 500 in Thailand.[8]

Sexual mixing patterns and the prevalence of persons who regularly have *multiple* and *concurrent* sex partners are the primary determinants of the rapidity and extent of epidemic sexual HIV transmission.[9,10] If sexually active persons have many different sex partners, but only one at a time for months or years (i.e., serial sex partner exchange, as in most developed countries), it would be difficult for HIV to spread rapidly in persons whose only risk of infection is through sexual intercourse. When multiple sex partners are usually concurrent, HIV or any other STI can spread rapidly and extensively.[11] Commercial sex is a prime example of having multiple and concurrent sex partners. Another major factor in epidemic sexual spread of HIV is the size and pattern of sex networks and the extent of mixing (or "overlap") between different networks. In populations with a high prevalence of sexual risk behaviors, there will invariably be a relatively high prevalence of STI and other facilitating factors that can greatly increase HIV transmission. These facilitating factors will be described in more detail later in this chapter. The risk of HIV transmission via anal intercourse is higher than via vaginal intercourse. Anal intercourse poses a higher risk because of the greater degree of tissue trauma that may occur. Still, the risk of HIV transmission via anal intercourse is relatively low, especially when compared with other STI such as syphilis and gonorrhea that may be as high as 20 to 40 percent per coital act.

Patterns of Sexual HIV Transmission

Several distinct epidemiologic patterns of sexual HIV transmission have been observed. Understanding these different patterns of sexual HIV transmission is essential for the development of effective HIV prevention strategies.

1 Explosive or rapid epidemic ($R_0 > 1$ in less than 1 year) transmission pattern. This epidemic pattern requires frequent, almost daily sex partner exchange within large open sex networks. MSM in gay bathhouse settings who may have had up to 10 to 20 different sex partners in a single day/night and FSW

---

[*] Any factor that can cause lesion(s) in the genital or rectal epithelium (i.e., concurrent STD, especially ulcerative STD, "dry sex," traumatic sex, lack of male circumcision, etc.) can be a facilitating factor.

in large brothel type establishments are prime examples of this explosive epidemic HIV transmission pattern.

2 Slow epidemic (R_0 >1 over many years) transmission (non-explosive) pattern. This requires having unprotected sex with multiple and concurrent sex partners within small sex groupings or networks that overlap with each other. A varying proportion of different populations have this pattern of sex partner exchange. It is found in a very large proportion of MSM and from 20–40 percent of sexually active adults in many SSA populations but usually in only a small percent of most other populations.

3 Nonepidemic (R_0 <1) transmission pattern. In most developed countries a fairly large percent of adolescents and adults (up to 20 percent) have, during their lifetime, multiple sex partners, but generally sex partner exchange is serial (one after another) and not concurrent (i.e., having several different sex partners within the same time period). When sex partner exchange is on a monthly or annual basis and the pattern of exchange is serial rather than concurrent, no epidemic HIV transmission can be expected in such populations.

4 HIV transmission from an HIV-infected person to his/her regular sex partner, i.e., among HIV-discordant couples. The annual risk of sexual HIV transmission from an infected person to his/her regular sex partner is usually less than 10 percent, but the cumulative risk is very high over many years. A large percent, most likely the majority, of these regular sex partners do not have any significant HIV risk behaviors. As a result they are not involved with any further HIV transmission and they should be included in the nonepidemic (R_0 <1) pattern of HIV transmission. This distinct nonepidemic pattern of sexual HIV transmission will invariably follow after all HIV epidemics. As of late-2006, this pattern of HIV transmission is probably the predominant mode of HIV transmission globally, including SSA, where the problem of HIV-discordant couples is highly prevalent.

These fairly distinct epidemiologic patterns of sexual HIV transmission have been described above. But in reality, there is a continuum of HIV risk ranging from the highest risk sex partner exchange pattern (concurrent versus serial) with the highest number of different sex partners to the lowest or no risk in persons who are mutually monogamous and who never had sex with anyone other than their spouse/regular sex partner as presented in Table 5.1.

Table 5.1 Gradient of risk for sexual HIV transmission

Annual number of sex partners (Frequency of exchange)	Pattern of sex partner exchange	Potential R_0 (time period)	Examples
1 or none (no exchange)	Monogamous or abstinent	Zero or close to 0	Majority or large percent of all heterosexuals
>1 to <10 (Months/years)	Mostly serial	<1	Up to 20% of adults in some Western countries
>1 to <100 (Weekly/monthly)	Mostly concurrent	>1* (many years)	Up to 20–40% of adults in some SSA countries

Continued

Table 5.1 (Continued)

Annual number of sex partners (Frequency of exchange)	Pattern of sex partner exchange	Potential R_0 (time period)	Examples
>100 to <1000 (Daily/weekly)	Mostly concurrent	>1* (< 1 year)	FSW (direct and indirect) and small MSM networks
>1000 (Daily)	Concurrent	>1* (< 1 year)	Brothel based FSW and MSM in bathhouses

* The reproductive number (R_0) of HIV, i.e., on average how many other persons will an HIV-infected person infect, is directly correlated to increasing numbers and frequency of *sex partner exchanges* and increasing prevalence of *facilitating factors* for sexual HIV transmission. Condom usage will reduce the potential R_0 of HIV and circumcised males are at lower risks of transmitting or acquiring an HIV infection via unprotected sexual intercourse.

Primary Determinants of Epidemic Heterosexual HIV Transmission

An evaluation of all populations where epidemic (R_0 >1) heterosexual HIV transmission has occurred as of late-2006 makes it clear that such epidemics have occurred only when the following patterns and prevalence of heterosexual risk behaviors are present.

1 A sexual mixing pattern of concurrent and/or overlapping sex partners.
2 A high frequency of sex partner exchange (daily or weekly sex partner exchange).
3 A high prevalence of factors that result in lesions in the genital/rectal epithelium that can greatly facilitate sexual HIV transmission. These are not cofactors since they are not required for HIV transmission, but they can greatly facilitate sexual HIV transmission. A low prevalence of protective factors such as male circumcision and consistent condom use will also "facilitate" epidemic sexual HIV transmission.

These and other major determinants of epidemic heterosexual HIV transmission are described in detail in the following section.

New (incident) HIV Infections

Individuals newly infected with HIV are much more infectious compared with individuals who have passed the acute period. Exactly how infectious or how much of a facilitating factor this may be is not clear, but some modelers have estimated it to be high. This factor might account for up to a 20-fold increase in the infectivity of HIV during the first few months after acquisition of infection.[12] Studies of HIV epidemics – in MSM in the USA,[13] heterosexuals in SSA, and heterosexuals in Thailand[14] – all indicated that large numbers of new (incident) infections were a major factor that contributed to the initial rapid spread of HIV.

Other STI

It is generally accepted that other STI, especially those that cause ulcerative lesions such as genital herpes, chancroid and syphilis, increase or facilitate HIV transmission. It is clear from epidemiologic studies[15,16] that if an individual has an ulcerative genital lesion, the risk of transmission may be increased by from five to tenfold or more. Genital herpes virus, type 2 (HSV-2) is the major STI associated with genital lesions. The median recurrence rate after a symptomatic first episode of HSV-2 is four to five episodes per year, and severe first episodes are associated with even higher recurrence rates.[17,18] Results of a retrospective cohort study in 1993–2000 of 2732 HIV negative patients at STD clinics in Pune, India appears to confirm that HSV-2 is a major independent risk factor for HIV infection. The study suggests that recent HSV-2 infection is independently associated with a 3.64-fold increased risk of primary HIV infection. Most significant, perhaps, this supports the hypothesis that mucosal infection from acute HSV-2 may be a key biological mechanism that facilitates HIV acquisition. A study of risk factors influencing the incidence of HIV infection in a rural African population concluded that HSV-2 infection was the most important risk factor.[19]

Lack of Male Circumcision (MC)

Many epidemiological studies[20,21,22,23] have shown that male circumcision is associated with a reduced rate of HIV acquisition. Some of these studies support the hypothesis that protection derives from the removal of the foreskin that contains cells with HIV receptors that may serve as an entry point for HIV. However, these findings may, in part, be confounded by fundamental differences between populations in rates of male circumcision and in social-sexual patterns and prevalence of high sexual risk behaviors. Since this hypothesis was first suggested over a decade ago, increasing documentation to support it has accumulated: the findings of the 2003 DHS survey in Kenya presented in Figure 5.2 indicate that circumcised males have a much lower HIV infection rate (3 percent) compared with uncircumcised males (13 percent).

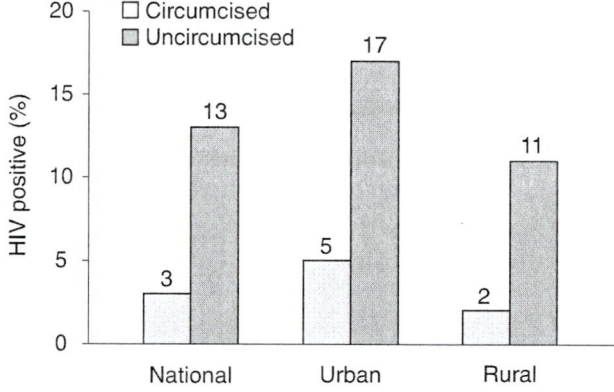

Figure 5.2 Male HIV prevalence by circumcision status (Kenya – 2003 DHS Survey).

Because MC is associated with other culturally related behaviors that may in turn influence HIV infection (i.e., confounding variables), more definitive evidence that MC itself can reduce risk was needed. Also, more information on the short-term risks of surgery and long-term risks (especially the possibility that men would feel more protected and adopt riskier sexual behaviors after circumcision, a phenomenon labeled "disinhibition") was needed. To meet these needs, three randomized clinical trials were started in SSA. Each trial randomly assigned uncircumcised HIV negative men either to be circumcised or not and then followed them for 18 to 24 months to determine what proportion got infected with HIV or other STD and what complications of MC were observed. These trials, designed to detect a 50 percent reduction in risk, were launched in Kenya, Uganda, and South Africa. The Uganda trial also planned to include HIV+ men to examine the safety of MC in infected men. These trials were expected to last 3 to 5 years. The South African trial was stopped half-way through by its ethical review board in February 2005 because the protective effect of MC was found to be so high (estimated at about 60 to 70 percent) it was considered no longer ethical to withhold MC from the control group. These latter men were contacted to see if they wanted to be circumcised.

"Dry Sex"

In many parts of SSA[24] and some areas of Southeast Asia, some women apply astringent substances into their vaginas to limit their vaginal secretions. Such "dry sex" can be much more traumatic and cause lesions in the vagina that can lead to an increase in HIV transmission rates. Paradoxically, nonoxynol-9, touted as a vaginal spermicidal lubricant that might also prevent HIV infection, turned out to be abrasive to the vaginal epithelium when used frequently and may have facilitated rather than prevented HIV infection.[25]

Condom Use

A high level of condom use can have a major effect in reducing HIV transmission. However, condom use was generally very low during the initial period of HIV introduction in almost all countries and still remains low in most countries with current low prevalence. Thus, it is unlikely that condom use accounts for the differences in prevalence between countries with high or low heterosexual HIV prevalence. However, the marked increase in condom use in commercial sex settings in Thailand, and in heterosexuals with multiple sex partners in Uganda has almost certainly been instrumental in leveling and even decreasing new infections in these countries during the latter half of the 1990s. Some faith-based organizations have criticized the recommendation by most public health programs for routine use of condoms to prevent sexually transmitted infections, including HIV, because they insist, without any scientific support, that condoms are not very effective for the prevention of HIV. However, an official from the United Evangelical Lutheran Church of Argentina, in response to this criticism, said: "unfortunately faithful relationships have a much higher failure rate compared to condoms!"

The following factors are believed by some, without any supportive data, to increase heterosexual transmission.

HIV Subtype

Some laboratory studies have shown that HIV subtypes C and E infect and replicate more efficiently than subtype B in Langerhans cells present in the vaginal mucosa, cervix and the foreskin of the penis but not on the wall of the rectum.[26] These laboratory data have led to a hypothesis that subtypes E and C may have a higher potential for heterosexual transmission than other HIV subtypes. However, there is no epidemiologic support for this hypothesis. The presence of subtypes E and C – designated as "heterosexual" subtypes – in many countries with low heterosexual HIV prevalence has not been correlated with any marked increase in heterosexual prevalence. Nevertheless, there are still some laboratory scientists who cling to this hypothesis.

Poverty

The contention that poverty is a primary factor responsible for high rates of HIV transmission and AIDS is a politically and socially attractive hypothesis. However, there is no scientific basis to support the contention that poverty is the primary or even a major factor responsible for the high rates of HIV and AIDS in SSA, a few countries in the Caribbean "region" and in South and Southeast Asia! Epidemiologic studies of HIV transmission in MSM during the early-to-mid-1980s clearly showed a direct correlation of high HIV prevalence rates with high sex partner exchange rates. MSM with very high sex partner exchange rates had the highest HIV prevalence rates whereas those rates in MSM who tended to be mutually monogamous were low or zero. Poverty was not and is not considered a factor for high HIV prevalence rates in MSM populations. In the 2003 DHS+ survey in Kenya, it was clearly shown that persons in the wealthiest 20 percent of the population had HIV infection rates 2 to 3 times the infection rate of persons in the lowest wealth quintile as shown in Figure 5.3. Almost identical findings were reported from the 2003–2004 DHS+ study in Tanzania.[27]

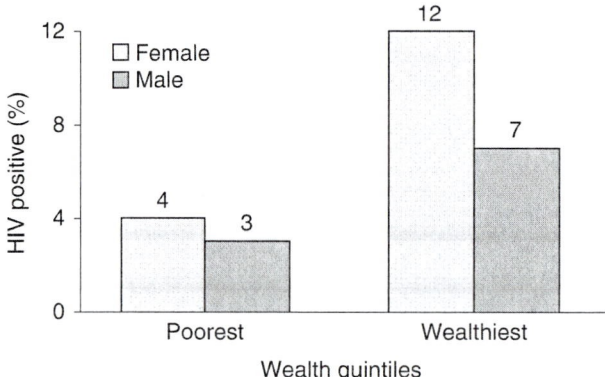

Figure 5.3 HIV prevalence by economic status (Kenya – 2003 DHS Survey).

Epidemiologic studies in SSA have consistently showed that both males and females in the highest socioeconomic class also had the highest HIV prevalence rates as the 2003 data in Figure 5.3 indicates. This result was attributed to the finding that persons in the highest socioeconomic class in SSA also tended to have the highest number of sex partners.

In addition, countries with the highest HIV prevalence rates in SSA – Botswana, Zimbabwe, and Swaziland – are not the poorest countries in SSA, and many of the poorest countries in Africa have some of the lowest HIV prevalence rates as shown in Figure 5.4. Furthermore, most of the poorest countries in the world outside of SSA have the lowest prevalence rates. Epidemic heterosexual HIV transmission has not and will not occur in most of the poorest countries in Latin America, North Africa, Middle East, most Central Asian countries, and most of the poorest countries in the Asia-Pacific region because the general pattern and prevalence of heterosexual risk behaviors are not sufficient to enable R_0 of HIV to get close to 1.

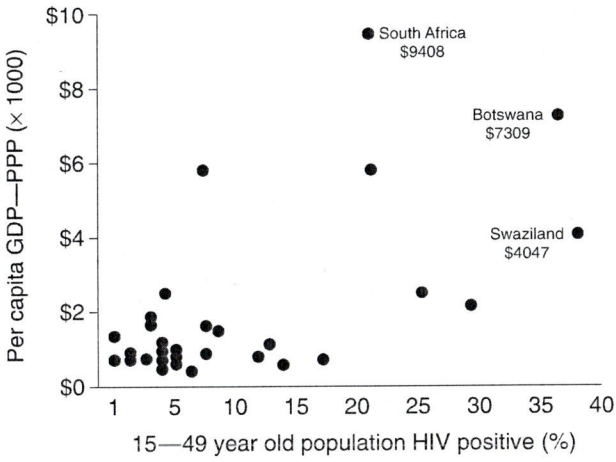

Figure 5.4 Correlation of HIV prevalence with per capita GDP.

Poor nutrition caused by poverty has been proposed as a major factor responsible for the higher mother-to-infant HIV transmission in SSA mothers compared with mothers in developed countries. However, it is now accepted by UNICEF and UNAIDS that about 25 to 30 percent of HIV-infected pregnant females will transmit HIV infection to their infants. There is no significant difference in mother-to-infant transmission of HIV in poorly nourished SSA mothers compared with mothers in developed countries that is not fully explained by the known differences in breastfeeding. Another false assertion is that because of poor nutrition due to poverty most Africans have an "undermined" immune system that makes them more susceptible to HIV infection and to the development of AIDS. This assertion has been based primarily on anecdotal reports or flawed studies. A review[28] of the largest cohort studies that followed HIV-infected persons from about the time of their infection to death in Uganda, Thailand, and Haiti concluded that the median period from HIV infection to development of severe immune deficiency is the same in developing countries (including SSA) as in developed countries – about 7 to 8 years. However, a significant difference was found in the median survival interval from severe immune deficiency to death in developing countries compared with developed countries. This latter difference is attributed primarily to the lack of anti-HIV therapy in developing countries and not to "undermined" immune systems.

The conclusion that poverty is not a major factor responsible for high HIV prevalence in MSM and heterosexual populations in SSA, and a few countries in the Caribbean and in South and Southeast Asia, should not be interpreted to suggest that poverty plays no role in the current AIDS pandemic. Poverty plays no significant role as a biologic determinant of HIV transmission, nor does it affect the natural progression from HIV infection to AIDS. In countries where the pattern and prevalence of heterosexual risk behaviors are "low," no significant epidemic heterosexual HIV transmission can be expected regardless of whether the country is rich or poor. However, poverty can clearly increase the number of females who place themselves at risk for HIV infection because they have to sell sex to survive. In addition, poverty, along with other social factors, can contribute to the large number of IDU who are at risk of acquiring HIV by sharing their drug injecting equipment. Poverty was also a major factor that induced poor peasants in China to sell their blood: many were infected with HIV as a result of contaminated plasma collection equipment. Outside of SSA, the major risk behaviors that led to HIV epidemics were the sharing of injection equipment by IDU and extensive use of FSW by a large proportion of males. The major determinants of these risk behaviors in addition to poverty include cultural, social, and religious factors that collectively may be more important than poverty alone. UN Secretary-General Kofi Annan in late 2002 said: "[HIV/AIDS] has exacerbated the problems of poverty, discrimination, malnutrition and sexual exploitation of girls and women..." Secretary-General Annan's statement is right on the mark. However, too many AIDS program advocates and activists have incorrectly concluded that these factors – poverty, etc. – are major determinants of high HIV prevalence.

Patterns and Measurement of Heterosexual Risk Behaviors

HIV is primarily a sexually transmitted infection (STI). As with all STI, the major driving force of the pandemic is heterosexual transmission because heterosexuals comprise the vast majority of all populations. Although high HIV infection rates (50 percent and higher) have been found and may still occur in susceptible pockets of IDU and MSM, more than 90 percent of the global total of adult infections have been and will continue to be due to heterosexual transmission. The patterns and prevalence of heterosexual risk behaviors are not the same in all the world's populations. Cultural, social, religious, economic and many other factors may influence and determine the patterns and prevalence of unprotected sex outside of mutually monogamous relationships. There are different patterns of sexual risk behaviors outside of traditional marital relationships as well as major differences in the proportion of the sexually active population who routinely engage in such behaviors. These differences are of paramount importance in determining the extent of HIV transmission that may occur in any heterosexual population.

Several datasets are available to quantify the prevalence of heterosexual risk behaviors in different populations. A couple of these datasets are measurements of STD that should also serve as good indicators of sexual risk behaviors. The other datasets are sexual risk behavior surveys that were carried out by GPA/WHO over a decade ago as part of large scale Knowledge, Attitudes, Behaviors and Practices (KABP) surveys.[29]

Estimated Prevalence Rates of STD as an Indicator of Sexual Risk Behaviors

Are the patterns and prevalence of sexually transmitted diseases (STD) the same in all populations? The obvious answer to this question is that STD prevalence can and does vary markedly from one population to another. The primary reason for such differentials is the varying patterns and prevalence of sexual risk behaviors present in different populations. However, many AIDS "experts" review and evaluate STD data collected from STD clinics and come to the politically correct conclusion that STD prevalence is "high" and not markedly different in different populations. There have been scant population-based surveys of STD prevalence to enable any meaningful comparison of STD prevalence in different countries and regions. A few years ago WHO's HIV/STI unit in Geneva prepared detailed estimates of the prevalence of several curable STD in the different WHO global regions: these estimates give a more objective assessment of STD prevalence in different "general" populations compared with the use of STD clinic data only.

Table 5.2 Estimated regional HIV and STD prevalence[x]

Region	Adults 15–49 millions	Number of HIV+ millions	HIV+ rate percent	Number of STD millions	STD rate percent	STD index
Sub-Saharan Africa	273.5	23.40	8.56	32.0	11.9	17.0
Caribbean & Latin America	269.0	1.55	0.58	18.5	7.1	10.1
South & SE Asia	993.5	5.80	0.58	48.0	5.0	7.1
"Western" countries	359.4	1.43	0.40	7.0	1.9	2.7
E Europe & Central Asia	197.7	0.41	0.21	6.0	2.9	4.1
N Africa & Middle-East	171.9	0.21	0.12	3.5	2.1	3.0
East Asia & Pacific	821.7	0.64	0.08	6.0	0.7	1.0[*]
TOTALS	**3086.7**	**33.34**	**1.08**	**116.5**	**3.8**	

[x]Prevalence of the following curable STD – Chlamydia, Gonorrhea, Syphilis, and Trichomoniasis
[*]The East Asia and Pacific region had the lowest STD rate, and all the other regions are multiples of this lowest rate – i.e., the STD rate in sub-Saharan Africa is 17 times greater than the STD rate in East Asia & Pacific region. The Spearman rank-difference correlation coefficient for HIV and STD prevalence in the seven world regions is +0.88.

HIV prevalence estimates in Table 5.2 were those published by UNAIDS/WHO in the July, 2002 Global report on HIV/AIDS.[30] Estimates of several curable STD were developed by the HIV/STI unit of WHO for 1999.[31] Table 5.2 shows a general concordance between HIV prevalence and a calculated STD index. The East Asia-Pacific region has the lowest STD prevalence rate, the lowest STD index as well as the lowest estimated HIV prevalence rate, while SSA had the highest values for these rates. The estimated STD prevalence rate in SSA was 17 times greater than the estimated STD prevalence rate in East Asia and the Pacific region. This indicates that sexual risk behaviors in SSA are significantly higher than in East Asia and the Pacific and so suggests that HIV prevalence in this latter region will not reach the high levels currently present in many SSA countries. The combined Caribbean and Latin America region in this table obscures the probably higher STD rates in the Caribbean; the STD rate in Eastern Europe may be overestimated. If STD rates in Eastern Europe are really that high, extensive heterosexual HIV spread may be expected if these STD rates are accurate and remain high.

These regional STD estimates do not include those STD with genital ulcerative lesions – chancroid and genital herpes. Both of these latter STD are known to be highly prevalent in SSA populations compared with most other populations. As described below, a high prevalence of genital herpes is a good objective indicator of a high prevalence of sexual risk behaviors. In addition, genital lesions from this viral infection that may recur four to five times annually can greatly facilitate sexual HIV transmission.

Genital Herpes Virus as an Indicator of Sexual Risk Behavior

The prevalence of genital herpes virus (HSV-2) infection as measured by antibody to HSV-2 is considered an objective indicator of sexual risk behaviors. An individual who has been infected with HSV-2 acquired infection either from having multiple sex partners, one of whom had a HSV-2 infection, or from his/her regular sex partner who must have had at least one other sex partner infected with HSV-2. Serologic surveys of HSV-2 antibody have consistently shown that persons with high sexual risk behaviors, such as STD patients and FSW, have very high HSV-2 prevalence while persons with little or no sexual risk behaviors have low or zero prevalence of HSV-2 antibody.

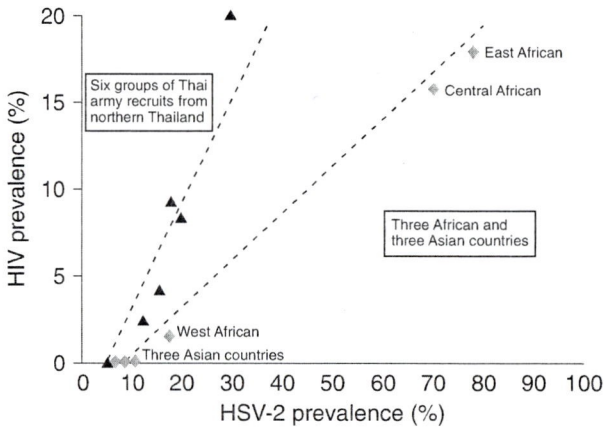

Data provided by Dr. John Moran (CDC)

Figure 5.5 Correlation of HIV and genital herpes antibody prevalence.

The line on the left in Figure 5.5 presents the correlation between HIV and HSV-2 prevalence in six groups of Thai army recruits[32] from different areas of northern Thailand. Recruits with low HSV-2 prevalence had no HIV infection but recruits with the highest prevalence of HSV-2 antibody also had the highest HIV prevalence. These data indicate that even within a region such as northern Thailand with the highest HIV prevalence in the country, sexual risk behavior as measured by infection with both HIV and HSV-2 can vary markedly.

The line on the right of Figure 5.5 shows the correlation between HIV and HSV-2 prevalence in three SSA and three Asian populations. These data were collected from either antenatal clinic (ANC) attendees (20–24 years of age) or in community-based surveys of 20–24 year old females. Thus it was assumed that the findings might be representative of sexually active females or at least not biased by large numbers of females with the highest sexual risk behaviors. HIV prevalence was virtually zero in Asian females and these females had low HSV-2 prevalence – none exceeded 10 percent. In contrast, there was a positive correlation between HIV and HSV-2 prevalence in females from the three African countries. East African females had the highest levels of HSV-2 and HIV and West African females had the lowest values of both viral infections.

These data indicate that Asian women have lower prevalence of sexual risk behaviors among 20–24 year olds compared with Africans in the same age group. This conclusion is also supported by data presented in the preceding section on estimated STD in different global regions and by surveys carried out by GPA/WHO over a decade ago as part of their large scale KABP surveys.

Behavioral Surveys of Sexual Risk Behaviors

During the early to mid-1990s, several Kenyan social research centers collected sexual risk behavior data on Kenyan youth.[33,34,35,36] Their major findings listed below showed very high levels of heterosexual risk behaviors in adolescent boys and girls.

1 Over 50 percent of Kenyan youths aged 15–19 had started sexual activity.
2 Close to 66 percent of boys and 40 percent of girls were sexually active by age 20.
3 In several rural districts, 75 percent of girls had sexual intercourse before the age of 16 and 27 percent before the age of 15.
4 In one district, both boys and girls began their sexual activity at an average age of 13.5.
5 A study of unmarried churchgoing youth (mostly 16–19) found 64 percent of males and 33 percent of females were sexually active. Thirty percent of the boys reported having had more than five different sex partners.

These Kenyan surveys confirmed and supported the results of the behavioral surveys (KABP) carried out by GPA/WHO in the late 1980s and early 1990s.

The pattern(s) and prevalence of heterosexual risk behaviors described in the GPA/WHO KABP surveys showed marked differences between the SSA countries and the Asian countries surveyed. Among the many parameters of sexual behavior surveyed were the following:

1 median age of first sexual intercourse
2 percent of young males and females who engaged in premarital sex

3 percent of sexually active males and females who had non-regular and commercial sex and

4 percent of males and females in regular sex partnerships (married or otherwise) who reported having sex partner(s) outside their regular sex partnership (i.e., the extent of infidelity).

These surveys showed a consistently larger percent of Africans (up to 50 percent or higher), especially African females, who reported sexual risk behaviors compared with their Asian counterparts. Of special note, these surveys indicated that single women in Thailand, Sri Lanka, Singapore, and the Philippines reported rates of sexual intercourse far lower than their African counterparts.

The KABP surveys found high sexual risk behaviors in youths in several SSA countries but a much lower prevalence in Asian youths, as shown in Figure 5.6. The KABP surveys showed that from 33 to 69 percent of boys in the six SSA countries surveyed reported sexual intercourse within the last 12 months and from 16 to 56 percent of adolescent girls had sexual intercourse. Among Asians in this young age group the prevalence of sexual risk behaviors was markedly different: almost no girls reported sexual intercourse and from 1 to 29 percent of Asian boys indicated they had sexual intercourse in the last 12 months.

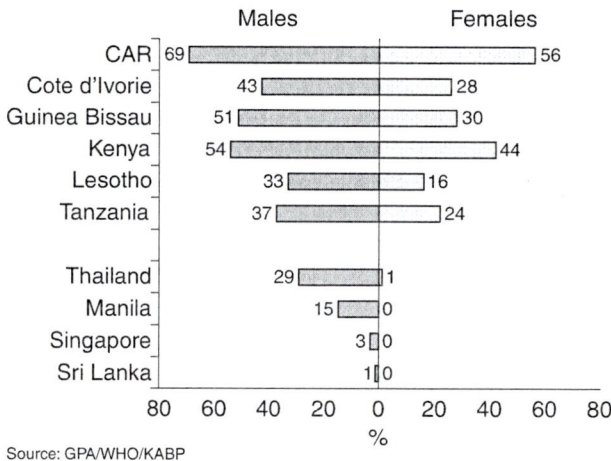

Source: GPA/WHO/KABP

Figure 5.6 Percent of 15–19 year olds who reported sexual intercourse in the last 12 months.

These findings and other research on sexual behavior suggest for Asia (in contrast to Africa, North America, and Europe) that cultural and social norms restrict female premarital and extramarital sex. In most Asian countries, sexual relations before marriage are strongly condemned by religious and social teachings. In countries such as Thailand, Cambodia, and Myanmar, where the difference in sexual risk behaviors between boys and girls is very great, it is almost the social norm for young males to seek out sex workers and older women who are already sexually experienced. Studies of sex networking in Southeast Asia have classified heterosexual multi-partner relationships into three types: commercial sex only, non-commercial sex only and a combination of commercial and non-commercial sex.

Figure 5.7 presents the median age at first sexual intercourse for the six SSA and the four Asian countries. African youths have their sexual debut at a much earlier age than Asian youths. Of special note are the relatively old ages for the sexual debut of males and females in Singapore and the very late age (27 years) for males in Sri Lanka. Also of special note is that the median age for sexual debut for Thai males is close to that of African males.

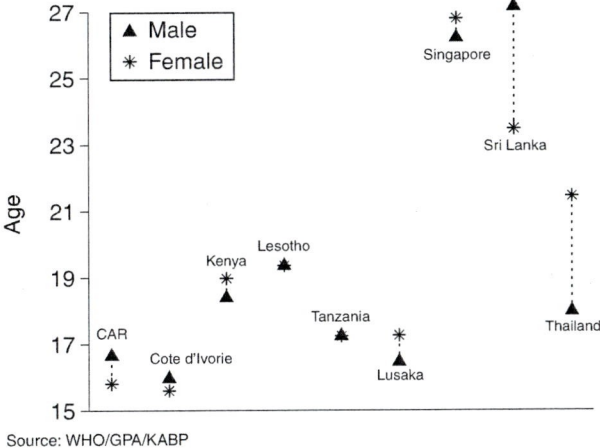

Source: WHO/GPA/KABP

Figure 5.7 Median age of first sexual intercourse.

The KABP survey of sexual risk behaviors in the 15–49 year old populations of these countries also shows that the sexual risk behaviors of youth continue into adulthood. Figure 5.8 presents the percent of males and females in rural and urban areas who had non-regular or commercial sex in the last 12 months. In the KABP surveys, casual or non-regular sex was defined as sex with a person who is not a spouse or a regular partner.

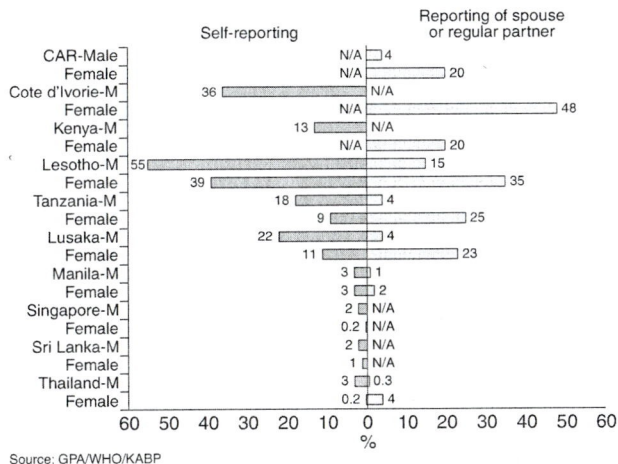

Source: GPA/WHO/KABP

Figure 5.8 Reported sex outside of regular sex relationship.

In most of the African countries, a higher prevalence of non-regular and commercial sex is consistently found in urban areas compared with rural areas, but the differences are not very large. Urban areas are associated with less family control of adolescent sexual behavior, more social mixing and opportunities for casual sex pairings, and more exposures to modern lifestyles. Again, only a small percent of Asian females report casual sex encounters in the last 12 months, but 40 percent of urban Thai males report having casual or more probably commercial sex in the last 12 months.

Figure 5.8 presents the percent of males and females who report either having sex outside of their marriage or regular sex relationship, or who report that their spouse or regular sex partner had sex with another partner in the last 12 months. Very high percents of males (55 percent in Lesotho) report having sex outside their regular relationship; a relatively high percent (48 percent in Cote d'Ivorie) of females report that their spouse or regular sex partner had other sex partners in the last 12 months. Only a few percent of Asian males and females report sex outside their regular relationship by themselves or their spouse/regular sex partner. All these findings show that the patterns and prevalence of sexual risk behaviors are significantly higher in the African populations compared with the Asian populations surveyed.

HIV Transmission Dynamics in Populations with Different Patterns and Prevalence of HIV Risk Behaviors

The epidemic potential of HIV in a region, sub-region or country should be evaluated based on the pattern(s) and extent of commercial and other sex networks; the prevalence of STD (especially untreated and ulcerative STD); the percent of the male population who use FSW on a regular basis; sex partner exchange rates; the percent of uncircumcised males; and the percent of consistent condom use for casual and commercial sex encounters. It is inappropriate to use one uniform set of prevention strategies with the same level of support for all countries, when an assessment based on STD and behavioral data can identify the highest potential HIV epidemic situations.

HIV transmission patterns and dynamics in any country or large population are dependent on the existing patterns and prevalence of HIV risk behaviors. Initial introduction of HIV-infected persons or HIV-infected blood products into populations can result in epidemic or nonepidemic sexual HIV transmission depending on the different types and levels of HIV risk behavior(s) in the recipient population.

I Introduction of HIV into a Population with Low or Minimal HIV Risk Behavior(s)

No epidemic HIV transmission can be expected, but there will be nonepidemic sexual transmission to the regular sex partner(s) of HIV-infected persons, i.e., R_0 of HIV will be <1.

Examples – The vast majority of heterosexual populations throughout the world. A specific example was the importation in the mid-1980s of HIV-infected blood products for the treatment of thousands of male hemophilia patients in Japan. The result was high infection rates in the patients who received the infected blood products and only limited transmission to some of the regular sex partners of these patients.

2 Introduction of HIV into MSM Populations with Multiple and Concurrent Sex Partners

If the MSM sex network is large, extensive epidemic (R_0 >1) transmission can be expected, but if the network is small, epidemic transmission will be accordingly be more limited. Such epidemic sexual transmission will be followed by nonepidemic sexual transmission to the regular sex partner(s) of these high risk MSM. The regular sex partners may be male or female, but further HIV spread will not occur unless the regular sex partners also have multiple and concurrent sex partners.

Examples – Many major cities in Western countries and to a more limited extent in many other major cities in Latin America and in Asian Pacific countries or cities.

3 Introduction of HIV into IDU Populations Who Regularly Share Needles and Syringes

The size of needle sharing IDU networks and the extent of overlapping or intersections between these networks will determine whether limited or widespread HIV epidemics can be expected to develop in IDU populations. Epidemic HIV transmission will be followed by nonepidemic sexual transmission from infected IDU to their regular sex partner(s). Most regular sex partners of IDU may not have HIV risk behaviors so no further HIV transmission from these regular sex partners will occur. However, some male and female IDU will become sex workers to support their drug use and some regular sex partners of infected male IDU may be FSW. In such situations, limited epidemic sexual HIV transmission may occur, but the extent of epidemic spread will depend on the prevalence of facilitating and protective factors and on the size of and levels of sex partner exchange rates in the heterosexual networks. Sustained epidemic heterosexual HIV transmission has not resulted from any epidemic in an IDU population. The one possible exception is Thailand, but the patterns and levels of heterosexual risk behaviors in Thailand were sufficient to support epidemic heterosexual HIV transmission without any epidemic in the Thai IDU population.

Examples – There have been over 100 HIV epidemics in IDU populations throughout the world. They have occurred in many major cities in Western countries and in several Latin American countries starting in the 1980s. In the 1990s, HIV epidemics were noted in several countries in Eastern and Southern Europe, in several Middle Eastern countries and in many Asia-Pacific countries. All HIV epidemics in IDU have been followed by nonepidemic heterosexual transmission to the regular sex partners of infected IDU. Some focal epidemic HIV transmission has occurred from FSW because they were IDU or the regular sex partners of infected IDU.

Table 5.3 presents the findings from a study of FSW and their male clients in Yunnan, China where there has been a high HIV prevalence (up to 25 percent) in the IDU population during the past decade. Public health officials have been concerned that HIV-infected male IDU would infect many FSW who then would transmit HIV to their clients. This study found over 10 percent of FSW to be

HIV+, but all HIV-infected FSW had a history of IDU and the 213 FSW who denied drug use were all HIV negative. In addition, none of the male clients of FSW in this study were found to be HIV+. This study provides support for the relatively low infectivity of HIV via heterosexual intercourse.

Table 5.3 HIV prevalence in female sex workers and truck drivers in Yunnan, China, 1999–2000

Group	Number	Number HIV+	Percent HIV+
Truck drivers	550	0	0.0
FSW denying drug use*	213	0	0.0
FSW admitting drug use**	292	52	17.8
Total FSW	505	52	10.3

* In a prior Yunnan study, HIV prevalence in underground FSW not using drugs was found to be 2.2%.
** HIV prevalence in IDU tested in detention camps in Yunnan in 2000 was about 25%.

4 Introduction of HIV into Heterosexuals with Different Sexual Risk Behaviors

Table 5.1 on p.64 summarizes the potential R_0 of HIV via sexual intercourse based on the patterns of sexual mixing and annual numbers of different sex partners. Only in populations where there is a pattern of multiple and concurrent sex partners as well as a high prevalence of facilitating factors can R_0 of HIV become >1.

Examples – Epidemic (R_0 >1) heterosexual HIV transmission has occurred predominantly in SSA populations where up to 20–40 percent of sexually active adolescents and adults have multiple and concurrent sex partners and a very high prevalence of other STI, especially ulcerative STI such as HSV-2. To a lesser extent epidemic HIV transmission has occurred in many countries in the Caribbean and a few countries in South and Southeast Asia. In these latter countries, commercial sex networks are large and characterized by brothel-type establishments.

There is no epidemiologic disagreement that there is a direct correlation of sexual risk behaviors with HIV prevalence. However, there are many health professionals who believe that, in addition to the facilitating factors and protective factors previously described, there must be some, as yet unidentified, factor(s) that may be important or required to account for the wide range of HIV prevalence in SSA populations – from the lowest of less than 5 percent of the 15–49 year old population to over 30 percent. I do not agree that any additional factors other than patterns, prevalence, and frequency of sex partner exchanges and prevalence of multiple facilitating factors and protective factors are needed to explain the differences in HIV prevalence in SSA. However, with some infectious diseases (hepatitis B, adenovirus disease in military recruits, Ebola virus, and SARS) there is the phenomenon of "super-spreaders" who transmit the infectious disease agent to many persons. Thus, it is possible that just as there is a small proportion of HIV-infected persons who do not progress from HIV infection to AIDS, there may be a small proportion of HIV-infected persons who are "super-spreaders." There have been some reports of HIV-infected persons infecting up to a dozen sex partners and these cases may represent HIV "super-spreaders," and they may play a major role in some SSA epidemics. In addition, the role of social/sexual venues such as bars and nightclubs in SSA towns and cities where young adults gather for social and potential sexual mixing has not been systematically studied as potential venues for amplifying the spread of HIV, analogous to the bathhouse venue for MSM and large brothel-type establishments in some Asian cities.

Summary/Conclusions

Understanding the epidemiologic definition of epidemic (R_0 >1) versus nonepidemic (R_0 <1) spread of an infectious disease agent and understanding the different transmission dynamics of HIV are needed to fully understand the current and most probable future of different patterns and prevalence of HIV/AIDS in different populations. It needs to be fully accepted that HIV is usually very difficult to transmit sexually because such transmission requires the exchange of a significant amount of blood or semen that contains HIV. Epidemic sexual HIV transmission can occur only in those populations where there are large numbers of persons who have unprotected sex with *multiple* and *concurrent* sex partners. How high HIV prevalence may reach in these populations depends on: the prevalence of *facilitating factors* such as ulcerative STD (chancroid and genital herpes) that can greatly increase the amount of blood and sexual fluids exchanged during intercourse; and the prevalence of *protective factors* such as male circumcision and consistent condom use.

Sexual mixing patterns (serial or concurrent) and the frequency of sex partner exchanges are the primary determinants of the rapidity and extent of epidemic sexual HIV transmission. Another major factor in epidemic sexual spread of HIV is the size and pattern of sex networks and the extent of mixing (or "overlap") between different networks.

Several distinct epidemiologic patterns of sexual HIV transmission have been observed. **Understanding these different patterns of sexual HIV transmission is essential for the development of appropriate and effective HIV prevention strategies.**

1 Explosive or rapid epidemic (R_0 >1 in less than 1 year) transmission pattern requires frequent, almost daily sex partner exchange within large open sex networks. MSM in gay bathhouse settings and FSW in large brothel-type establishments are prime examples of this explosive epidemic transmission pattern.
2 Slow epidemic (R_0 >1 over many years) transmission (non-explosive) pattern requires having unprotected sex with multiple and concurrent sex partners within small (3 to 12 persons) sex groupings or networks that overlap with each other. This pattern of sex partner exchange is found in a very large proportion of MSM and from 20–40 percent of sexually active adults in many SSA populations but usually in only a small percent of most other populations.
3 Nonepidemic (R_0 <1) transmission pattern. In most developed countries a fairly large percent of adolescents and adults (up to 20 percent) have, during their lifetime, multiple sex partners, but sex partner exchange is usually serial and not concurrent. When sex partner exchange is on a monthly or annual basis and the pattern of exchange is serial rather than concurrent, no epidemic HIV transmission has been detected or should be expected.

4 HIV transmission from an HIV-infected person to his/her regular sex partner, i.e., among HIV-discordant couples. This distinct nonepidemic pattern of sexual HIV transmission will invariably follow after all HIV epidemics. As of late-2006, this pattern of HIV transmission is probably the predominant mode of HIV transmission globally, including SSA.

A UNAIDS press release in mid-2005 describing the current status of the AIDS pandemic, said: "Studies have failed to determine why the AIDS pandemic has been most severe in southern Africa and why certain countries, like the Philippines and Sri Lanka, have low infection rates." How UNAIDS could make such a statement is hard to believe when, as described in this chapter, all of the available studies in the past couple of decades on the patterns and prevalence of sexual risk behaviors and the prevalence of STD show quite clearly that these factors – that are of paramount importance for the sexual transmission of HIV – are from 1 to 2 orders of magnitude* higher in most SSA populations compared to countries such as the Philippines and Sri Lanka. There is no disagreement within the public health community that high HIV prevalence rates in MSM and IDU populations throughout the world can be attributed to their high HIV risk behaviors. Still UNAIDS continues to declare that poverty, gender inequity, discrimination and stigma, and lack of access to healthcare are the major determinants of high HIV prevalence in SSA populations. These social and public health issues are important and need to be addressed aggressively by the international health community because they create major barriers to effective HIV prevention and treatment programs, but they are not the primary or even major determinants of high HIV prevalence.

---

* An order of magnitude is not a small or subtle difference – 1 order of magnitude is 10 times greater and two orders of magnitude are hundreds of times greater!

Appendix 1

This appendix provides several specific examples of how the reproductive number of HIV is calculated, as well as how the annual risk of acquiring an HIV infection is calculated. I emphasize to my students that they need to critically evaluate the assumptions used and the values used for each of the needed parameters. It is clearly not rocket science and can easily be calculated by hand or with a simple calculator. Any of the assumptions used and the value(s) used can be changed, but any change must be supported by data and not arbitrarily changed because one believes that some of the values are too high or too low.

Reproductive Number (R_0) of HIV in Female Sex Workers (FSW) in the Philippines

The average *annual* number of HIV infections that an HIV-infected FSW might transmit to her male clients depends on the following parameters:

1 probability of HIV transmission per coital act [**r**]
2 *annual* number of unprotected sex contacts with male clients [**n**].

r – Published studies of the risk of HIV transmission from an infected female to a susceptible male indicate that this risk is usually less than one per several thousand (**r** = <0.001 or about 1 per 2–3 thousand) unprotected coital acts. However, this low risk was estimated from regular sex partner studies and for this scenario, it will be assumed that the average risk is increased several fold to 1/500 (**r** = 0.002) because of the presence of some facilitating factors in the commercial sex population.

n – Behavioral surveillance studies in the Philippines indicate that the average FSW has less than one male client per day. FSW will thus have on average about 300 male clients per year. Reported condom use with FSW in the Philippines has reached about 75 percent, but for this calculation it will be assumed that at least 50 percent (**p** = 0.5) of male clients of FSW use a condom.[*] Thus, the average FSW in the Philippines will have about 150 unprotected sexual encounters annually with male clients.

$$R_0 \text{ HIV} = \mathbf{r} \,[0.002] \times \mathbf{n} \,[150] = 0.3$$

Conclusion

For every 100 HIV-infected FSW in the Philippines, about 30 male clients can be expected to be infected annually. As of late-2006, the estimated number of FSW in the Philippines is less than 200 000 and according to HIV sentinel surveillance data, about one per thousand are estimated to be HIV-infected. These most recent estimates yield from 200 to 300 HIV-infected FSW and collectively they would transmit HIV infection to less than 100 of their male clients.

However, it should be emphasized that the above calculations were for the *annual* reproductive number. If the average "professional" lifespan of a FSW in the

---

[*] Behavioral surveillance findings in the Philippines indicate that condom use with clients of FSW in 2005 was just a bit over 50 percent.

Philippines is arbitrarily estimated at 10 years, then the lifetime R_0 for HIV-infected FSW in the Philippines is dependent on when the FSW acquired her HIV infection. If she acquired her HIV infection early, she might infect 2 to 3 clients during her professional lifespan but if she acquired her infection in the last year or so then she might not infect any of her clients. This slow rate of HIV increase probably would not be sufficient to compensate for the annual 5–10 percent decrease in HIV-infected FSW and infected male clients that would be expected from AIDS deaths and from the normal "retirement" of FSW from commercial sex work.

The above calculations used the most likely values for each parameter based on available data. However, a best case and worst case scenario using the lowest plausible values (best case) compared to the highest plausible values (worst case) to calculate the R_0 for HIV-infected FSW are as follows:

Best case: $R_0 = \mathbf{r}\ [0.0005] \times \mathbf{n}\ [100] = 0.05 =$ five new HIV-infected male clients annually for every 100 HIV-infected FSW. For 200 to 300 HIV-infected FSW, 10 to 15 male clients will be infected annually.

Worst case: $R_0 = \mathbf{r}\ [0.002] \times \mathbf{n}\ [400] = 0.8 =$ eighty (80) new HIV-infected male clients annually for every 100 HIV-infected FSW. For 200 to 300 HIV-infected FSW 160 to 240 male clients will be infected annually.

Annual Risk of Acquiring HIV Infection (P) in Female Sex Workers in the Philippines

The annual probability [**P**] or risk for a FSW in the Philippines of becoming HIV-infected via her sex contact with male clients is dependent on the following parameters:

Probability that a sex partner is infected with HIV, i.e., the prevalence in a specific sex network [**p**]

Probability of HIV transmission per coital act [**r**]

Annual number of unprotected sex contacts with male clients [**n**]

$$\mathbf{P} = (\mathbf{p} \times \mathbf{r} \times \mathbf{n})$$

Based on the available data and some conservative assumptions, the following values are assigned for each of the above parameters to calculate **P** for a basic FSW scenario.

p – HIV sentinel surveillance (HSS) findings for the prevalence of HIV in FSW in the Philippines have since the early 1990s been consistently about 1 per thousand (**p** = 0.001). There are no HSS data for male clients of FSW, but from 2000 to 2004, the National Voluntary Blood Service reported 68 HIV positive blood samples out of over 1.5 million donors tested (**p** = 0.00004). It is doubtful that HIV prevalence in male clients of FSW is as low as 1/25 000 or as high as in FSW (1/1000 or **p** = 0.001), and for this calculation an HIV prevalence of 1/2000 (**p** = 0.0005) or half of the FSW prevalence will be used for male clients of FSW.

r – Several published studies of the risk of HIV transmission from males to females indicate that this risk is about 1/1000 (**r** = 0.001) unprotected coital acts. However, this low risk was estimated from regular sex partner studies and for this scenario, it will be assumed that the average risk is doubled to 1/500 (**r** = 0.002) because of the presence of some facilitating factors in the commercial sex population.

n1 – Behavioral surveillance studies in the Philippines indicate that the average FSW has less than one male client per day. FSW will thus have about 300 male client contacts per year. Reported condom use with FSW in the Philippines has reached about 75 percent, but for this calculation it will be assumed that at least 50 percent (**p** = 0.5) of male clients of FSW use a condom. Thus, the average FSW in the Philippines will have about 150 unprotected sexual encounters annually with their male clients.

$$P = (p\ [0.0005] \times r\ [0.002] \times n1\ [150]) = 0.00015$$

According to these calculations, one FSW out of 6667 will acquire an HIV infection annually via sexual contact with male clients. Thus, for every 100 000 FSW in the Philippines there may be about 15 new HIV-infected FSW annually. If there are 200 000 FSW in the Philippines, about 30 new HIV infections in FSW may be expected.

Conclusions

The current (2006) annual probability (**p**) of FSW in the Philippines acquiring an HIV infection from their male clients is very low because of the very low prevalence of HIV infection in their male clients and the low infectivity of HIV.[*] However, if an HIV epidemic in male IDU in the Philippines occurs and HIV prevalence in male clients of FSW suddenly increased to about 1 percent (**p** = 0.01) or a 20-fold increase from the current estimate, this would increase the risk of annual HIV infection in FSW to **P** = 0.003 – and instead of 30 new infections annually in an estimated population of 200 000 FSW, the annual number of new HIV infections in FSW could rise to about 600! Effective prevention of HIV transmission in the Philippines requires primary public health interventions such as needle exchange for IDU, prevention and/or prompt treatment of other STDs, as well as keeping condom use high for all commercial sex encounters to keep HIV prevalence low in FSW.

Annual Risk of Acquiring HIV Infection in Male Clients of FSW in the Philippines

The annual probability [**P**] for a male client of FSW in the Philippines to become HIV-infected is dependent on the following parameters:

Probability that a FSW is infected with HIV [**p**]
Probability of HIV transmission per coital act [**r**]
Annual number of unprotected sex contacts with FSW [**n**]

$$P = (p \times r \times n)$$

Based on the available data and some conservative assumptions, the following values are assigned for each of the above parameters to calculate **P** for male clients of FSW.

p – HIV sentinel surveillance (HSS) findings for the prevalence of HIV in FSW in the Philippines have since the early 1990s been consistently about 1 per thousand (**p** = 0.001).

---

[*] In addition, the vast majority of Filipino males are circumcised and male circumcision has been associated with low sexual HIV transmission rates.

r – Several published studies of the risk of HIV transmission from an infected female to a susceptible male indicate that this risk is about 1 per several thousand unprotected coital acts. However, this low risk was estimated from regular sex partner studies and for this scenario, it will be assumed that the average risk is increased to 1/500 (**r** = 0.002) because of the presence of some facilitating factors in the commercial sex population.

n1 – Behavioral surveillance studies in the Philippines indicate that the average male client of FSW has about 2 visits per week. Male clients will thus have about 100 visits per year. Reported condom use with FSW in the Philippines has reached about 75 percent, but for this calculation it will be assumed that at least 50 percent (**p** = 0.5) of male clients of FSW use a condom. Thus, the average male client of FSW in the Philippines will have about 50 unprotected sexual encounters annually with FSW.

$$\mathbf{P} = (\mathbf{p}\ [0.001] \times \mathbf{r}\ [0.002] \times \mathbf{n1}\ [50]) = 0.0001$$

According to these calculations, one male client out of 10 000 will acquire an HIV infection annually via sexual contact with FSW. Thus, for every 100 000 male clients of FSW in the Philippines there may be about 10 new HIV-infected FSW annually, and for a million male clients, about 100 new HIV infections can be expected annually.

Conclusions

The current (2006) annual probability (**p**) of male clients of FSW in the Philippines acquiring an HIV infection is very low because of the very low prevalence of HIV infection in FSW and the low infectivity of HIV. Thus, if there are from 3 to 4 million male clients of FSW annually in the Philippines, each averaging 50 unprotected sex contacts with a FSW, then about 300 to 400 new HIV infections may be expected. Effective prevention of HIV transmission in the Philippines requires primary public health interventions such as needle exchange for IDU, prevention and/or prompt treatment of other STDs, as well as keeping condom use high for all commercial sex encounters to keep HIV prevalence low in FSW. The fact that the vast majority of the male population is circumcised just prior to puberty is also an important "protective" factor against epidemic sexual HIV transmission in the Philippines.

Appendix 2

The President of Uganda, Yoweri K Museveni, at the opening ceremony of the Tenth International Conference on AIDS in Africa held at Kampala in December 1995, eloquently described the AIDS epidemic in Africa in the following words: "AIDS is really like a wildfire. If you can visualise a fire in the bush – that is how I think of the spread of AIDS. If a spark of fire drops on wet grass, there will be no fire, but if it drops on dry grass, the fire will spread. I think this was the problem here in Africa. There was dry grass and it assisted the spread of the fire."

During the past decade, I have also used the analogy of a forest fire to describe the potentials for epidemic heterosexual HIV transmission.

The Potential for Heterosexual HIV Epidemics or How Dry are the Trees?

The gathering or impending storm analogy for AIDS in many developing countries is not an accurate description of the probable future scenarios of HIV/AIDS. A better example or a more apt analogy to describe the potential for epidemic HIV transmission in populations where no HIV epidemics have occurred would be to liken the potential for epidemic HIV transmission with the potentials for a large forest fire. Using such an analogy – with the dryness or wetness of the forest equated with the patterns and prevalence of heterosexual HIV-risk behaviors – the potential for extensive or epidemic HIV spread in populations where epidemic HIV transmission has not occurred can be better understood.

Table 5A2.1 Factors needed for a forest fire and their counterparts for epidemic HIV transmission

Forest fire	Epidemic HIV transmission
1. A source – some spark, lightning, a match, a discarded cigarette, etc.	1. Importation of an HIV-infected person(s) or importation of HIV-infected blood products
2. Kindling and dry brushes to ignite the trees	2. Extensive HIV spread in the highest HIV-risk groups – FSW, IDU
3. Location/spacing/amount of the kindling and brushes	3. Patterns, prevalence and the social dynamics of sex and IDU networks
4. Forest fire potential – are the trees wet or dry?	4. Prevalence of HIV-risk behaviors in the population, dry = high, wet = low
5. Wind and other factors such as total neglect until the fire is out of control	5. Facilitating factors – other STD, recent infections, "dry sex," traumatic sex, lack of male circumcision, etc.
6. The heat intensity of a raging forest fire can ignite wet trees that would not be consumed by a smaller fire.	6. The high HIV prevalence in an explosive HIV epidemic can increase the risk of HIV transmission in persons with low HIV risk behaviors.

In virtually all large "general" populations, it is difficult if not impossible to get a "generalized" HIV epidemic (a large forest fire) started. This is because the patterns and prevalence of heterosexual risk behaviors, especially the pattern and size of sex networks in the general or total heterosexual population, are insufficient to sustain any extensive HIV transmission outside of the highest HIV-risk behavior groups such as MSM, IDU, and FSW and their male clients, or to use the forest fire analogy, most of the trees in the forest are wet!

In most populations, in addition to a general lower prevalence of heterosexual HIV-risk behaviors (i.e., the forest is wet), most of the factors that facilitate sexual HIV transmission are either not present or present in relatively small amounts. In some raging forest fires, the intense heat generated by the fire will consume some "wet" trees that ordinarily would be difficult to ignite. Many persons with lower heterosexual risk behaviors might get infected in an African HIV epidemic situation because of the high prevalence of HIV infections and a high proportion of facilitating factors and very recent and therefore very infectious HIV infections. Persons with identical heterosexual risk behaviors would not be at any significant risk of acquiring an HIV infection from having multiple and serial sex partners in populations where HIV prevalence is very low.

The strategies and methods for fighting a raging forest fire are markedly different from what are needed in most forest fire prevention programs. For prevention of a forest fire, it is not a very high priority to constantly wet down all the trees, rather the top priority is to clear out the dry brush and kindling as much as possible to prevent them from igniting and possibly starting a forest fire.

The forest fire analogy and epidemiologic observations of HIV prevalence trends in Thailand from 1989 through 2004 can be used to describe the past, present, and future of HIV/AIDS in Thailand. It can be concluded that although much of the dry brush and kindling (IDU and FSW) in Thailand have burned and some of the surrounding forest has been singed, no generalized forest fire has occurred primarily because most of the forest is wet! The Thai HIV sentinel surveillance data show very clearly that extensive HIV transmission has essentially been limited to their highest HIV-risk behavior groups (RBG) and from these RBG to some of their regular sex partners. However, since the mid-1990s, HIV prevalence trends in heterosexuals outside of the highest RBG have been steadily decreasing. This indicates that HIV can and does spread to a limited extent from infected male clients of FSW to their regular sex partners and from infected IDU to their regular sex partners, but not much further. In countries such as the Philippines and Indonesia, despite the presence of thousands of HIV-infected persons during the past decade, the dry bushes and kindling (IDU and FSW) in these countries have not yet ignited into flames, but continue to smolder. The potential for extensive HIV spread to suddenly erupt in the highest RBG is constantly present and as with any good fire protection program, such potentials should be reduced as much as possible before these dry bushes and kindling burst into flames!

In Figure 5A2.1, annual findings from ANC attendees in Francistown, Botswana, where epidemic heterosexual HIV transmission has been occurring since the early 1980s, has been added to the Thai HSS findings to show the marked difference between a raging forest fire in a SSA population compared to the brush and kindling fires in Thailand.

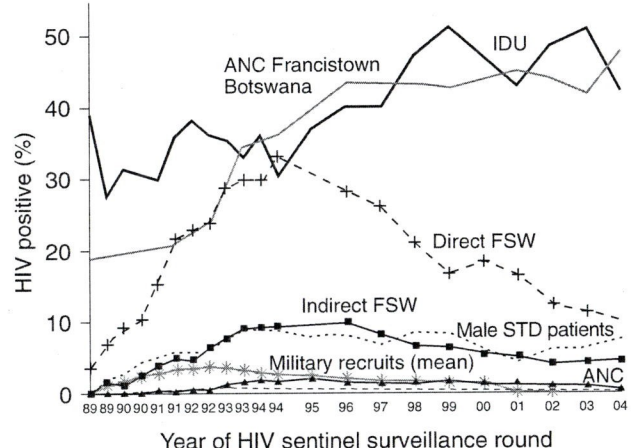

Figure 5A2.1 HIV sentinel surveillance – Thailand.

References

1 Fumento M (1990) *The Myth of Heterosexual AIDS*. Basic Books, New York.

2 Center for Disease Control and Prevention (1995) Case-control study of HIV seroconversion in health-care workers after percutaneous exposure to HIV infected blood – France, United Kingdom, and United States, January 1988 – August 1994. *MMWR*. **44**: 929–33.

3 Royce RA, Sena A, Cates W and Cohen MS (1997) Sexual transmission of HIV. *N Engl J Med*. **336**: 1072–78.

4 Padian NS, Shiboski SC, Glass SO and Vittinghoff E (1997) Heterosexual transmission of human immunodeficiency virus (HIV) in northern California: results from a ten-year study. *Am J Epidemiol*. **146**(4): 350–7.

5 Nicolosi A, *et al*. for the Italian Study Group on HIV Heterosexual Transmission (1994) The efficiency of male-to-female and female-to-male sexual transmission of the human immunodeficiency virus: a study of 730 stable couples. *Epidemiology*. **5**: 570–75.

6 De Vincenzi I, for the European Study Group in Heterosexual Transmission of HIV (1994) A longitudinal study of human immunodeficiency virus transmission by heterosexual couples. *N Engl J Med*. **331**: 341–46.

7 Gray RH, *et al*. and the Rakai Project Team (2001) Probability of HIV-1 transmission per coital act in monogamous, heterosexual, HIV-1-discordant couples in Rakai, Uganda. *Lancet*. **357**: 1149–53.

8 Mastro TD and Kitayaporn D (1998) HIV type 1 transmission probabilities: estimates from epidemiologic studies. *AIDS Res Hum Retrovirol*. **14**(Suppl 3): S223–7.

9 Chin J, Bennett A and Mills S (1998) Primary determinants of HIV prevalence in Asian-Pacific countries. *AIDS*. **12**(Suppl B): S87–91.

10 May RM and Anderson RM (1987) Transmission dynamics of HIV infection. *Nature*. **326**: 137–42.

11 Anderson RM (1991) The transmission dynamics of sexually transmitted diseases: the behavioral component. In: JN Wasserheit, SO Aral, KK Holmes, *et al*. (eds). *Research Issues in Human Behavioral and Sexually Transmitted Diseases in the AIDS Era*. American Society for Microbiology, Washington DC.

12 Pilcher C, Tien H, Stewart P, *et al*. (2002) Estimating transmission probabilities over time in acute HIV infection from biological data. Ninth Conference on Retroviruses and Opportunistic Infections, Feb 24–28; Poster 366-M.

13 Jacquez JA, Koopman JS, Simon CP and Longini IM (1994) Role of the primary infection in epidemics of HIV infection in gay cohorts. *J Acq Imm Def Syn*. **7**: 1169–84.

14 Satten GA, Mastro TD, Longini IM Jr (1994) Modeling the female-to-male HIV transmission probability in an emerging epidemic in Asia. *Statistics in Medicine*. **13**: 2097–106.

15 Simonsen JN, Cameron DW, Gakinya MN, *et al*. (1988) Human immunodeficiency virus among African men with sexually transmitted diseases. *N Engl J Med*. **319**: 274–8.

16 Laga M, Nzila N and Goeman J (1991) The interrelationship of sexually transmitted diseases and HIV infection: implications for the control of both epidemics in Africa. *AIDS*. **5**: S55–63.

17 Benedetti JK, Corey L, Ashley R, *et al*. (1994) Recurrence rates in genital herpes after symptomatic first episode infection. *Ann Intern Med*. *121*(11): 847–54.

18 Benedetti JK, Zeh J and Corey L (1999) Clinical reactivation of genital herpes simplex virus infection decreases in frequency over time. *Ann Intern Med*. **131**(1): 14–20.

19 Todd J, Grosskurth H, Changalucha J, *et al*. (2006) Risk factors influencing HIV infection incidence in a rural african population: a nested case-control study. *JID*. **193**: 458–66.

20 de Vincenzi I and Mertens T (1994) Male circumcision: a role in HIV prevention? *AIDS*. **8**(2): 153–60.

21 Halperin DT and Bailey RC (1999) Male circumcision and HIV infection: 10 years and counting. *Lancet*. **354**: 1813–15.

22 Weiss HA, Quigley MA and Hayes RJ (2000) Male circumcision and risk of HIV infection in sub-Saharan Africa: a systematic review and meta-analysis. *AIDS*. **14**(15): 2361–70.

23 Bollinger R, *et al*. (2004) Male circumcision and risk of HIV-1 and other sexually transmitted infections in India. *Lancet*. **363**(9414): 1039–40.

24 Beksinska ME, Rees HV, Kleinschmidt I and McIntyre J (1999) The practice and prevalence of dry sex among men and women in South Africa: a risk factor for sexually transmitted infections? *Sex Transm Infect*. **75**(3): 178–80.

25 Centers for Disease Control and Prevention (2000) CDC Statement on study results of product containing nonoxynol-9. *MMWR*. August 11. **49**(31): 717.

26 Soto-Ramirez LE, Renjifo B, McLane MF *et al*. (1996) HIV-1 Langerhans' Cell Tropism Associated with Heterosexual Transmission of HIV. *Science*. **271**: 613–17.

27 Shelton JD, Cassell MM and Adetunji J (2005) Is poverty or wealth at the root of HIV? *Lancet*. **366**: 1057–8.

28 UNAIDS Reference Group for Surveillance, Estimation and Projection of HIV/AIDS numbers (2001) Consultation to determine criteria for estimating adult and child mortality for country-specific estimates of HIV/AIDS, Le Cottage, Talloires, France, 17–19 July.

29 GPA/WHO (1995) Knowledge, Attitudes, Behaviors, and Practices (KABP) surveys, published as: J Cleland and B Ferry (eds). *Sexual Behaviour and AIDS in the Developing World*. Taylor & Francis, London.

30 UNAIDS (2002) *Report on the Global HIV/AIDS Epidemic*. www.who.int/hiv/pub/epidemiology/pubepidemic2002/en/

31 WHO/HIV/AIDS/STI (1999) Global prevalence and incidence of selected curable sexually transmitted infections. www.who.int/hiv/pub/sti/who_hiv_aids_2001.02.pdf

32 Dobbins JG, Mastro TD, Nopkesorn T, *et al*. (1999) Herpes in the time of AIDS: a comparison of the epidemiology of HIV-1 and HSV-2 in young men in northern Thailand. *Sex Transm Disease*. **26**(2): 67–74.

33 Tetea Vijana (1995) National Council for Population and Development and the John Hopkins Population Communications Service/Population Information Program, Nairobi.

34 Illinigumugabo A, Njau PW and Rogo K (1994) *The Socio-Cultural and Medical Outcomes of Adolescent Pregnancies: a survey report of four rural districts.* Centre for African Family Studies, Nairobi.

35 Kiruhi M and Simalane ON (1993) *Communication of Information on Sexuality and Sex Behavior with Young People: a case study of patterns of communications in sex with youths in Nyeri District.* Centre for African Family Studies, Nairobi.

36 Kiiti N, Dortzbach D, Guturo F and Wangai A (1995) *AIDS Prevention and Kenya's Churched Youth: an assessment of knowledge, attitudes and sexual practices.* Presented at the Third USAID HIV/AIDS Prevention Conference, Washington DC, August 21–24.

Chapter 6

Understanding HIV/AIDS Numbers

It has often been said that if you knew what sausages are made of, you wouldn't eat them. Similarly, if you knew how most HIV/AIDS numbers are generally "cooked," you would surely use them with extreme caution! Chapter 4 described AIDS and all the evidence supporting HIV as the cause of AIDS. This chapter describes how public health epidemiologists try to measure and monitor the patterns (distribution) and prevalence (numbers and/or rates) of HIV-infected persons and AIDS cases and deaths (HIV/AIDS). In Chapter 4, it was made very clear that reported AIDS cases in most developing countries are totally unreliable and thus unusable as any meaningful measure of how many AIDS cases have occurred or may be occurring. In most developed countries, reported AIDS cases are reasonably accurate for monitoring the distribution and prevalence of AIDS in the population after adjustments for incomplete and delayed reporting. The numbers of HIV-infected persons and/or AIDS cases have been estimated using what are considered the more reliable datasets. In developed countries, this entails the use of reported AIDS cases for estimating HIV incidence and prevalence. In contrast, developing countries use findings from HIV serosurveys to estimate past and current AIDS cases and deaths. The last section of this chapter will focus on methods and models for the projection of HIV/AIDS numbers and an appendix to this chapter describes how EPIMODEL, a simple computer model, is used for estimation and short-term (less than 5 years) projection of AIDS cases and deaths. The topics and questions addressed in this chapter include:

- What is public health surveillance; is surveillance of HIV infections and AIDS cases (HIV/AIDS) different from surveillance of other infectious agents and diseases?
- What HIV/AIDS numbers are needed for HIV/AIDS programs and why are they needed?
- What methods and assumptions are used to estimate HIV/AIDS numbers; how accurate are these methods and assumptions?
- The uses and limitations of EPIMODEL, a simple computer program developed to estimate annual AIDS cases and deaths based on estimates of HIV prevalence.

Only with a more complete and better understanding of all the different HIV/AIDS numbers and how they are determined can we begin to review and evaluate the relative accuracy of HIV/AIDS estimates and projections and to place these numbers in proper perspective.

Public Health Surveillance of HIV/AIDS

There are many definitions of public health surveillance, but the one I use is:

> Public health surveillance is the routine collection, analysis, and dissemination of all data relevant to the prevention or control of a public health problem.

The general methods used for public health surveillance of HIV/AIDS are, in general, no different from those used for other diseases and infections. However, the methods used have to be adapted to the unique epidemiology, wide variation in prevalence levels, and the very long incubation period from HIV infection to the development of AIDS. In addition, the severity of AIDS and the extreme social and personal implications of identifying HIV-infected persons make surveillance of HIV/AIDS much more difficult and make issues such as anonymity and confidentiality of paramount importance. The need for confidentiality of personal data is universally accepted. However, anonymity in the public health management of any infectious or communicable disease has not been readily accepted by public health epidemiologists, especially in developing countries. It is important to recognize that public health surveillance of HIV infections and AIDS cases does **not** mean a program for finding and identifying individuals with these conditions, i.e., it is **not** a method for case finding. Public health surveillance is designed to systematically monitor the general pattern(s), prevalence, and trends of HIV/AIDS in populations where it is or may be occurring.

Public health surveillance of infectious diseases has traditionally relied primarily on a passive system of disease reporting. Most countries have established by law or regulation a list of diseases that are required to be reported by the medical community. However, it is common knowledge that most reportable diseases are not well reported. The accuracy and completeness of communicable disease reporting may vary from a few percent for most reportable diseases to over 90 percent for some diseases in developed countries. Much lower levels of reporting are generally found in developing countries.

I was responsible from 1987 to 1992 for receiving and tabulating national reports of AIDS cases submitted to WHO in Geneva and I know the general validity of reported AIDS case data to WHO. Reported AIDS cases from most developing countries are grossly underdiagnosed and those cases that may come to medical attention are also grossly under-reported. I consider reported AIDS case data from most developing countries to be one of the *most accurate tabulations* of the *most inaccurate and incomplete data* collected and distributed by WHO! However, I always tried to spend at least 5 minutes a month reviewing the officially reported AIDS cases and that was usually 5 minutes wasted each month. Because AIDS case ascertainment and reporting are so poor in developing countries, especially in sub-Saharan Africa (SSA), other methods and data that rely primarily on HIV seroprevalence surveys or HIV sentinel surveillance sampling must be used to estimate AIDS cases and deaths. By contrast, in most developed countries, AIDS case reporting, although not complete, is generally fairly good: up to 80 percent or more of diagnosed AIDS cases are reported. In addition, many developed countries carry out special studies to estimate the percent of under-reporting and late or delayed reporting. Although public health epidemiologists are well aware of the limitations of reported disease data, especially from developing countries, this knowledge has not been effectively communicated to the public and policy makers. There is a need to inform the public and policy makers about the virtual uselessness of reported disease and death data from most developing countries.

HIV/AIDS Numbers

As of late-2006, there continues to be tremendous misunderstanding by the public, policy makers, news reporters and even most HIV/AIDS program workers about HIV/AIDS numbers. Part of this misunderstanding is the confusion of HIV infection with AIDS that was described in the previous chapters: additional misunderstanding relates to not knowing the difference between incidence and prevalence numbers and the different rates that can be calculated for HIV infections, AIDS cases and deaths. The epidemiology of a "classical" infectious disease such as measles is not difficult to understand because the difference between infection and disease is minimal. However, for an infectious disease such as tuberculosis (TB), where primary infection with the tubercle bacillus is often undetected and the development of overt clinical pulmonary tuberculosis may not occur for many decades, if at all, epidemiologists must measure TB incident infections and incidence rates separately from TB disease cases and case rates. Similarly, HIV infections and infection rates have to be kept separate from AIDS case and death numbers and rates. The following sections will describe in detail all of the different HIV/AIDS numbers and rates used by public health programs and how they are estimated and projected. The confusion between HIV incidence and HIV prevalence continues to obscure measurements of the status of HIV epidemics because of the very long interval from HIV infection to the development of AIDS (median period estimated to be 7 to 8 years). As a result, HIV prevalence will not begin to decrease until almost a decade after HIV incidence peaks and begins to decline!

Epidemiology and Rates

Epidemiologists have the unique responsibility of counting cases of a disease or a condition in populations. Case counts are the core component of disease surveillance and are of paramount importance in any investigation of an old or new disease. However, case counts must be placed in proper perspective by using rates to quantify the risk of a specific disease in a specific population. One of the most important epidemiologic methods or tools is the calculation and use of rates in order to compare diseases or conditions in different populations. Although the concept of rates is simple, consistent and appropriate use of rates is what separates epidemiologists from nonepidemiologists. We will see that failure to define the disease or condition (the *numerator*) clearly, as well as failure to define the population at specific risk of the disease or condition in question (the *denominator*), has and continues to confuse the public and policy makers about most HIV/AIDS numbers and rates. The following table lists and defines all HIV/AIDS numbers and rates used by public health programs and describes how each of these numbers and rates are measured or estimated. In developed countries, the annual number of reported AIDS cases, after adjustments for incomplete and delayed reporting, is accepted as the total number of AIDS cases that developed during the year. However, in most developing countries, estimated HIV prevalence is used instead as the primary input parameter to a simple model (EPIMODEL or similar model) to estimate by back-calculating AIDS cases and deaths.

Table 6.1 HIV/AIDS numbers and measurements

HIV/AIDS Number	*Definition*	*Method(s) for Measurement or Estimation*
HIV prevalence	Number or rate of persons in the 15–49 year old population alive with an HIV infection at a specified time period – usually at the beginning or end of a year	(1) Estimated by a back-calculation method based on annual reported AIDS cases or (2) extrapolated from HIV serosurvey data. Estimated HIV prevalence is the major **input** parameter of EPIMODEL.
Annual HIV incidence	Number or rate of new HIV infections in the 15–49 year old population during a specific year	Difficult to measure directly. Usually calculated by a model such as EPIMODEL where it is a primary **output** parameter
Cumulative HIV incidence	Cumulative number of HIV infections in the 15–49 year old population	The total of annual incidence – calculated by EPIMODEL – an **output** parameter
Annual AIDS incidence	Number or rate of new AIDS cases in the 15–49 year old population during a specific year	Developed countries use annual reported AIDS cases after adjustments for incomplete reporting; developing countries use estimated HIV prevalence in a model such as EPIMODEL to calculate annual AIDS cases
AIDS prevalence	Number or rate of persons in the 15–49 year old population alive with severe immune deficiency due to HIV at the beginning or end of a year	Estimated by calculating the estimated annual incidence of AIDS cases and the average survival period from onset of AIDS to death – calculated by EPIMODEL – an **output** parameter
Cumulative AIDS incidence	Cumulative number of AIDS cases that have developed in the 15–49 year old population	The total of annual AIDS incidence – calculated by EPIMODEL – an **output** parameter
Annual AIDS deaths	Number of AIDS deaths in the 15–49 year old population during a specific year	Developed countries can use reported annual AIDS deaths after adjustments for incomplete reporting. In developing countries calculated by EPIMODEL – an **output** parameter
Cumulative AIDS deaths	Cumulative number of AIDS deaths in the 15–49 year old population	The total of annual AIDS deaths – calculated by EPIMODEL – an **output** parameter

The basic HIV/AIDS information needed by public health include the following items.

Incidence and Prevalence of HIV Infections

How many new HIV infections are occurring and what is the annual rate of increase or decrease of these new infections? In epidemiologic terms, new infections constitute *HIV incidence*, which is usually expressed or measured on an annual or 12-month basis. Annual incidence data provide valuable information on whether HIV infections are increasing or decreasing. However, direct measurement of new infections in any population is generally not possible and HIV incidence is usually estimated by using a spreadsheet or computer model.

How many persons are currently infected and living with HIV? In epidemiologic terms this value is defined as *HIV prevalence*. This information is essential to public health programs and public health planning because it provides data about the severity or extent of the HIV epidemic in a specific population. HIV prevalence (the total number of persons living with HIV infection) is the total number of HIV infections (i.e., cumulative incidence) minus the total number of AIDS deaths. HIV prevalence is usually calculated at the end of a year from estimates of:

1 HIV prevalence at the beginning of the year – i.e., the number of persons living with HIV at the beginning of the year
2 plus the number of new HIV infections during the year and
3 minus the number of AIDS deaths during the year (*see* Figure 6.1).

The methods and problems related to estimating HIV prevalence will be described in detail later in this chapter.

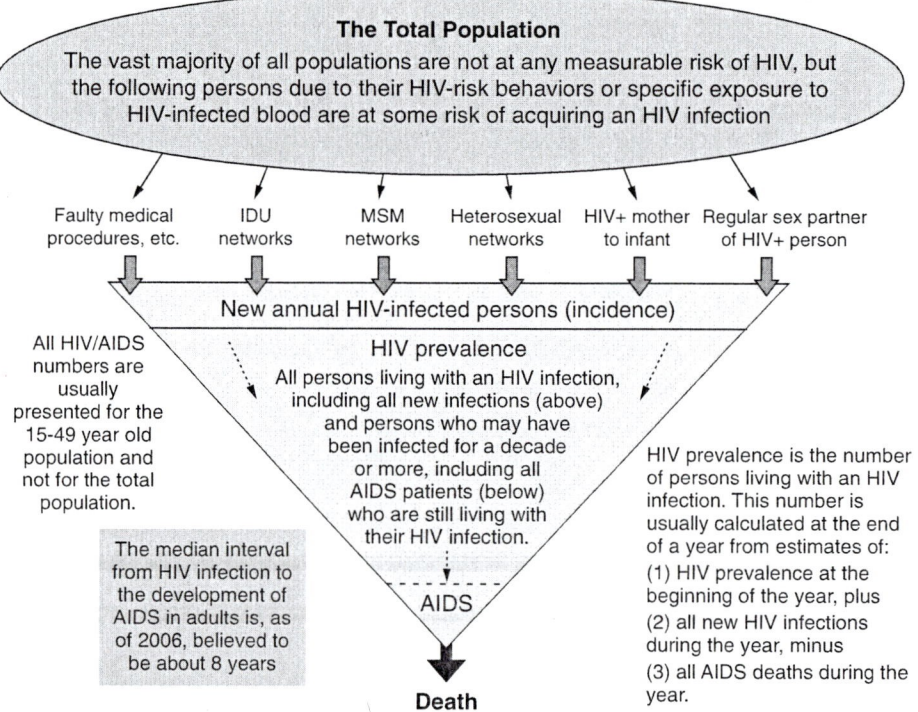

Figure 6.1 HIV transmission and natural history.

A conclusion drawn by some public health workers that the annual number of reported or detected HIV infections represents the annual HIV incidence is misleading and inaccurate. Annual HIV screening or testing of different population groups identifies HIV-infected persons, but most of these *newly detected* infections are not *newly infected* persons. Annual sampling of different population groups identifies prevalent HIV infections in these groups and not annual HIV incidence. The number of HIV infections *detected* annually depends on the total number of persons tested. As shown in Figure 6.1, there are six major separate modes or routes of HIV transmission and the annual number of new HIV infections in any population will depend on the patterns and prevalence of HIV risk behaviors and on HIV incidence for each of the risk behavior groups.

The prevalence of AIDS (number of persons living with AIDS) in any population is a dynamic and constantly changing number because this value depends on how many of the total HIV-infected persons have had their immune system sufficiently damaged so that they can be classified as an AIDS case and how many have died. In developing countries, most AIDS cases in the absence of anti-HIV treatment will die within a few months after developing "full blown" AIDS. In Figure 6.1, HIV-infected persons are exiting the pool of infected persons by dying shortly after developing AIDS. How many AIDS deaths may have occurred during the past years and how many AIDS cases and deaths can be expected this year and in future years? These numbers are estimated and projected via the use of models since death reporting in most developing countries is grossly inaccurate and incomplete.

The continuing confusion between *annual HIV incidence* (new infections during a year) and *HIV prevalence* (the total number of persons living with an HIV infection at the end of a calendar year) by the news media and many health professionals as well as the general public was highlighted by the uproar created by the release in 2005 of the official 2004 HIV prevalence estimate for India. The Minister of Health was misquoted or misinterpreted as saying that there were only 28 000 "additional" HIV infections in 2004 compared with more than 500 000 "additional" HIV infections included in the 2003 prevalence estimate. What he actually said was: "In comparison to the 2003 estimates, there has been an additional 28 000 infections in 2004 as compared to 52 lakh[*] [520 000] additional infections in 2003." What he meant was that in 2004 there had not been any significant change in the total number of persons living with an HIV infection (i.e., HIV prevalence) from the year 2003. He did not mean that that there were only 28 000 new HIV infections in 2004. The annual number of new HIV infections cannot be directly measured, but can be estimated using a model such as EPIMODEL. *If* HIV prevalence in India at the end of 2003 or 2004 was about 5 million and if significant HIV transmission started in India in the mid-to-late 1980s, then according to EPIMODEL calculations, there had to be close to 500 000 annual AIDS deaths in India in both 2003 and 2004. Therefore, in order to keep the total number of persons living with an HIV infection (HIV prevalence) level at 5 million, this required an annual HIV incidence of about 500 000. Many NGOs and some AIDS "experts" in India refused to believe that there were only 28 000 new HIV infections in India in 2004 because they were seeing a marked increase in the numbers of HIV-infected persons seeking treatment. However, although they were correct that there had to be more than 28 000 newly infected persons in 2004, they need

---

[*] One lakh is 100 000.

to realize that most HIV-infected persons who are now seeking treatment were infected many years to a decade or more ago. Very few, if any, of the probable hundreds of thousands of persons who acquired an HIV infection in 2004 are even aware that they have been infected and almost all of the persons infected in 2004 have not yet developed severe immune deficiency. UNAIDS chief Peter Piot said at the end of 2005 that: "the Health Ministry's report that new infections dropped from 520 000 in 2003 to 28 000 in 2004 was impossible." Yes, this was indeed impossible, but Peter Piot should know that the difference between annual HIV prevalence estimates cannot be considered to be the annual incidence of new HIV infections!

The dynamics of annual HIV incidence, prevalence, and AIDS deaths might be better understood by comparing these numbers with the dynamics of a water reservoir. The volume of water in the reservoir at the end of a year is equivalent to HIV prevalence (number of persons living with HIV at the end of a year), the annual flow of water into the reservoir is equivalent to the annual incidence of newly infected persons, and the annual outflow of water from the reservoir is equivalent to annual AIDS deaths. Thus, if the volume of water in the reservoir is about the same at the end of 2004 (5 million gallons) as it was at the end of 2003 (about 5 million gallons), this means that if the annual outflow from the reservoir in 2004 was about 500 000 gallons, then the annual water inflow to the reservoir in 2004 had to be about 500 000 gallons in order to keep the total volume of water at about 5 million gallons.

At the start of public health surveillance for HIV/AIDS in the early to mid-1980s, no distinction was made between prevalent and cumulative numbers of HIV infection and/or AIDS cases. However, with time and the progression of HIV infection to AIDS and death, the constant widening difference between the prevalent number of HIV infections and the cumulative number became very obvious. By mid-to-late 1990s, cumulative numbers of HIV infection and/or AIDS cases were not commonly used except to put HIV/AIDS epidemics into historical perspective. Public health programs now almost exclusively use prevalent and incident numbers. However, in the last couple of years, some AIDS program advocates are beginning to use cumulative numbers again to highlight the fact that about half of the cumulative number of HIV-infected persons have died: the estimated cumulative number of HIV infections is 70–80 million; and 30–40 million AIDS deaths have been estimated during the last three decades.

As of late-2006, confusion is still also present about the basic population rate of HIV infection used by virtually all HIV/AIDS programs. Since HIV is primarily a sexually transmitted infection, HIV prevalence is most frequently presented for those aged 15–49 – the most sexually active age group – and not for the total population. HIV prevalence can be a number or rate of persons living with an HIV infection. Thus, if there are 2000 HIV infections in a population of 10 000 15–49 year olds, the prevalence of HIV in this 15–49 year old population is 2000 or 20 percent (2000 divided by 10 000). If there are 500 HIV infections in persons outside of the 15–49 year old age group and there are 15 000 persons in these other age groups, the HIV prevalence for the total population would be 2500 or 10 percent (2500 divided by 25 000). This latter HIV prevalence rate is rarely presented but when it is, this may be confusing to the public and policy makers who usually see the prevalence rate for this 15–49 year old population as 20 percent. Similarly, annual HIV incidence or incidence rates are usually presented only for the 15–49 year old population. When presenting data for pediatric AIDS or for maternal AIDS orphans, the age group may be 1–5, or 1–15, or 1–18 years.

This general misunderstanding was highlighted in early 2005 when the results of the 2004 Botswana AIDS Impact Survey (BAIS) were released. The headlines in the news media read: "**Botswana HIV rate at 17, not 40 percent**...the 2004 BAIS has documented the scale of the AIDS pandemic in the country. Contrary to widespread belief and reference, the HIV prevalence rate in Botswana is not close to 40 percent, but now stands at 17.3 percent..." However, these headlines actually obscured the most important finding of the 2004 BAIS. As described above, WHO and UNAIDS have been consistently estimating HIV prevalence for the population aged 15–49 and not for the total national population. In Botswana, the 2003 national HIV prevalence estimate for 15–49 year olds (derived primarily from ANC data) was 330 000 (37.3 percent). The 2004 BAIS presented a national HIV prevalence estimate (all HIV infections [287 000] estimated divided by the total population of 1.7 million = 17.1 percent). What was almost totally ignored was the new estimated HIV prevalence of 25.3 percent for those aged 15–49 (who numbered close to 900 000). Thus, HIV infections in this age group were estimated by the BAIS to be about 225 000 while the UNAIDS estimate of 37.3 percent gave a total of 330 000, an overestimate of almost 50 percent! This general problem of HIV overestimation in the 15–49 year old population will be reviewed in detail in the next chapter.

Source of HIV/AIDS Numbers

The accuracy of HIV/AIDS numbers can vary markedly depending on the source of the data and the expertise of those reporting or estimating these numbers. Public health workers collect reports of HIV infections and AIDS cases, but usually these reported numbers are "adjusted" to take account of delays and incompleteness inherent in the reporting system. As described in the section on public health surveillance, the completeness and reliability of *reported numbers* of HIV infections and or AIDS cases varies markedly from country to country and even within any country, there may be marked temporal variations in the accuracy of these reports. *Official numbers* of HIV/AIDS may be either reported cases or in some instances estimated cases (i.e., reported cases after "adjustment" may then become the official numbers). *Estimated numbers* may be derived by a government appointed expert group or can be the estimate of an individual or an agency. Estimated numbers should be evaluated with care since many AIDS organizations and agencies tend to uncritically accept high estimates to strengthen their advocacy efforts. All estimates depend on the available data, the specific assumptions used, and the value(s) used for these assumptions. Thus, the result can represent a reliable working estimate of the actual HIV/AIDS numbers or may represent gross overestimation or underestimation of these numbers. *The actual or real numbers* represent the "Holy Grail" for public health epidemiologists. The best approximation of the actual or real numbers can be derived via *an objective process* that use the *best data available*, reasonable or *defendable assumptions*, and methods that will be described in the last section of this chapter.

Estimation and Projection of HIV/AIDS Numbers

The difference between estimation and projection needs to be clarified. Some statisticians believe that projections are estimates but I use estimation for measuring past and current numbers and projection or forecasting for estimating future numbers and trends. The methods for HIV/AIDS estimation or projection are limited and remain more of an art than a science since there are still some vital aspects of the natural history of HIV and of the different patterns and prevalence of HIV risk behaviors that remain unclear and must be assumed and/or approximated. For example, since the late 1990s, the accepted median interval from HIV infection to development of AIDS has been reduced from 10 to about 8 years: this decreased interval has resulted in an increase of 10 to 20 percent in modeled cumulative HIV infections and close to a 50 percent difference in modeled cumulative AIDS deaths in SSA during the 1990s. It is still possible that the median interval for progression from infection to AIDS may be even shorter! This problem will be described and presented in detail in the last section of this chapter and in an appendix that will describe how EPIMODEL calculates past, present, and future AIDS cases and deaths.

In general, HIV prevalence in developing countries is estimated or extrapolated from available HIV seroprevalence data: most other HIV/AIDS numbers, including projections or forecasts are derived from modeling or development of scenarios. Methods used by epidemiologists to estimate HIV/AIDS numbers differ greatly between developed countries and developing countries because the reliability of the available HIV/AIDS data is so different. In developed countries, reported AIDS case data are considered sufficiently reliable (especially after "adjustments" for incomplete and delayed reporting) so that AIDS case data can be used in "back-calculation" models to estimate HIV incidence and prevalence needed to generate the annual AIDS cases that have been reported. Thus, in developed countries the accuracy of HIV/AIDS estimates depends primarily on the accuracy of reported AIDS cases. The back-calculation model also requires some estimate of what year or time period significant HIV infections first began to occur, as well as use of annual progression rates from HIV infection to development of AIDS. If a relatively short median interval of 6–7 years is used compared with a much longer median interval of about 9–10 years, the result will be higher estimates for HIV incidence in order to compensate for the higher numbers of AIDS deaths during the same time period.

In most developing countries the reliability of reported AIDS cases is so poor that these data cannot be used to estimate HIV incidence, prevalence and annual AIDS cases and deaths. During the late 1980s, my unit* within GPA/WHO developed guidelines for HIV sentinel surveillance (HSS). Using these guidelines, most developing countries began developing a system of sentinel sites to monitor HIV prevalence trends in selected populations considered at high or low risk of HIV infection. Although HSS was not designed to collect HIV data that could be used to estimate national prevalence, most AIDS programs used whatever HIV serosurvey data they could access, including HSS data. In developing countries, national prevalence estimates are made by using available HIV serosurvey

---

* Surveillance, Forecasting, and Impact Assessment (SFI) unit.

data. All estimates or projections of AIDS cases and deaths are made by using a model – EPIMODEL or similar models.

Methods for HIV/AIDS Estimation

WHO and UNAIDS have, since the early 1990s, prepared periodic reports of HIV prevalence estimates in the 15–49 year old population[*] by region and for individual countries. As already noted, estimation of HIV infections and/or AIDS cases can be considered more of an art than a science. With the known vagaries inherent in HIV/AIDS data and the limitations of the data, methods, and assumptions used, estimation and projection of HIV/AIDS numbers cannot be precise. Even though HIV prevalence estimates are not precise, the available data can be used to reliably group HIV prevalence rates by orders of magnitude into low, moderate, high, or very high levels.[†] The available data can also be used to monitor prevalence trends in sentinel populations. I will first describe how HIV risk behaviors in any population can be simply grouped into low, moderate, and high and how the number of HIV-infected persons (HIV prevalence) can be calculated based on available HIV serosurvey data.

Estimating Populations at Risk of HIV

For infections such as a feared pandemic human influenza virus that can be transmitted easily from person to person via the respiratory route, virtually everyone who has any human contact will be at high to moderate risk of infection. HIV infection requires the exchange of infected blood or body fluids such as semen and therefore the risk of acquiring or transmitting an HIV infection varies significantly in any population from high risk to very low or no risk. All populations can be arbitrarily divided into those who:

1 have very low to no risk
2 have a moderate risk and
3 have a high risk for HIV infection.

To illustrate, let us first ignore any potential HIV transmission in healthcare settings and focus on the risk of HIV in the 15–49 year old population from all other routes of HIV transmission in a hypothetical country X. All 15–49 year olds in country X who do not have risk behaviors such as having unprotected sex with multiple sex partners or sharing drug injecting equipment with other drug users can be considered to be at low or no risk of acquiring an HIV infection. This group usually comprises the vast majority of all "general adult populations" throughout the world and in country X this group is estimated to be about 70 percent of the 15–49 year old population. Persons whose regular sex partner may have high HIV risk behaviors can be considered to be at moderate risk of acquiring an HIV

---

[*] When I arrived at WHO in early 1987, this age group was called the *sexually active* age group. One of my greatest accomplishments at GPA was to change the name to the *most sexually active* age group since I was able to assure everyone that I personally could attest to the fact that there is sex after the age of 50!

[†] *Low* (< 1 HIV infection per 1000 of the 15–49 year old population, i.e., < 0.1 percent); *moderate* (> 1 per 1000, but < 1 percent); *high* (> 1 percent, but < 10 percent); and *very high* (> 10 percent).

infection and they are estimated to be about 15 percent of the adult population of country X and finally persons with high HIV risk behaviors constitute about 15 percent of all adolescents and young to middle aged adults in country X.

Before we start to estimate the number of HIV-infected persons in country X, we need to be aware that the risk of HIV infection in those persons considered at high risk because of their HIV risk behaviors is not uniform or equal in this "group." Again, we can sub-divide this group considered at high risk into three arbitrary sub-groups: those at the highest risk; those at moderate risk; and those at the lowest risk. We need to be acutely aware of this arbitrary sub-grouping because this will be a very important factor that can and has contributed to overestimation of HIV prevalence. In addition, there has also been gross over-estimation of the total numbers of MSM and IDU. Even without any consideration of specific sexual risk behaviors and/or the pattern of and frequency of needle sharing, estimation of the total numbers of sexually active MSM or needle sharing IDU in any specific population (national, provincial, city, etc.) is difficult and some of these estimates can be different by several folds depending on whether the estimate is made by AIDS program advocates or by more conservative government agencies.

Major Problems in Estimating HIV Prevalence

In a small population it may be physically possible to test everyone regardless of whether they have any HIV risk behaviors or not, but in large populations it is simply not feasible. Thus, public health epidemiologists use whatever HIV sero-survey data may be available and have to make assumptions as to how representative of the specific population the collected serosurveys may be. For example it has been estimated that there are a total of 100 000 IDU in country X, and sero-surveys of IDU in country X's drug abuse clinics consistently find half or 50 percent HIV positive. However, these findings probably are representative of IDU with the highest risk patterns and prevalence of needle sharing with other IDU. Many AIDS "experts" will simply extrapolate such HIV serosurvey results to the total estimated IDU population and thereby grossly overestimate the number of HIV-infected IDU. If the highest risk IDU group represented by those in the drug abuse clinics comprise only a quarter (25 percent) of the total IDU population and HIV prevalence is 10 percent in the remaining 75 percent of IDU in country X, then the number of HIV-infected IDU is 50 percent of 25 000 (12 500) plus 10 percent of 75 000 (7500) for a total of 20 000. However, if the 50 percent infection rate is applied to the total IDU population of 100 000, the estimated number of HIV-infected IDU in country X is inflated to 50 000 or more than double the actual number of 20 000! This has been the most prevalent error in the development of HIV prevalence – the application of high HIV prevalence rates found in persons with the highest HIV risk behaviors to the total population of persons with lower levels of risk behaviors.

A similar problem in overestimating HIV prevalence in most sub-Saharan African (SSA) populations has been the insufficient attention paid to the urban/rural HIV prevalence differential. There is known to be a marked urban to rural HIV prevalence differential and thus there were attempts to measure HIV prevalence in rural populations. However, HIV prevalence rates found in peri-urban ANC attendees were frequently used as representative of all rural ANC attendee women. HIV prevalence in peri-urban ANC populations is generally much higher compared with truly rural ANC populations and this has been the major cause of gross overestimation of most national HIV prevalence estimates in SSA.

Specific Methods That Have Been Used for Estimating HIV Prevalence

A simple "forced" Delphi or bracketing method was used during the mid- to late-1980s to develop a crude working estimate of the possible number of HIV-infected persons in a specific population. This method asked persons who had the most up-to-date information from HIV surveys and reported AIDS cases in a specific population to guess both the highest and lowest possible number of HIV infections that could be supported with the limited data. I refer to this method as a forced Delphi because I used this method to force participants at a meeting convened by GPA/WHO in Strbske Pleso, Slovakia in 1988 to develop working HIV prevalence estimates. For those national AIDS experts who were hesitant to estimate HIV prevalence, I would start them off with the lowest possible number as more than one and the highest possible number as less than one million. I would then gradually get them to increase the lowest number and decrease the highest number until they were "satisfied" with the estimated range. I then recommended that they take the midpoint of this range to use as an initial working estimate to be revised and refined as more data became available to justify any change. This was essentially the method used to derive the Coolfont prevalence estimate in the USA in 1986. Estimates made in the late 1980s with this crude method were in general gross overestimates when compared with estimates made a decade later when more data were available.

Prior to the advent of effective drug therapy that delays or prevents the relentless progression from HIV infection to development of AIDS, most developed countries considered reported AIDS cases to be sufficiently reliable for estimating HIV prevalence by using a *back-calculation method*. The back-calculation method use annual progression rates from HIV infection to AIDS and reported annual AIDS cases (usually after adjustments for incomplete and delayed reports) to calculate how many annual HIV infections would have been needed to generate the annual number of AIDS cases. This method appears to be relatively reliable, but requires fairly complete reporting of AIDS cases.

A *"ratio" method* that used an estimated ratio of prevalent HIV infections to prevalent AIDS cases was used in the late 1980s and early 1990s to estimate HIV prevalence. Like the back-calculation method, the ratio method required reliable estimates of AIDS cases, which were generally not available. Further, most users of the ratio method did not realize that in all HIV epidemics the ratio of prevalent HIV infections to prevalent AIDS cases changes rapidly over time. This ratio falls from many thousands to one during the first few years of an epidemic, to less than ten to one after the first decade. This decline occurs whether HIV incidence is increasing or decreasing because in the absence of effective treatment, virtually all HIV-infected persons progress to AIDS. Thus, at the start of any HIV epidemic there are virtually no AIDS cases in the first few years so that the HIV to AIDS ratio is almost all HIV and no or few AIDS cases. As the HIV epidemic continues, almost all HIV infections will progress to AIDS and the HIV to AIDS ratio will gradually decrease. In a hypothetical situation where all new HIV transmission is stopped, the HIV to AIDS ratio will eventually decrease to almost 1:1 because virtually all HIV infections eventually progress to AIDS. Another major problem with using this simple ratio method was that this method was inappropriate for populations where epidemic HIV transmission had not occurred. This was because virtually all of the detected HIV infections or AIDS cases in such situations were imported from another country where there was some epidemic transmission, and thus, there was no sound epidemiologic basis to multiply the detected number of HIV/AIDS by a factor of 50 or 100, or whatever. This was the problem with the initial estimate of HIV prevalence in the Philippines where the minister of health multiplied the 50 detected HIV/AIDS cases by 1000 to derive an estimate of 50 000!

In the absence of either reliable AIDS estimates or data, epidemiologists have estimated HIV prevalence by *using the results of HIV serological surveys* and extrapolating from these data to the total 15–49 year old population. This has been and continues to be the primary method used in developing countries. Major problems with this method are the limited number of HIV seroprevalence studies that may be representative of specific populations or subgroups, and the wide variability in estimates of the size of important HIV risk behavior groups (RBG), such as female sex workers (FSW), injecting drug users (IDU), and patients seen in sexually transmitted disease (STD) clinics. Nevertheless, epidemiologists have derived reasonable working estimates of the prevalence, general distribution, and trends of HIV infection for many countries by an objective and detailed analysis of all HIV serosurvey data combined with demographic data on population sizes and distribution.

Estimation of HIV Prevalence by Using HIV Serological Data

As described earlier in this chapter, the strategy for HSS relied on routine and consistent collection of data from sentinel groups that may be considered representative of their group's risk for acquiring HIV infection. The basic purpose of HSS is to detect changes (i.e., trends) in HIV prevalence in the sentinel groups selected. If various sentinel groups can be monitored consistently over time at selected sites, the data collected should provide reliable infection trends in these groups. These data should be sufficient to design and direct prevention and control programs. The sentinel populations selected should, to the extent possible, include all major HIV risk behaviors known to be present in any given population and/or area. Virtually all HSS systems developed by national AIDS programs in Africa and Asia focused on *urban* sentinel sites where the *highest HIV prevalence* might be found. HSS was not designed to make national prevalence estimates, but when countries needed HIV data to make prevalence estimates, HSS data were routinely used because they were available.

HIV/AIDS programs have routinely used HSS data to estimate HIV prevalence in the major sentinel groups. HIV prevalence in the total 15–49 year population has been calculated according to the following general formulas:

1 number of HIV infections in each of the major high risk groups = estimated HIV seroprevalence rate (from HSS data) multiplied by the estimated members in the high risk group (estimated for a specific population or a province) and
2 number of HIV infections in the "general" 15–49 year population = estimated HIV seroprevalence rate in ANC attendees in the province (from HSS data)

multiplied by the estimated number of 15–49 year olds in the province (from census estimates).

Major sources of potential error when using this general method include:

1 The poor quality of the data and the possibility that the usual grab samples collected for most HSS systems are not representative of the target population can result in large estimation errors. However, no systematic attempts to quantify the probable range of error(s) related to these data quality issues were carried out until 2001 when there were some studies that compared prevalence estimates derived using HSS data with prevalence estimates from population-based serosurveys.

2 Errors in estimating the size of specific HIV RBG such as MSM, IDU and FSW can be quite large – up to several folds higher or lower. Estimates of IDU populations can vary by an order of magnitude between non-governmental organizations (NGO) or government units. In addition, the proportion of drug users who are IDU and who regularly share their injection equipment can vary markedly by time and place. This makes estimating the number of IDU who are truly at risk of an HIV infection very difficult. Similar difficulties are encountered in estimating MSM and FSW in a specific population or area.

3 The heterogeneity of HIV risk behaviors, even within any specific RBG, is well known, but frequently findings from sentinel HIV sites that capture persons from RBG with the highest or very high risk behaviors are then extrapolated to the total RBG. This obviously makes for higher HIV prevalence estimates.

4 A major assumption used in this method is that HIV prevalence found in ANC attendees can be used as a surrogate for HIV prevalence in the total 15–49 year population. This assumption, used in sub-Saharan Africa, is supported by limited community-based HIV serosurveys. However, this assumption has not been validated for populations outside of SSA.

5 The male to female (M/F) ratio of HIV infections has been measured or estimated by using a variety of methods and assumptions. In SSA, a slight excess of infected females to males (about 1.2:1) has been consistently found. In most other regions there has been a consistent and fairly large preponderance of infected males to females. This is so because the predominant HIV transmission outside SSA is related to MSM, IDU and commercial sex networks that result in a very large male preponderance. Many countries outside SSA do not factor in an M/F ratio in estimating their national HIV seroprevalence and this could result in a gross underestimation if ANC data are used alone without adjustment for the higher infection rate in males.

6 In heterosexual HIV epidemics in SSA, a marked urban to rural differential of up to ten-fold or more was noted in the early phase of HIV spread. This differential narrowed markedly with time and after 10 years or more had, in some countries, been reduced to less than 1- or 2-fold. A frequently used assumption in Asia is that changes in the urban to rural HIV prevalence differentials follow the same general course as that observed in SSA. It is quite possible (and indeed probable) that in Asia, heterosexual transmission may remain more localized in the highest RBG in urban centers and may penetrate or diffuse much more slowly (if at all) into most rural populations. However, in the absence of any substantive prevalence data collected from truly rural populations, the assumption that no significant urban to rural prevalence differential

exists in Asian populations, has resulted in very large and unsupported HIV prevalence estimates.

The methodology and assumptions used for estimation of national HIV prevalence in developing countries have been evolving, as HIV epidemiology is better understood, the quality of HIV surveillance data improves, and the methods and models for estimation improve. As a result, UNAIDS/WHO has cautioned that recent estimates of national HIV prevalence should not be directly compared with previous or possibly future estimates. UNAIDS has, as of the new millennium, developed more detailed guidelines and a newer model for estimation and projection of HIV/AIDS – the **Estimation and Projection Package (EPP)**. This new package is used to estimate and project adult HIV prevalence from surveillance data in countries with "generalized" epidemics, i.e. HIV epidemics primarily in SSA countries. The major inputs to EPP are data collected from ANC attendees at urban and rural sites. EPP uses a simple epidemic model (similar to EPIMODEL) to fit a curve from data that are considered representative of urban or rural populations. EPP appears to be easy to use, but it cannot assure that the input data derived from ANC samples are truly representative of the population modeled. In the next chapter we will see that use of EPP in many SSA countries did not prevent overestimation of HIV prevalence by up to 100 to 200 percent!

The majority of African populations are rural as noted earlier. Thus, it was essential that the urban/rural differential be taken into consideration when a national HIV prevalence estimate was made. The urban/rural HIV prevalence differential began to narrow in recent years, but still most countries in SSA continue to have urban rates from 1 to 3 fold higher than rural rates. Lack of attention to urban/rural HIV prevalence differentials has been the major problem contributing to the gross and systematic prevalence overestimation in most developing countries and will be reviewed in detail in the next chapter.

Demographic and Health Surveys (DHS) are nationally-representative household surveys with large sample sizes (usually between 5000 to 30 000 households). DHS surveys provide data for a wide range of monitoring and impact evaluation indicators in the areas of population, health, and nutrition. Typically, DHS surveys are conducted every 5 years, to allow comparisons over time. Many countries in SSA and the Caribbean have since the new millennium completed DHS that have included HIV testing (+). The DHS+ findings indicate that current prevalence estimates in many of these high HIV prevalence populations have been overestimated by an average of 50 percent. These overestimates are due primarily to the use of sentinel surveillance data heavily biased by urban sentinel sites. It was not until DHS that included HIV testing in some African countries, notably in Zambia in 2001/2002, that the extent of this overestimation was fully appreciated. UNAIDS was initially reluctant to accept the DHS+ data as more accurate than estimates based on HSS data, but since DHS samples are more representative of the total population than are HSS samples, the greater accuracy of the DHS data is now accepted. UNAIDS has not accepted the results of some population-based surveys because of the very high (up to 40 percent or more) refusal rates encountered in some of these surveys. In low HIV prevalence populations, participation bias of persons with high risk behaviors was found to significantly lower the estimated prevalence from these surveys. However, a study in Malawi in 2005[*] has shown that less than 10 percent of persons who think they may be infected with HIV are in fact infected. In a population with high HIV prevalence (5–10 percent or more of the 15–49 year old population infected), the refusal by persons who believe they may be infected to participate in a HIV survey may not significantly lower the survey estimate of prevalence. There are many reasons for refusal to participate in DHS type studies in SSA populations, but unless there are data to indicate that HIV prevalence in those who refuse to participate are significantly higher or lower than those who participate, the results of DHS+ surveys should be accepted as reasonably representative of HIV prevalence in the survey population.

Estimation of AIDS Cases and Deaths

Annual AIDS cases and deaths are estimated from:

1 estimated HIV prevalence or
2 reported AIDS cases

depending on which of these two datasets are considered to be more reliable. With the advent of effective anti-HIV treatment, modeling of annual AIDS deaths will have to take into account the percent of HIV-infected persons on such treatment. There was some confusion regarding the increased deaths in TB patients infected with HIV during the late 1980s and early 1990s. Many of these deaths were attributed to TB and some to AIDS. The Tenth Revision of the International Statistical Classification of Diseases and Related Health Problems (ICD-10) was approved by WHO in 1990 and has been available for implementation since 1993. According to ICD-10, deaths are attributed to the primary underlying cause: in persons infected with HIV whose immediate cause of death is TB, the death should be coded to AIDS on the basis that TB was the fatal "opportunistic" infection in a person with AIDS.

HIV/AIDS Projection (Forecasting)

Since recognition of AIDS in the early 1980s, the pandemic's future trends and ultimate dimensions have been shrouded in uncertainty. This uncertainty persists because of the difficulties in measuring the prevalence and incidence of HIV/AIDS in a given population with any substantial degree of precision. As a result, investigators have used many methods and models in attempts to understand the dynamics and interrelationships of the major determinants of HIV transmission, and to develop reliable estimates and projections of HIV and AIDS. However, the methods and models used need to be examined critically and understood before their outputs are accepted and used for public health programs or policy decisions.

There is an ancient Arabic saying – *those who predict the future, lie, even if they think they are telling the truth*! This saying succinctly sums up the great uncertainty in projecting the future, especially for a complex problem such as HIV transmission.

---

[*] Bignami-Van Assche S, Chao LW and Anglewicz P (2005) *The Validity of Self-reported HIV Infection Among the General Population in Rural Malawi.* Presented at the 2005 Meeting of the International Union for the Study of Population (IUSSP), 18–23 July, Tours, France.

Nevertheless, attempts to predict future trends and prevalence of HIV have been carried out with a very wide range of errors and uncertainty. From my perspective, the biggest problem that has and continues to confront most AIDS modelers is that in general they do not fully understand HIV transmission dynamics and they spend most of their efforts trying to fit mathematical curves to inaccurate and/or unrepresentative data and thereby develop models that can reproduce with precision a biased or flawed simulation of what they assume to be reality. With this brief introduction, the following is my critical review of the methods that have been used for HIV/AIDS projections or forecasts and for scenario building or development.

Delphi Method

The simplest and, in the opinion of most AIDS modelers, the least scientific method for predicting future HIV/AIDS numbers is the Delphi method. The Delphi method was developed in the 1950s by the RAND Corporation to make forecasts on relatively uncertain situations as well as to provide a means of quantifying such judgments. The Delphi method was originally systematized in the 1960s for use in developing business management policies and was first applied to the health field in the 1970s.* Essentially, the Delphi method obtains educated guesses from selected experts in a reiterative fashion, and then uses the average and range of the Delphi responses as projections. Major advantages of the Delphi method are speed and low cost. However, it is difficult to select truly knowledgeable experts (i.e., experienced quantitative epidemiologists who are familiar with the epidemiology of HIV and general demographics of a specific country or population) to develop reliable estimates or projections of the number of HIV infections. Furthermore, estimates and projections made by the Delphi method may have extremely wide ranges. This method should be used only for populations where no or scant HIV/AIDS data are available! During the late 1980s, the simplest and most understandable method for predicting or guessing the potential numbers of global HIV infections was to use the Delphi survey method. In 1989, GPA/WHO developed global HIV projections to the year 2000 using a Delphi survey and concluded: "The WHO Delphi projections should be considered the first of many attempts to develop planning estimates for the HIV/AIDS pandemic over the next decade. All of the WHO estimates and projections on HIV/AIDS presented need to be periodically reviewed and revised as additional data suggest that changes are warranted."†

HIV/AIDS Models

Mathematical models have been used to develop short and long-range projections of HIV prevalence. However, any mathematical projection model is only as reliable as the assumptions and values used for all of the input parameters. Such models should be used primarily for hypothesis testing – not for making estimates and projections of annual HIV incidence for a specific country or population. That was the

---

* I recall participating in a CDC Delphi survey sometimes in the 70s or early 80s to develop recommendations for the use of live measles vaccine in children who had received inactivated measles vaccine and who may have developed "atypical" measles.

† Chin J, Sato P, Mann JM(1990) Projections of HIV infections and AIDS cases to the year 2000. *Bulletin of the World Health Organization.* **68** (1): 1–11.

conclusion of an expert committee that reviewed the HIV/AIDS modeling situation in the UK in 1994. This committee concluded that the general uncertainty of many of the needed input parameters, such as the size of the risk groups as well as reliable data on their current sex partner exchange rates, made estimation and projection of HIV/AIDS incidence and prevalence in the UK extremely uncertain. As a result, they stated clearly that model outputs should not be used for specific program or policy development. However, many international "experts" and international agencies have ignored this sage advice and as a result, some unrealistic prevalence estimates and projections have been developed by modelers. Some of these estimates and projections will be reviewed in the next chapter.

The results produced by any model should not be used to make program or policy decisions unless those making such decisions agree with the assumptions used, the values used for the input parameters, and understand how the model works. I have classified HIV/AIDS models into three types that range from the simplest to the most complex. The first two types are what I consider to be empirical and extrapolation models, while the last type has been called explanatory or deterministic. In general, the simpler extrapolation models are designed for short-term projections; the more complex models for evaluating determinants of the HIV/AIDS pandemic and for hypothesis testing.

Type I models use reported AIDS case data to make short-term (less than 5 years, usually 2–3 years) projections of AIDS cases. Such short-term projections have been made by statistical extrapolation and regression techniques applied to the observed temporal curve of reported cases. These models assume that after adjustment for reporting delays (and in some models, further adjustments for incomplete reporting) trends of reported cases during the next few years will remain essentially similar to those observed in the most recent past. However, the curve of reported AIDS cases could represent several distinct and separate epidemics and many mathematical curves might fit the data equally well. Not only is there no way to choose the "best" among the various curves, but the fitted curves may lead to widely divergent projections, particularly if they are used to make projections for periods longer than 2–3 years. These simple extrapolation models are not based on biological or behavioral data and thus they are limited in usefulness. These models should be used only for short-term projections in populations where case reporting is relatively reliable and complete.

Type II models use data on estimated HIV infections as well as progression rates from infection to AIDS to calculate the number of past cases and to provide short-term (3–5 years) projections. These models are very sensitive to the available HIV/AIDS data and also to the incubation function. EPIMODEL uses these variables and is a Type II model developed for use in areas where AIDS case reporting is known to be largely incomplete and unreliable. A variation of this approach is the "back calculation" method that uses AIDS case reports with annual progression rates from infection to AIDS to estimate the annual number of HIV infections. This method requires accurate, complete, and timely reporting of AIDS cases. However, because very few persons develop AIDS within two to three years after acquiring their infection, this method – even in areas where AIDS case reporting is considered reliable – cannot be used to estimate HIV infections that occurred during the past two to three years.

Type III models are more complex and incorporate biologic and behavioral variables that describe the transmission and natural history of HIV infection to simulate the entire disease process from infection, progression to AIDS, and death. Many mathematically sophisticated Type III models have been developed to project the future course of HIV/AIDS epidemics in different areas and populations. These models require, in varying degrees, extensive datasets on nearly all of the demographic, biologic, and behavioral variables considered to be important in the epidemiology and natural history of HIV infection. The major problem with these models, besides their complexity, is that most of the precise, detailed datasets they require to make reliable projections are not available, even in those countries with the best data collection systems. In addition, the values or even the plausible range of values for many of the important biologic and behavioral variables involved in HIV transmission are still unclear and different modelers use markedly different values for these important variables. The most important or sensitive input parameters for all epidemic AIDS models are the infectivity of HIV per unprotected sexual contact, patterns of sex partner exchange and sex partner exchange rates in any specific population. The greatest value of such complex mathematical models may be to test hypotheses and to help in understanding the dynamic interrelationships between important biologic and behavioral variables rather than for estimation and projection of HIV/AIDS prevalence. The Interagency Work Group (IWG) model developed by a US government agency at an estimated cost close to 10 million dollars is the most complex Type III model. This model requires over 350 separate datasets, most of which have to be distributed by age groups, gender, and urban/rural residence.

SFI/GPA and the UN Population Division convened a group of modelers in NYC in 1989 in an attempt to compare the outputs of different Type III models. This exercise asked six AIDS modelers to project the HIV prevalence rate in a hypothetical population over the succeeding 25 years. A standard set of demographic and epidemiologic variables was given to the modelers. A major problem was that not all of the models were designed to use the standard set of input parameters provided: furthermore, data required by some models were not included in the standard set of variables. The projected HIV prevalence ranged from a low of 2.8 percent to a high of 39.5 percent for a 14-fold difference, and the projected size of the modeled population ranged from a low of 236 million to a high of 427 million for an almost 2-fold difference. With such wide differences in model outputs, policy makers and health planners need to be very cautious in using any long-range model projections. However, most modelers staunchly defend their models and "garbage in, garbage out" has been transformed by most AIDS modelers to "garbage in, Gospel out"!

It needs to be realized that it is totally inappropriate to use an epidemic model for populations that have no significant patterns and prevalence of HIV risk behaviors that are needed to start and sustain epidemic HIV transmission. In Chapter 5, I described what patterns and prevalence of HIV risk behaviors are needed for epidemic HIV transmission. I am convinced that the majority of heterosexual populations outside of SSA do not have the necessary high risk patterns of and frequency of sex partner exchanges to drive or sustain significant epidemic heterosexual HIV transmission.

Scenario/Modeling of HIV/AIDS

When I was responsible for surveillance, forecasting, and impact assessment of the AIDS pandemic at GPA/WHO during the late 1980s and early 1990s, I developed a simple scenario/modeling method for estimation and projection of HIV infections and AIDS cases. This scenario/modeling method can be used for a global region, individual countries, or for selected populations within countries to provide working estimates and short-term projections of HIV related morbidity and mortality for policy development and public health planning. A scenario is an outline of any series of events, real or imagined. HIV/AIDS models can be considered highly structured scenario building machines. HIV/AIDS scenarios can be made up or constructed with or without models to "fit," or at least be consistent with, the observed data and trends. The following is a summary of the general methods used to develop working estimates and projections of HIV infections and AIDS cases and deaths for a specific country or population.

1 Assemble and analyze all available HIV seroprevalence data to estimate the most recent pattern(s), prevalence, and trends of HIV infection. The HIV/AIDS database compiled by the Center for International Research, US Bureau of the Census (USBOC) was and continues to be a valuable data source, but their computerized data should be supplemented with additional and unpublished national HIV data, when and if available.
2 Based on these data and other epidemiologic observations, different HIV patterns and prevalence levels (i.e., HIV scenarios) can be constructed for a decade or longer to "fit" the available data. Optimistic or "best-case" scenarios as well as pessimistic "worst-case" scenarios can be constructed for public health planning.
3 EPIMODEL, a Type II model, or any similar model can be used to derive annual incident, prevalent, and cumulative estimates and projections of AIDS cases, deaths, maternal AIDS orphans, and HIV-related TB cases based on the general HIV scenarios constructed.

In developing methods for the estimation and projection of HIV infections and AIDS cases and deaths in SSA, I realized, as I pointed out in the preceding chapters, that reported AIDS case data from developing countries (especially SSA) are so grossly underdiagnosed and under-reported that official case data are virtually useless. Thus I had to develop alternative methods for surveillance and estimation of HIV infections and AIDS cases and deaths. The methodology for HIV surveillance developed by my Surveillance, Forecasting, and Impact Assessment (SFI) unit focused on monitoring HIV prevalence trends in well-defined population groups. Earlier in this chapter, I described the methods for estimating HIV prevalence and even though the accuracy of HIV prevalence estimates can be questioned, these estimates are still far more reliable than most reported AIDS case data. Since I recognized that reported AIDS case data in most SSA countries may only represent a very small percent (usually less than 5 percent) of cases and deaths that occurred, I had to develop another method to estimate AIDS and AIDS deaths in SSA and that is why EPIMODEL was developed. EPIMODEL or similar models are still used widely to estimate annual AIDS cases and deaths for populations where AIDS case detection and reporting are largely incomplete and unreliable.

Estimation of Pediatric AIDS and Maternal AIDS Orphans

In developing countries, reliable data on pediatric AIDS cases and maternal AIDS orphans are not available for estimating and projecting the current and future numbers of these children. Two methods which do not rely on reported case data are available for estimating the number of infected and uninfected children born to HIV-infected women. The simplest method first estimates the percent of females of child-bearing age infected with HIV, and then applies this percent to total annual births to calculate births among HIV-infected women. Annual HIV-infected infants can then be obtained by applying an average mother to child transmission rate to total births of HIV-infected women. Uninfected infants born to HIV-infected women constitute potential maternal AIDS orphans. The CHILD module of EPIMODEL provides a more detailed method for estimating and projecting pediatric AIDS and maternal AIDS orphans. This module calculates the total number of children born to HIV-infected women – including those children born before these women were infected – and calculates the age of these children at the time their mothers die of AIDS, i.e., when they become maternal AIDS orphans.

Estimation of TB Cases Related to HIV

The basic module of EPIMODEL uses epidemiologically derived estimates of HIV prevalence and distributes this prevalence by annual HIV-infected cohorts back to the start of the HIV epidemic along a theoretical epidemic curve. EPIMODEL then applies annual progression rates from HIV infection to the development of AIDS to each of the annual HIV cohorts to calculate annual numbers of adult AIDS cases and deaths. The TB module of EPIMODEL provides estimates of the annual number of tuberculosis (TB) cases related to HIV infections.

Modeling of the interaction between HIV and *Mycobacteria tuberculosis* (*Mtbc*) infections provides useful estimates and projections of the additional TB cases that may be expected annually in different epidemiologic situations. In SSA high HIV prevalence rates (10 to 20 percent), and high *Mtbc* infection rates (>50 percent) are present in young and middle-aged adults (15–49 years of age). Although the adult prevalence of *Mtbc* infection in most Asian countries is relatively high (ranging from 25 percent to over 40 percent), HIV prevalence levels in Asian countries range from well less than 0.1 percent to over 2 percent.

Public health and healthcare systems must plan for the expected increase in TB cases that will result from the HIV epidemic. In SSA, this means the need to develop additional resources to cope with TB cases up to 10 times or greater compared to the pre-HIV epidemic level. In several Southeast Asian countries, HIV prevalence can be expected to double annual TB cases during the new millennium. Asian countries with relatively low HIV prevalence (<0.1 percent), as of the new millennium, will have only modest increases of TB cases related to HIV infection.

The appendix to this chapter provides a detailed description of the method used by WHO/UNAIDS to estimate annual HIV incidence and AIDS deaths. The appendix describes the epidemiologic basis of and the initial development of EPIMODEL. It then shows how it works by using EPIMODEL to estimate AIDS deaths in a hypothetical SSA country.

Summary/Conclusions

To fully understand HIV/AIDS numbers requires a basic understanding of the natural history of HIV infection and the clinical and public health definitions of an AIDS case, as well as the methods used to estimate the annual incidence and prevalence of HIV/AIDS. HIV/AIDS surveillance needs to be adapted to the specific patterns and prevalence of HIV risk behaviors in any given population. The general methods used for public health surveillance of HIV/AIDS are, in general no different from those used for other diseases and infections. However, the methods used must be adapted to the unique epidemiology, wide variation in prevalence levels, and the very long "incubation" period of HIV infection prior to the development of AIDS.

Recognition, diagnosis and reporting of HIV/AIDS is generally very incomplete so HIV infections and AIDS cases reported to health authorities throughout the world constitute a variable and usually only a small fraction of the estimated total, i.e., "the tip of the iceberg," especially in developing countries. The estimated completeness of AIDS case reporting varies from highs of up to 80 to 90 percent in the more developed countries to less than 5 percent in most developing countries. Reporting of HIV infections is usually much more incomplete and inaccurate than AIDS case reporting, even in those countries where HIV reporting is required. Therefore reported AIDS cases and HIV infections should serve only as a starting point for estimation of actual HIV infections and AIDS cases that have occurred. It needs to be realized that methods for the estimation of HIV prevalence in developing countries do not rely on reported HIV infections or reported AIDS cases.

Estimating HIV prevalence in any population requires reliable and representative HIV serosurvey data. Prior to the advent of effective drug therapy that delays or prevents development of AIDS most developed countries considered reported AIDS cases to be sufficiently reliable for estimating HIV prevalence by a back-calculation method. In the absence of reliable AIDS case data, the only other method for estimating prevalence was to use the results of serological surveys in specific populations. Major problems with this method were the limited number of seroprevalence studies that might be representative of specific populations or subgroups, and the wide variability in estimates of the size of important subgroups, such as female sex workers (FSW), injecting drug users (IDU), and patients seen in STD clinics.

From the beginning of the HIV/AIDS pandemic there has been a general tendency to overestimate HIV prevalence for many areas and populations. In some situations, overestimates rather than underestimates have been deliberately chosen for advocacy purposes. Many HIV estimates or projections have been criticized as being much too high or low, based not on an objective assessment of available data, but on whether the numbers were sufficiently high or low to affect attitudes and opinions of the public and policy makers. Although HIV sentinel surveillance (HSS) systems were not designed to provide data for making HIV prevalence estimates, they have been used for this purpose primarily because there are generally no other HIV data available. HSS data are heavily biased by inclusion of sentinel sites where the highest HIV prevalence might be found.

As a result of all of the vagaries inherent in the available HIV/AIDS data and limitations of the methods for estimating HIV prevalence, estimation of national HIV prevalence cannot be considered very precise. Nevertheless, if major over-estimation biases in many HIV datasets are taken into account, reliable working estimates of low (< 0.1 percent), moderate (> 0.1 percent and < 1 percent), high (> 1 percent and < 10%), or very high (> 10 percent) national HIV prevalence in the total 15–49 year old population can be made. These broad HIV prevalence levels along with some HIV prevalence trend data (stable, increasing or decreasing) for those in the highest HIV risk behavior groups should be adequate for developing and implementing appropriate public health policies and programs for the prevention and control of HIV/AIDS.

Mathematical models have been used to develop short and long-range projections of HIV prevalence. However, any mathematical projection model is only as reliable as the assumptions used and the values used for all of the input parameters, and such models should be used primarily for hypothesis testing and not for making estimates and projections of annual HIV incidence for a specific country or population. However, many international "experts" and several international agencies have used both complex and simple models to project the course of HIV epidemics in countries in Africa and Asia. As a result, unrealistic HIV prevalence estimates and projections have been inappropriately developed and used in some countries for program and policy development. It is inappropriate and wrong to use an epidemic model (even UNAIDS' improved and updated Asian epidemic model) in populations that have not had any significant heterosexual HIV epidemics and where there is no sound epidemiologic basis to expect any heterosexual HIV epidemic to occur.

Appendix

EPIMODEL

If the number of persons infected with HIV were known and in addition, the year when they were infected known, then by using what are accepted as annual progression rates from HIV infection to the development of AIDS and from AIDS to death, the annual number of AIDS cases and deaths expected from each of the annual cohorts of new HIV infections can be calculated. EPIMODEL was designed to make these calculations. Initially, in mid-1987, I started with hand calculations and then switched to a spreadsheet program, but spreadsheet programs in the late 1980s were cumbersome to use and it was very cumbersome to make minor changes to any of the input parameters. However, since I had decided to support the development of a newer version of Epi-Info,[*] I had Tony Burton, who I recruited from his position at CDC (Atlanta), arrange to bring Jeff Dean[†] to Geneva on a short-term contract to write version III of Epi-Info. Since I (SFI/GPA/WHO) was paying for his service, I also had Jeff write Epi-Map (Version 1) and while we had him chained to his chair, I had Jeff write the DOS program of EPIMODEL according to my specifications.

The methodology and assumptions used for estimating and projecting national HIV prevalence in developing countries have been evolving and changing. As HIV epidemiology in these countries is better understood and the quality of surveillance data improves, the methods and models for estimation and projection of HIV/AIDS improves. As a result, UNAIDS/WHO has cautioned that estimates of national HIV prevalence since 2003 should not be compared with previous or possibly future estimates. UNAIDS has, as of the new millennium, developed more detailed guidelines and a newer model (a variant of EPIMODEL) for estimation and projection of HIV/AIDS. The new Estimation and Projection Package (EPP) uses the same general input data and assumptions as EPIMODEL, but can handle more detailed as well as more datasets (i.e., age, gender, urban/rural, ANC, MSM, IDU, etc.) compared with a single 15–49 year old population used by EPIMODEL. Thus, to get the detailed output that EPP can provide, numerous EPIMODEL runs would have to be made for each of the variables. However, it should not be concluded that EPP provides any more accurate estimates and projections than EPIMODEL. The accuracy of EPP or EPIMODEL depends on the accuracy of the input parameters and assumptions used: these are or should be the same whether EPP or EPIMODEL is used.

The following section illustrates how EPIMODEL works by estimating annual AIDS deaths in a small hypothetical SSA country (XZ). According to this scenario, the total population of country XZ in 1990 was 2.2 million, with one million in the 15–49 year age group. HIV prevalence in the 15–49 year old population of

---

[*] Epi-Info is a relational database that was developed at CDC, Atlanta by Andy Dean (Jeff's father), Jeff Dean, and Tony Burton.
[†] Jeff Dean was one of the principal programmers for Epi-Info. Jeff eventually got his PhD from the University of Washington in computer science during the early 1990s and now is one of the millionaires working for Google in California.

country XZ was estimated to be 100 000 or 10 percent* in 1990 by a national expert committee. The number of reported AIDS deaths in country XZ in 1990 was 500, but it was clear that reported deaths were only a small percent of AIDS deaths that actually occurred. The Ministry of Health in country XZ needed a more reliable estimate of AIDS deaths that had occurred and might be expected during the next few years.

Table 6A.1 presents all of the input variables needed for EPIMODEL to calculate annual AIDS cases and deaths for country XZ.

Table 6A.1 EPIMODEL input variables/parameters for country XZ

Input Variables	*Comments*
Estimated HIV prevalence in the 15–49 year old population in 1990 (the reference year) – 100 000	This was estimated by a national expert committee and is the source of the largest potential error in the estimation of AIDS cases and deaths.
Year epidemic HIV transmission started – late 1970s – 1980	The exact year is not too important since annual HIV infections in the first few years are low.
Shape of HIV epidemic curve – a straight line or the left half of a gamma 5 curve	Requires some estimates of prevalence in years prior to the reference year.
Placement of reference year on curve – at or near the peak of the gamma 5 curve	Minimal effect on AIDS estimates for 3–4 years after the reference year, but will have major impact on AIDS projections of >5 years.
Population size – Total population 2.2 million in 1990 with 1 million in the 15–49 year old age group	Estimated by demographers – assumed to be accurate
Annual population growth rate – 2 percent	Estimated by demographers – assumed to be accurate.
Progression rates from HIV infection to AIDS – median interval selected – 8 years	EPIMODEL provides four median intervals to select: 6, 8, 10 and 12 years. The default interval is 10 years, but for this scenario an 8 year median was selected.
Progression from AIDS to death – less than 1 year	Assumed to be less than a year in the absence of HIV drug treatment – the default progression is 50 percent in the year that AIDS develops and the median interval from infection to death for this scenario is 8–9 years.

EPIMODEL provides default values for the last two input parameters considered in the late 1980s to be appropriate for modeling HIV/AIDS in a SSA population, but all input parameters for EPIMODEL can easily be changed to achieve a better "fit" for the specific population being modeled.

---

* Numerator/100 000 HIV infections in the 15–49 year old population divided by the denominator/1 million persons in the 15–49 year age group.

The primary input parameters for EPIMODEL's calculations of annual AIDS deaths in country XZ are

A an estimate of when extensive or epidemic HIV transmission started and
B the estimated HIV prevalence in a specific year – the reference year (Figure 6A.1).

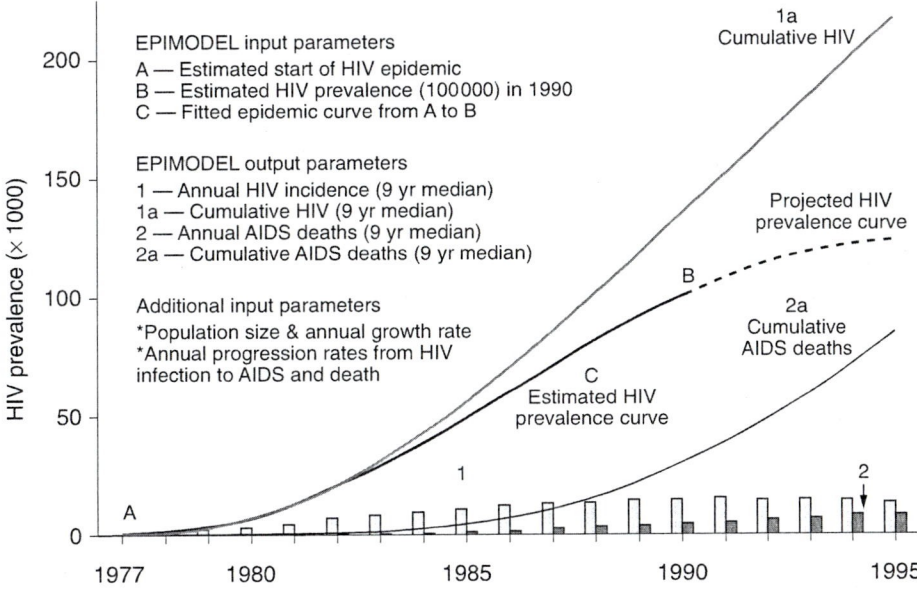

Figure 6A.1 EPIMODEL input and output parameters.

The exact year when extensive or epidemic HIV transmission started is not too important since annual HIV infections in the first few years are low. In this scenario, the estimated starting period is the late 1970s (A) but large numbers of HIV infections did not occur until about 1980: we will see that this is reflected in the epidemic curve selected (C) to fit the increasing prevalence from the starting period to the reference year – 1990 (B). EPIMODEL distributes the estimated HIV prevalence in 1990 back to the estimated start of the HIV epidemic by calculating annual cohorts of HIV incidence (1 – the light shaded bars in Figure 6A.1) according to the selected epidemic curve. EPIMODEL applies the selected annual progression rates (median interval of 9 years) from HIV infection to AIDS and death to each annual HIV cohort to calculate annual AIDS deaths (2 – dark shaded bars in Figure 6A.1). The user has to specify the shape of an epidemic curve from the starting year of epidemic spread to the reference year and also specify where on that epidemic curve the reference year should be placed. EPIMODEL's default HIV epidemic curve is S-shaped. Such a curve is characteristic of a single source epidemic with person-to-person transmission. A frequent criticism of EPIMODEL is that many curves can be "drawn" from the start of an epidemic through a single point (the HIV prevalence estimate for the reference year). While that argument is theoretically true, the epidemiologic basis upon which the model is formulated and the empirical data used rules out the majority of curves that can be drawn through the point chosen for the reference year. EPIMODEL assumes that the distribution of HIV infection over time in any population will be skewed with a long right tail. Of the many curves that could satisfy these assumptions, a simple gamma function was selected[*] to describe HIV incidence at time t. Parameter p defines the steepness of the epidemic curve. A value of p = 5 is used since this gamma distribution for HIV infections provided the best empirical fit to the reported AIDS case curves in countries with reliable reporting systems. This empirical fit was made to the left half of the curve (i.e., the epidemic phase). Whether the gamma 5 curve will "fit" any HIV epidemic curve after its peak (the right half of the curve) is unknown but EPIMODEL enables the user to switch to other curves to "fit" HIV scenarios where prevalence falls to an endemic level after its epidemic peak.

Where on the HIV epidemic curve should the HIV reference year be placed? This question can be answered only by analysis of all the available epidemiologic data. Such data and other observations may suggest that incidence is generally increasing or decreasing. If extensive HIV spread has been noted for less than five years, then it can be assumed that the epidemic is still in its early phase and has not yet peaked;[†] thus, the reference year should be somewhere on the left half of the epidemic curve. If epidemic spread has been noted for five to ten years, then the reference year may be shortly before, at, or shortly after the peak of the epidemic curve. If the epidemic is more than ten years old, then the reference year may be beyond the peak. For this modeling example, the prevalence estimate of 100 000 for the reference year (1990) was placed at the peak of the gamma 5 curve. However, any HIV prevalence estimate must underestimate cumulative incidence that occurred during the epidemic, since AIDS deaths would be omitted from the most recent prevalence estimate. EPIMODEL adjusts the prevalence estimate upwards by using the selected annual progression rates from HIV to AIDS to arrive at an estimate of cumulative HIV incidence from the time widespread transmission began to the prevalence estimate year (i.e., the reference year). HIV cumulative incidence (upper curve [1a] in Figure 6A.1) is then partitioned into annual cohorts of HIV-infected persons by use of the gamma 5 curve that was selected.

Another major source of significant "error" in producing estimates of AIDS deaths with EPIMODEL is the selection of the median interval period from HIV infection to death. This is because up to the new millennium progression rates were estimated primarily from cohort studies of MSM and hemophilia patients in the USA and western European countries. Progression rates from infection to AIDS and death were postulated to be more rapid in developing country populations because of the presence of many other infectious diseases which might place additional stress on the immune system. However, there were scant data to confirm or to refute this conclusion. In the early 1990s, several reports from female cohort studies suggested that progression rates to development of AIDS from initial infection were similar to those reported for men. Only age at time of HIV infection has been established as a host factor that may influence the rate of progression to AIDS. The average time from infection to AIDS for men with hemophilia who were infected at age 35 or over was about 7–8 years; while for those males who were infected when they were less than

---

[*] $t^{(p-1)}e^{-t}/(p-1)$

[†] This applies to national epidemic modeling. HIV epidemics in some IDU populations can peak in less than a year.

35 years old the average was approximately 12 years. Similar results were reported in 1992 for a cohort of women followed from year of infection to the onset of AIDS. As of late-2006, neither the proportion of HIV-infected adults who will ultimately develop AIDS nor are annual progression rates from HIV infection to AIDS known precisely.

Prospective cohort studies that followed HIV-infected homosexual men from initial infection showed that only about 3 percent developed AIDS within the first three years. After that, there appeared to be a steady 6–7 percent annual progression up to about year 10. In 1995, one of these cohort studies estimated that over 75 percent of young and middle-aged white men infected with HIV developed AIDS by year 17 after infection. The proportion or percent of nonprogressors (HIV-infected persons who may never progress to AIDS) is still not known. Some investigators believe that from 5–10 percent of all infected persons may be nonprogressors, but NIH suspects that the actual percent of nonprogressors is very small and may be at most 1–2 percent. For modeling purposes, EPIMODEL conservatively assumes that 90 percent of HIV-infected adults will develop AIDS and die within 20 years after infection.

A review of several cohort studies in Uganda, Thailand, and Haiti in 2001 suggests that the median interval from HIV infection to AIDS is about 7–8 years. This median period has been accepted by WHO and UNAIDS to calculate annual HIV incidence and AIDS* in most developing countries. However, there is a consensus that the survival period from the development of AIDS to death is much shorter in most developing countries compared with developed countries where the advent of HAART therapy has significantly increased patient survival. The median interval from HIV infection to AIDS death may be about 8–9 years in developing countries.

During the 1990s, most AIDS models, including EPIMODEL, used a default median from HIV infection to AIDS of 10 years. This resulted in a median interval from infection to death of 11 years. The change, since the new millennium, from the 11-year median survival period to the 9-year median results in much higher cumulative HIV infections. In addition, use of a 9-year median survival period results in a higher number of annual AIDS deaths. This increase in annual and cumulative AIDS deaths is needed to compensate for the increase in cumulative HIV infections. These differences are shown in Table 6A.2 and Figure 6A.2.

Table 6A.2 EPIMODEL outputs using a 9 or 11 year median from HIV infections to AIDS and death

Year	HIV Prevalence	Cum HIV 11yr median	Cum HIV 9yr median	Cum AIDS Deaths – 11yr	Cum AIDS Deaths – 9yr
1985	49 500	50 500	**55 400**	3100	**4800**
1990	100 000	122 400	**134 300**	19 700	**30 200**
1995	125 000	197 800	**217 200**	56 800	**85 500**

* Consultation to determine criteria for estimating adult and child mortality for country-specific estimates of HIV/AIDS 17–19 July 2001, Le Cottage, Talloires, France. UNAIDS Reference Group for Surveillance, Estimation and Projection of HIV/AIDS numbers.

In 1990, estimated HIV prevalence in persons age 15–49 years was 100 000 and if the median interval from infection to death was 11 years, cumulative HIV infections in 1995 were calculated by EPIMODEL to be about 198 000 (1b in Figure 6A.2); if the median interval of 9 years was used, the cumulative number of HIV infections in 1995 increased to over 217 000 (1a) for a difference of about 10 percent. The cumulative AIDS death total in 1995 with use of the 9-year median is about 86 000 (2a in Figure 6A.2) and if the 11-year median is used it is about 50 percent lower at about 57 000 (2b in Figure 6A.2).

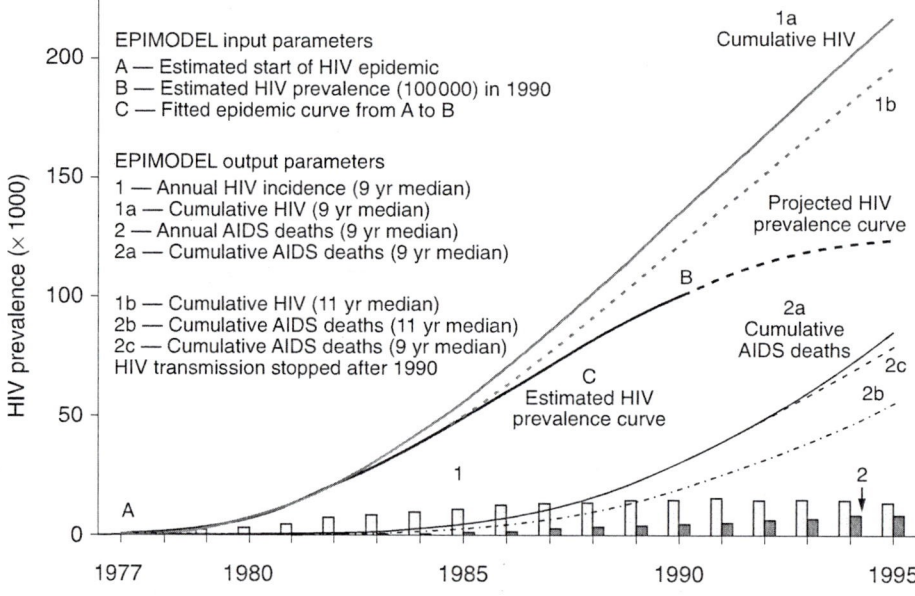

Figure 6A.2 EPIMODEL input and output parameters.

EPIMODEL was *not* designed to provide projections of HIV infection. However, short-term projections of AIDS cases and deaths are not greatly affected by stopping or continuing HIV transmission after a specific year. This is because 80–90 percent of AIDS cases/deaths that will occur 3–5 years after a reference year will be in persons who were infected up to the reference year. However, major sources of potential error in this simple model must be constantly reviewed. Projections of AIDS cases for periods longer than 3–5 years can be produced by EPIMODEL by assuming that annual HIV infections beyond the reference year will continue along the curve selected for use. However, longer term projections of AIDS cases using EPIMODEL, or any other model, are less reliable because they depend on accurate projections of future HIV infections. If HIV transmission was stopped after 1990, cumulative AIDS deaths in 1995, using the 9-year median interval, would be about 81 000 (2c in Figure 6A.2) compared with the almost 86 000 (2a in Figure 6A.2) if transmission continued after 1990.

Because EPIMODEL is a very simple program and easy to use, i.e., input a couple of numbers and press a key and EPIMODEL generates all the needed HIV/AIDS numbers, it has been used by many AIDS workers who do not have a good understanding of the basic epidemiology and natural history of HIV infection. It must be emphasized that the greatest potential error in estimating AIDS deaths with EPIMODEL is the accuracy of the HIV prevalence estimate that is the key *input* **parameter** and not an *output* **parameter**. EPIMODEL makes calculations based on input parameters supplied by the user. Just as a calculator should not be held accountable for preparing an inaccurate tax return, EPIMODEL should not be blamed for inaccurate estimates of AIDS deaths. If HIV prevalence is overestimated, then EPIMODEL will overestimate AIDS deaths.

Chapter 7

How Credible are HIV/AIDS Estimates?

One of the major problems related to national HIV/AIDS estimates is the diverse perceptions that the public and policy makers have regarding estimated HIV/AIDS numbers. These perceptions range from total distrust of any "official" estimate to an almost blind, uncritical acceptance of high estimates from UNAIDS and many self-proclaimed AIDS "experts." When AIDS was first recognized in the early 1980s, there was an initial period of almost universal denial that AIDS (initially referred to as the "American disease of homosexuals and drug users") was present in any significant numbers in most developing countries. Since then there has been a general tendency to overestimate HIV prevalence for many areas and populations. As described in Chapter 6, overestimates of HIV prevalence during the 1980s were due primarily to overestimating the size of different subpopulations with high HIV risk behaviors and this was partly due to the limited data available. In the United States, from 1985 through 1992 official estimates of cumulative HIV infection remained consistently in the range of 1 to 1.5 million. As of 2006, the official CDC estimate of prevalent HIV infections in the USA remains at about 1 million, which clearly indicates that previous estimates were all high.

HIV serosurvey data have been collected by public health programs since the mid-to-late 1980s. Although questions remain about the quality of these data and how representative of the specific populations they may be, reasonably reliable descriptions of the basic patterns, general prevalence levels, and temporal trends of HIV infections in different global regions and in individual countries can be developed from an objective analysis of all HIV/AIDS data. This chapter will first describe the general patterns, prevalence levels, and trends of HIV/AIDS in all of the major global regions and in selected countries and then review and evaluate the problem of overestimation and projection of HIV prevalence in SSA and in several selected Asian countries.

Estimated Regional HIV Prevalence

Starting in the late 1980s, public health surveillance systems were developed to monitor HIV transmission patterns and to collect HIV data to estimate HIV prevalence in all major regions of the world. As noted in the previous chapter, because of the inherent vagaries of HIV data and the limitations of estimation methods, HIV prevalence estimates cannot be precise, but HIV prevalence in the 15–49 year old population (the most sexually active age group) in countries or regions can be confidently classified as:

- **low:** Less than 1 per 1000 of the 15–49 year old population (< 0.1 percent);
- **moderate:** More than 1 per 1000 and less than 1 per 100 (> 0.1 to < 1 percent);
- **high:** More than 1 per 100 and less than 1 per 10 (> 1 to < 10 percent);
- **very high:** More than 1 per 10 (> 10 percent).

Table 7.1 Estimated HIV prevalence in major regions – 2001 and 2005

Region	Adults (15–49)[*] Millions	Number HIV+[*] Millions	HIV+ 2001[*] Percent	HIV+ 2001R[**] Percent	HIV+ 2005[***] Percent	HIV+ 2005R[^] Percent	Major HIV Risk Behavior Groups
Sub-Saharan Africa	291.3	26.0	9.0	7.6	7.2	6.1	Heterosexual
Caribbean	17.2	0.4	2.3	2.2	1.6	1.6	Heterosexual
South & Southeast Asia	1031.5	5.4	0.6	0.6	0.7	0.6	FSW & IDU
Latin America	262.2	1.4	0.5	0.5	0.6	0.5	MSM & IDU
East Europe & Central Asia	209.0	1.0	0.5	0.4	0.9	0.8	IDU
"Western" Countries[****]	373.5	1.5	0.4	0.4	0.4	0.4	MSM & IDU
North Africa & Middle-East	180.5	0.5	0.3	0.2	0.2	0.2	–
East Asia & Pacific	833.1	1.0	0.1	0.1	0.1	0.1	IDU
Global Totals:	**3198.3**	**37.1**	**1.2**	**1.0**	**1.1**	**1.0**	

[*]Adapted from the UNAIDS Global report, July 2002. [**]Adapted from the UNAIDS Global report, July 2003. [***]Adapted from the UNAIDS Global report, December 2005. [****]Includes N American countries, Western European countries, Australia and New Zealand. [^]Adapted from the UNAIDS 2006 report on the global AIDS epidemic (May 30, 2006).

I will first present global and regional HIV prevalence estimates in 2001 and 2005 and describe HIV prevalence trends during this 5-year period. Table 7.1 presents UNAIDS estimated HIV prevalence (both number and rate as a percent) and the major modes of HIV transmission in major global regions for 2001 and 2005. Unless specified otherwise, all prevalence estimates are for the 15–49 year old population and not for the total population.

Regional Summaries: 2001–2005

It must be recognized that in any large geographic region that there is bound to be some major differences in the patterns and prevalence of HIV risk behaviors and accordingly some marked differences in the pattern and prevalence of HIV in some individual countries in the region. Even though any regional summary may obscure these differences, the general trends in different global regions are helpful in monitoring the HIV/AIDS pandemic.

Sub-Saharan Africa (SSA)

In 2001, UNAIDS estimated that this region had the highest mean HIV prevalence rate (9 percent), with 16 of the 44 countries in this region having an estimated prevalence of more than 10 percent. Two countries (Botswana and Zimbabwe) had estimated HIV prevalence rates of over 35 percent. Such a national prevalence rate meant that more than half of all persons 25–39 years old in urban areas were infected with HIV. HIV transmission in this region is predominantly heterosexual. However, the initial 2001 HIV prevalence estimates for SSA countries were overestimated on average by about 50 percent as will be described in detail later in this chapter. Based on better data and methods for HIV prevalence estimates, UNAIDS in 2003 revised the 2001 estimates for this region from 9 percent (26 million adults infected) to 7.6 percent (22 million infected). In 2005, the prevalence rate was estimated at 7.2 percent. HIV prevalence in this region has probably been gradually decreasing since the new millennium, but most of the decrease in estimated prevalence since 2001 may be related to reduction of previously overestimated prevalence levels. Analysis of all HIV serosurvey data and ANC data support the general conclusion that HIV incidence rates in this region peaked by the late 1990s and have been slowly decreasing since. UNAIDS in its mid-2006 report on the AIDS pandemic reduced its prior estimates of the HIV prevalence rate in the 15–49-year-old population in this region from 7.2 percent in 2005 to 6.1 percent. This most recent UNAIDS revision is now almost identical to my estimate of SSA adult HIV prevalence in 2005.

Caribbean

In 2001, this small region had the second highest estimated HIV prevalence rate – 2.3 percent. HIV prevalence estimates in this region ranged from lows of about one percent to highs of three to six percent (Bahamas and Haiti). Heterosexual transmission predominates. Cuba was and continues to be exceptional in that its estimated HIV prevalence is one of the lowest in the world – 0.02 percent or 1/5000 of the adult (15–49) population. In 2005, UNAIDS without providing many details estimated HIV prevalence in this region to be 1.6 percent and also retrospectively revised the 2003 prevalence estimate for this region sharply downwards to 1.6 percent even though the prevalence estimate in the *UNAIDS 2004 Global AIDS Report* was 2.3 percent.

South and Southeast Asia

HIV/AIDS numbers in this region are dominated by India (estimated close to 4 million HIV-infected adults in 2001) and high prevalence rates in Thailand, Cambodia, and Myanmar. In 2001, HIV prevalence rates in this large and diverse region ranged from lows of less than 0.1 percent (Iran, Bhutan and Afghanistan) to highs of 2.5 percent and 1.8 percent (Cambodia and Thailand). In 2005, HIV prevalence estimates in Cambodia and Thailand were reduced to 1.9 and 1.5 percent, respectively. Heterosexual transmission predominates in this populous region, but there are significant pockets of HIV transmission in IDU populations in India, Malaysia, Myanmar, Nepal, Vietnam, Pakistan and Thailand. From 2001 to 2005, HIV prevalence in this region has been decreasing, but there is considerable controversy about HIV prevalence estimates for India. Based on what data I have seen for India since 2000, it appears to me that HIV prevalence peaked in India during the late 1990s and has been relatively level or stable since then. Some population-based HIV surveys are planned and scheduled to be carried out in major States in India in 2006 and these surveys should be able to clarify whether HIV prevalence in India is closer to 3 million or to 6 million.

Latin America

HIV prevalence in this region ranged in 2001 from a low of 0.07 percent (Bolivia) to highs of 0.69 percent and 0.63 percent (Argentina and Brazil). Guyana is exceptional in that its estimated HIV prevalence was 2.13 percent and this country may be more appropriately grouped with Caribbean countries. Nonepidemic heterosexual transmission is increasing, but more than half of HIV infections in this "region" are attributed to MSM and IDU transmission. There has been little change in HIV prevalence estimates in this region from 2001 to 2005.

Western Countries (North America, Western Europe, and Oceania)

HIV prevalence in this "region" in 2001 ranged from lows of 0.01–0.02 percent or 1/10 000–1/5000 (Macedonia and Finland) to highs of 0.6 and 0.5 percent (USA and Portugal). Nonepidemic heterosexual transmission is increasing, but the majority of HIV infection in this "region" has been and continues to be attributed to MSM and IDU transmission. There also has been little change in HIV prevalence estimates in these countries since 2001 but the current stable HIV prevalence is attributed to major increases of HIV drug treatment programs that have greatly extended the lifespan of persons living with an HIV infection.

North Africa and the Middle East

HIV/AIDS numbers in this region in 2001 were dominated by southern Sudan (estimated 410 000 HIV infections – close to 90 percent of this region's total). Without Sudan, HIV prevalence in other countries of this region was 0.04 percent or about 1/2500. HIV prevalence rates in this region ranged from a low of less than 0.005 percent or 1/20 000 (Iraq) to a high of 2.6 percent (Sudan). Sudan, especially southern Sudan, should be classified in the SSA region. There has not been any major change in HIV prevalence estimates or trends in this region from 2001 to 2005.

Eastern Europe and Central Asia

HIV/AIDS numbers in this region were in 2001 dominated by the Ukraine (250 000 HIV infections) and Russia (700 000 HIV infections) – about 95 percent of the region's total. Without the Ukraine and Russia, prevalence in all of the other countries in this region was 0.05 percent or 1/2000. Most HIV infections were attributed to IDU transmission, with subsequent nonepidemic heterosexual transmission from infected IDU to their regular sex partner(s). There is no question that significant IDU epidemics have occurred in several countries in this region, but HIV prevalence in these countries may be overestimated. From 2001 to 2005, overall HIV prevalence was estimated to have almost doubled as a result of unabated HIV epidemic transmission in IDU populations.

East Asia and the Pacific

HIV/AIDS numbers in this region was and continues to be dominated by China (estimated 850 000 HIV infections in 2001 – about 90 percent of this region's total). Without China, HIV prevalence in other countries of this region was

0.018 percent or about 1/5000. HIV prevalence rates ranged from a low of less than 0.005 percent or 1/20 000 (North Korea) to a high of 0.7 percent (Papua New Guinea – PNG). A large proportion (about 90 percent) of HIV infections in China are attributed to transmission in IDU populations and to faulty plasma collection in paid plasma donors that occurred during the early to mid-1990s. Since 2001, HIV prevalence has been steadily increasing in PNG, but not increasing in other countries in this region, including China. However, as will be described later in this chapter, many AIDS "experts," without any sound epidemiologic basis, have projected that HIV prevalence in China will reach 10 to 20 million by the year 2010. The 2005 HIV prevalence estimate for China that was released in early 2006 was 650 000, a much reduced estimate compared to the 2003 estimate of 840 000.

For each of the global regions summarized above, Figure 7.1 presents the three countries with the highest estimated HIV prevalence rates in 2003. The tremendous differences in prevalence are clear when the country with the highest HIV prevalence in SSA (Swaziland) is over 50 times greater than countries with the highest HIV prevalence in Latin America and Western countries and is close to 400 times greater than China, the country with the second highest estimated prevalence in East Asia and the Pacific.

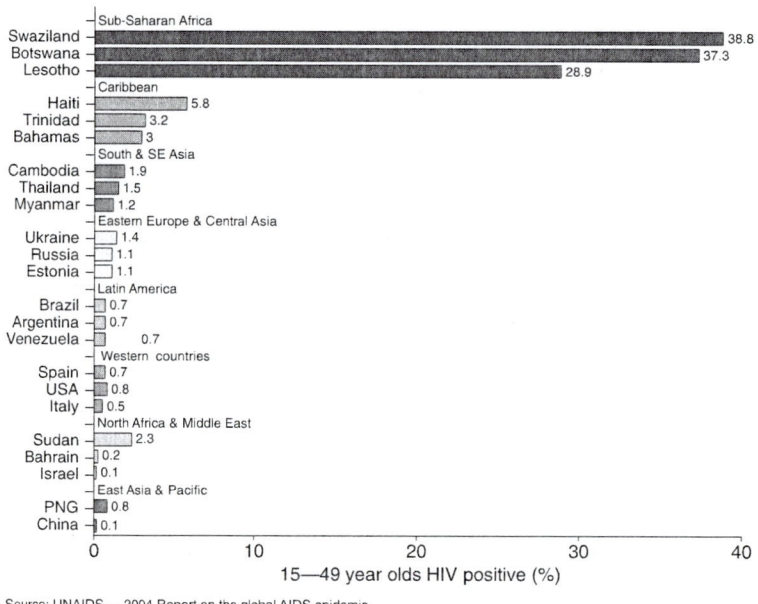

Source: UNAIDS — 2004 Report on the global AIDS epidemic

Figure 7.1 Countries with the highest estimated HIV prevalence in different global regions – 2003.

This tremendous difference in estimated HIV prevalence levels should help to put the AIDS pandemic in proper perspective. These data reinforce the differences in the epidemiologic patterns of HIV transmission present in different countries and regions. The relative independence of HIV epidemics in MSM, IDU, and heterosexuals with multiple sex partners is suggested by the relatively low prevalence (less than 1 percent) in countries with IDU and/or MSM epidemics but no epidemic heterosexual transmission. Prevalence rates (up to 50 percent or more) can be found in some MSM and IDU populations but because these populations are relatively small compared with the general adult population, national HIV prevalence will not get close to 1 percent of the 15–49 year old population unless there is some epidemic heterosexual transmission. It should be noted that even if some national prevalence estimates were overestimated or underestimated by plus or minus 100–200 percent that this would usually not be sufficient to change a country with moderate HIV prevalence to one with high HIV prevalence. If HIV prevalence in China were doubled or tripled, countries with the highest HIV prevalence in SSA would still be at least 100 times greater than China.

Figure 7.2 presents the estimated percent of HIV infection compared with the percent of the 15–49 year old population for each region. It shows that SSA has close to two-thirds of global adult HIV prevalence but less than 10 percent of the global population whereas East Asia and the Pacific (mostly China) has over a quarter of the global adult population but less than 3 percent of the global total of adult HIV infection.

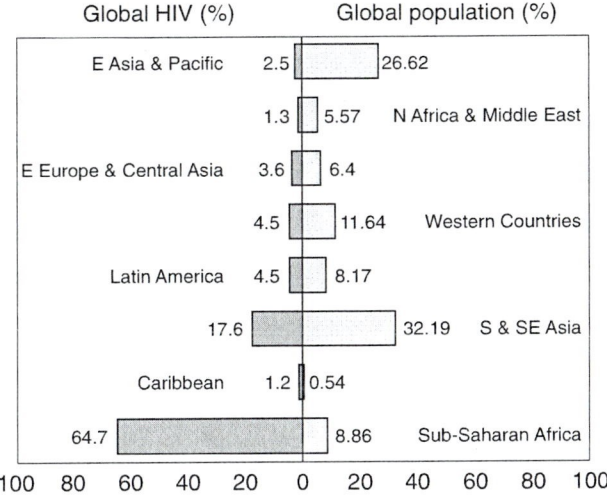

Figure 7.2 Distribution of adult HIV infection with adult population – 2003.

As large as these national and regional prevalence differentials are, the country differences in HIV prevalence in female populations are even greater and are thousands of times higher in Swaziland compared to most low HIV prevalence countries as shown in Table 7.2.

Table 7.2 Estimated HIV prevalence in 10 000 15–49-year-old females – 2003[1]

Country	Number	HIV Transmission
Swaziland	4300	Primarily heterosexual
Haiti[2]	700	Primarily heterosexual
Cambodia	120	Primarily heterosexual
Thailand	100	Mostly heterosexual & IDU
Russia	75	Primarily IDU

Continued

Table 7.2 (Continued)

Country	Number	HIV Transmission
USA	30	Mostly MSM & IDU
Mexico	20	Mostly MSM & IDU
Malaysia	15	Primarily IDU
China	5	Focul IDU and faulty plasma collection
Philippines	1	No epidemic HIV spread
Republic of Korea	<1	No epidemic HIV spread
Bangladesh	<1	No epidemic HIV spread
Egypt	<1	No epidemic HIV spread

[1]Based on UNAIDS estimates (2004) and/or the most recent "official" national estimate.
[2]The 2005 UNAIDS HIV prevalence estimate was reduced by about half – down to 300 to 400.

HIV Prevalence Trends

Regional prevalence trends can obscure some individual country trends, but are nevertheless useful to monitor trends of the HIV/AIDS pandemic. To derive the prevalence trends shown in the following figures, assumptions were made as to when epidemic transmission started in each region; then a curve was fitted to the prevalence estimates published by UNAIDS/WHO. Figure 7.3 presents HIV prevalence numbers and Figure 7.4 presents HIV prevalence rates. Both figures clearly show the increasing prevalence in the adult population in SSA that began prior to the 1980s up through the year 2001.

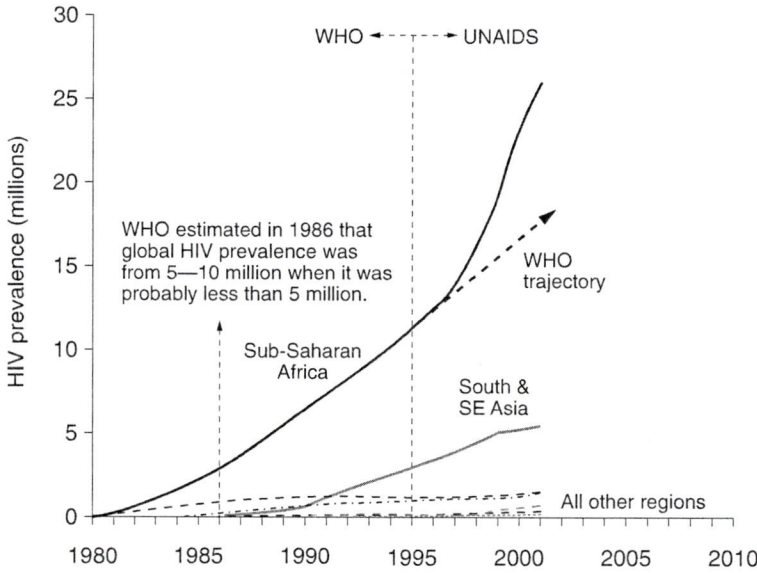

Figure 7.3 Estimated regional HIV prevalence numbers – 1980–2001.

In 2001 SSA had by far the highest estimated prevalent number (26 million) and highest prevalence rate (9 percent). The region with the second highest number of HIV-infected adults is South and Southeast Asia (primarily because of the estimated 4–5 million in India) and the region with the second highest prevalence rate is the Caribbean (over 2 percent).

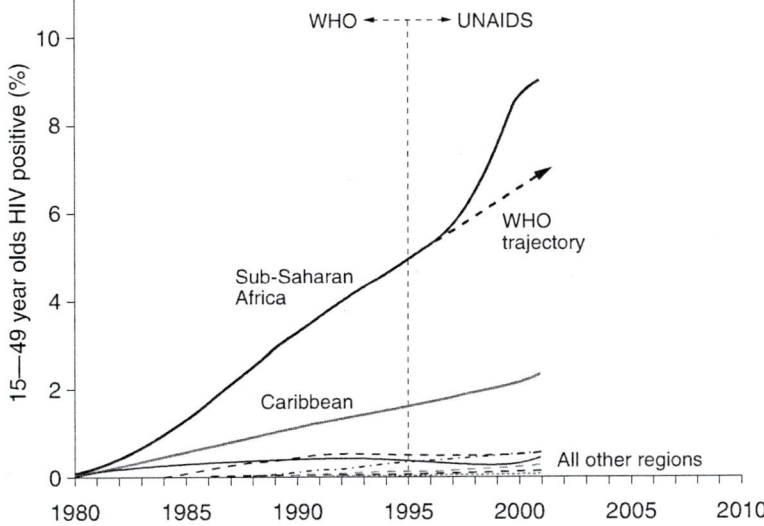

Figure 7.4 Estimated regional HIV prevalence rates – 1980–2001.

In reviewing these temporal trends, it appears that HIV prevalence in SSA increased steadily almost on a straight line from 1980 to shortly past 1995: then during the late 1990s, the slope of the prevalence curve for SSA took a sharper upward climb. One obvious conclusion is that HIV transmission in SSA increased markedly during the late 1990s to account for this shift in the rate of increase noted in the HIV prevalence curve for SSA. Another possible, and what I believe is the more probable, explanation for this sharp increase is that there were significant changes in calculating annual HIV prevalence estimates for SSA by UNAIDS in the late 1990s. These differed from annual HIV prevalence estimates developed by GPA/WHO up to the mid-1990s. HIV prevalence estimates developed when I was with GPA/WHO from the late 1980s up to the early 1990s were deliberately conservative. Estimates made by WHO after I resigned from WHO in early 1992, up to the mid-1990s continued to be conservative. After the mid-1990s, UNAIDS assumed responsibility for developing global and regional HIV/AIDS estimates. As can be seen in Figures 7.3 and 7.4, HIV prevalence estimates for SSA took a marked upward turn during the late 1990s and reached a high of 26 million (9 percent) in 2001.[*]

Revision of UNAIDS' 2001 HIV Prevalence Estimates

Until about 2001, HIV sentinel surveillance (HSS) data collected from ANC populations were routinely used to estimate national prevalence in SSA

---

[*] I was told by a colleague involved with developing HIV prevalence estimates for UNAIDS that there was a clear administrative decision made in 1997 to use the higher range of HIV estimates rather than the lower or mid-range that were used by GPA/WHO.

countries. It was initially assumed, based on limited comparisons of HIV prevalence in ANC samples with prevalence found in community surveys of both males and females, that prevalence in pregnant females could be used as a reasonable surrogate of HIV prevalence in the total 15–49 year old population. However, it was also noted from the very beginning that HIV prevalence in urban populations was much higher than in rural populations. Thus, when some of the initial national prevalence estimates were made for SSA countries, I used an arbitrary and conservative ratio of urban to rural HIV prevalence of 10:1, if there were no rural ANC data to indicate that this ratio was either too high or too low.

Since 2001, UNAIDS has been recommending the collection of more accurate or representative HIV serologic data for developing national HIV prevalence estimates in SSA populations. As a result, many countries in SSA and in the Caribbean region have in recent years completed national Demographic and Health Surveys (DHS)* that included HIV testing (+). The general DHS(+) findings indicate that current prevalence estimates in some of these high HIV prevalence countries were too high by up to over 200 percent primarily due to the use of HIV sentinel surveillance (HSS) data that were heavily biased by urban sentinel sites. For example, the national HIV prevalence estimate of 21.5 percent for Zambia in 2001 was based primarily on HSS data from antenatal clinics. In 2001, a population-based DHS that included HIV testing was carried out in Zambia (ZDHS+) and the national HIV prevalence was estimated to be much lower at 16.7 percent. Analysis of the different sampling methods used by these two national surveys led to the conclusion that the HIV prevalence rate estimated by the 2001–2002 ZDHS+ is about the same as the prevalence rate estimated by ANC surveillance **when adjusted for the *biased geographic coverage* of the ANC surveillance system**.

Based on the DHS+ and/or population-based surveys whose findings were available by mid-to-late 2003, UNAIDS had to reduce some of their initial 2001 HIV prevalence estimates by up to 50 percent or more – the 2001 estimate for Kenya was 2.3 million and the revised 2001 estimate was 1.2 million an overestimate of more than a million or close to 100 percent. It should be noted that there is a significant difference between reductions in prevalence estimates compared with overestimations of prevalence. For example, prevalence in Kenya was reduced from 2.3 million to 1.2 million for a reduction of almost 50 percent. If we accept that 1.2 million is the more accurate prevalence, then HIV prevalence in Kenya was overestimated by about 100 percent. The 2001 HIV prevalence estimate for those aged 15–49 in SSA was reduced from the initial 26 million to 22 million in the July 2004 Global AIDS Report. However, since release of the revised estimate, additional population-based HIV serosurveys have been carried out (Botswana, South Africa, Cameroon, Burkina Faso, Angola, Ghana, Sierra Leone, and Tanzania); collectively they indicate that the revised estimate of 22 million for 2001 should have been reduced even more – probably by at least several million more. This is

---

* DHS are nationally representative household surveys that focus on reproductive and child health. Typically, DHS consist of interviews with between 4000 and 12 000 women aged 15–49 years living in households that are sampled in a multiple-stage cluster design.

especially likely since there are still about a dozen SSA countries that have not had population-based surveys that might force significant reductions in current HIV prevalence estimates that are derived primarily from urban or peri-urban sentinel ANC data.

When the UNAIDS revised estimates for 2001 are compared with the 2003 estimates, more than two thirds of SSA countries showed either no change or slight decreases. For less than one third of SSA countries there was an estimated increase in prevalence from 2001 to 2003, but the increase was minimal and/or the estimated prevalence was relatively low. Thus, the HIV prevalence trend in SSA according to the UNAIDS revised 2001 and 2003 estimates is level or mostly decreasing: there is not a continuing unabated increase as shown in Figures 7.5 and 7.6 that presents HIV prevalence trends from 1995 up through 2005. As already noted, the most recent (2005) UNAIDS estimate for SSA is still probably too high. Figures 7.5 and 7.6 present three different levels and trajectories of the SSA prevalence curve. The highest is the initial UNAIDS 2001 estimate of 26 million (9 percent); an intermediate level is the UNAIDS' revised 2001 estimate of 22 million (7.6 percent); and the lowest is my estimate of 19 million (6.5 percent) in 2001. As will be described later, long-term demographic projections (up to 50 years) of the impact of AIDS in SSA are markedly different depending on what is accepted or used as the prevalence in 2001 and whether the prevalence curve continues to increase or begins to level off and slowly decrease after 2001.

In mid-2006, UNAIDS finally acknowledged that many HIV prevalence estimates for SSA countries were grossly overestimated and reduced their HIV prevalence rate for the 15–49-year-old population in this region from 7.3 percent in 2003 to 6.2 percent and for 2005 it was reduced from 7.2 percent to 6.1 percent. These revised estimates are almost identical to the rates I used for my SSA HIV scenario – I used 6.5 percent in 2001 and 6.15 percent in 2005.

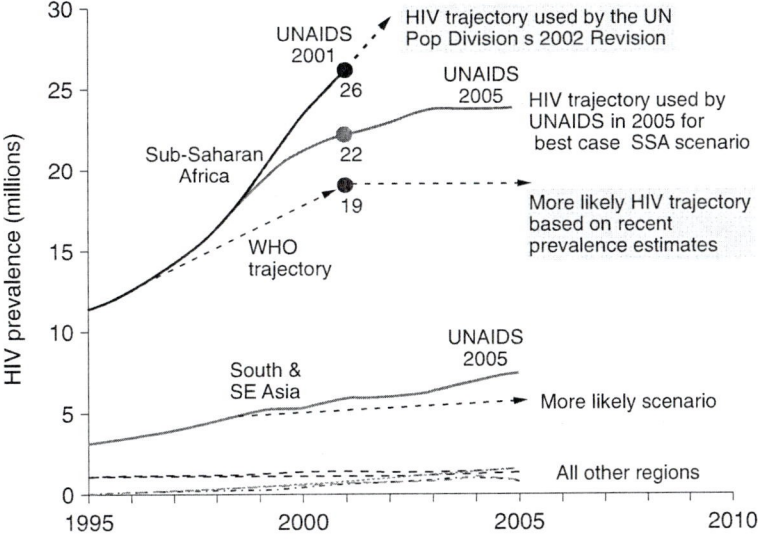

Figure 7.5 Estimated regional HIV prevalence numbers – 1995–2005.

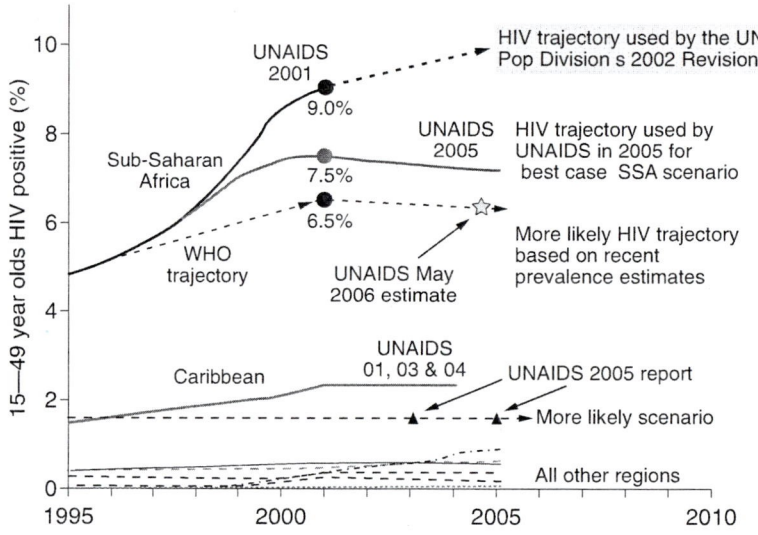

Figure 7.6 Estimated regional HIV prevalence rates – 1995–2005.

Estimation and Projection of HIV Prevalence in Selected Asian Countries

Five Asian countries were selected by UNAIDS for HIV/AIDS modeling. They included the three countries that had estimated HIV prevalence of more than 1 percent – Cambodia, Thailand, and Myanmar – and the two largest countries in the world, India and China. The latter two countries were selected because of their sheer size and the fact that even low increases in HIV infection rates in either country translate into millions of infected persons. In Asia during the past decade, estimation of national HIV prevalence has been carried out by a variety of agencies and methods. Many countries, with the support of donor agencies, have organized national meetings and workshops to develop national prevalence estimates. These national meetings have usually included a group of national experts, along with some external consultants,* to review all available HIV/AIDS data.

Figure 7.7A presents unadjusted national prevalence estimates for the five Asian countries selected. The methodology and assumptions used for estimation of national HIV prevalence in these countries have been evolving and changing, as the epidemiology of HIV in the region is better understood and as the quality of surveillance data has been improving. All the national annual HIV prevalence estimates, except for China, are shown as dotted or dashed lines and are unadjusted prevalence curves. The official Chinese prevalence estimates are shown as the dark bars at the bottom of the figure.

---

* I have been directly involved with national estimation meetings/workshops in all of these countries although as of late-2006 I have never been shown any of China's HIV data.

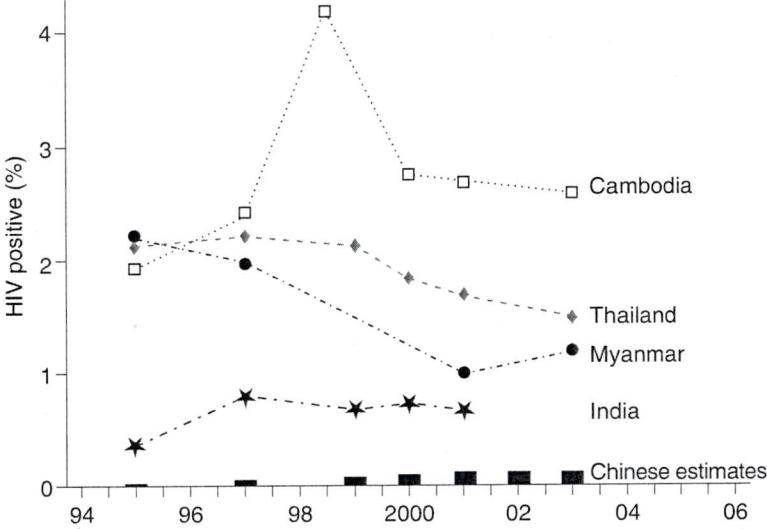

Figure 7.7A Unadjusted HIV prevalence estimates in selected Asian countries.

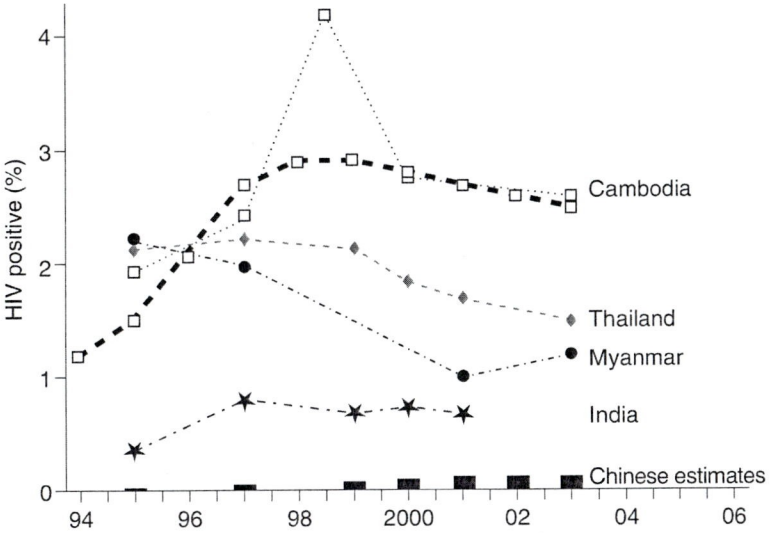

Figure 7.7B Unadjusted and an adjusted HIV prevalence estimate in selected Asian countries.

In Figure 7.7B, UNAIDS prepared an "adjusted" HIV prevalence curve for Cambodia (the thicker dashed line) by using the most recent HIV surveillance data to "fit" and back-calculate a prevalence curve. They assumed that, compared with previous years, the most recent data were more accurate. The adjusted HIV prevalence curve for Cambodia was smoothed with the use of a curve-fitting model and the highest unadjusted annual prevalence in 1999 (over 4 percent) was reduced to less than 3 percent to provide a better fit with the decreasing prevalence trend in recent years.

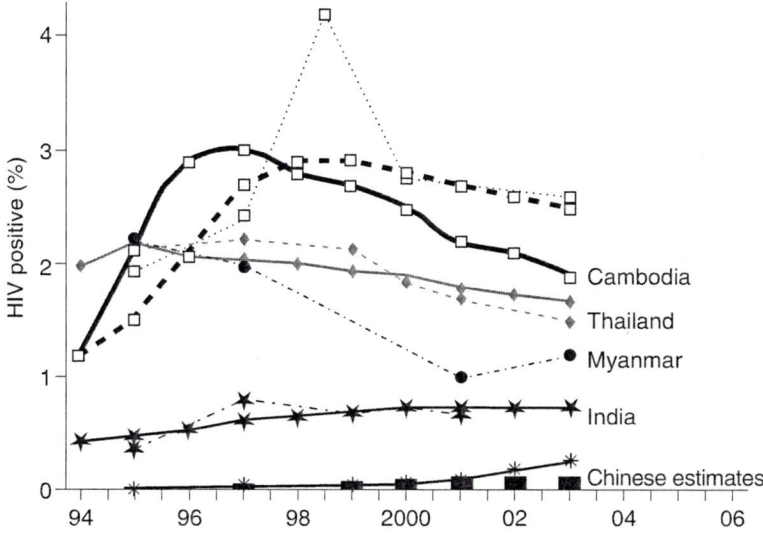

Figure 7.7C Adjusted HIV prevalence estimates in selected Asian countries.

UNAIDS developed adjusted or modeled HIV prevalence curves for all these countries except Myanmar. The Myanmar prevalence curve was not "adjusted" but will require adjustment because the most recent prevalence estimate was derived by using urban and rural ANC data, while previous estimates were derived by using only urban ANC data. HIV prevalence in India appears to have peaked in 1997 and has remained steady at the same general level since 1999. However, India is a very large country with marked heterogeneity in the patterns and prevalence of HIV risk behaviors in individual states. UNAIDS elected not to make a specific prevalence estimate for India in 2003 but prepared a minimum/maximum range for 2003. UNAIDS used the official Chinese estimates up through the year 2001 to fit an HIV epidemic curve. It also should be noted that the most recent HIV prevalence estimate for Cambodia in 2003 was 1.9 percent and either UNAIDS and/or the national AIDS program in Cambodia has readjusted the HIV prevalence curve according as shown in Figure 7.7C. The most recent estimate for Cambodia indicates that prior estimates were grossly overestimated.

For both Cambodia and Thailand, the prevalence trends have clearly been decreasing starting around the mid-1990s. The prevalence trend for India appears to be level starting in the late 1990s and the official Chinese estimates have remained low over the past decade and have not increased significantly as the UNAIDS modeled curve projects. As mentioned above, it is difficult to estimate the prevalence trend in Myanmar because of the marked changes in the ANC data used for estimation. **From these estimated trends, there are no indications of any expanding HIV epidemics in any of these Asian countries.**

At the end of 2005, the Chinese AIDS program updated their 2003 national HIV prevalence estimate of 840 000. Using the most recent data and the recommended UNAIDS spreadsheet method for estimating national HIV prevalence they came up with an estimate of 650 000 that was significantly lower than the 2003 estimate. Since this most recent estimate was carried out as objectively as possible with the most recent data it is considered more accurate compared to the

2003 estimate – that may have been an overestimate. Nevertheless, the Chinese AIDS program was severely criticized by an American AIDS "expert" and many NGOs working on AIDS in China, who were convinced that the Chinese government was deliberately reducing their national HIV prevalence to minimize a very severe national problem. Most NGOs, who do not know how the latest Chinese estimate was made, have automatically rejected the latest estimate. When told that the estimate was made as a collaborative effort of several external agencies and staff that included UNAIDS, WHO, CDC (Atlanta), working with local and national AIDS workers and did not rely much on reported HIV or AIDS cases, most of these NGOs are still skeptical since UNAIDS and the Global Fund have been projecting huge HIV prevalence increases for China.

Similarly, in 2005, Richard Feachem, the executive director of the Global Fund for AIDS, Tuberculosis and Malaria, was quite critical and skeptical of the Indian prevalence estimate of about 5 million that he considered to be much too low. I have been involved with several Indian meetings for development of their national HIV prevalence estimate, and I can attest to the openness and collegial atmosphere in all these meetings. I know that there has not been any deliberate bias or manipulation of data to minimize the Indian HIV prevalence estimate. To the contrary, I'm convinced that rather than underestimating HIV prevalence, some of the Indian assumptions used for estimating HIV ratios have resulted in an overestimation.

Epidemiologic Significance of Current HIV Prevalence Trends

All infectious disease epidemics can be divided into different phases or stages such as:

1 early, when epidemic transmission (R_0 >1) gets started and incidence of new infections are increasing
2 mid or peak when the rate of increase of new infections slows and reaches a peak level and
3 when the incidence of new infections begin to decrease after reaching the highest or peak level.

For a simple or "classical" infectious disease agent like a pandemic influenza virus there is virtually no difference in the incidence and prevalence of influenza infection and disease since the time from infection to disease and then recovery or death is usually very short, within days or weeks or at most within a few months. For HIV/AIDS, the epidemic curves are more complex because of the long interval from HIV infection to the development of AIDS and then death. The median[*] interval from HIV infection to AIDS in adults has been accepted to be about 7–8 years, and in the absence of effective anti-retroviral treatment (ART), the median time from AIDS to death is about a year or less.

For epidemics of simple infectious diseases, there is usually no question about when infection and disease peak and decline. But, for HIV/AIDS we need to

---

[*] The median interval is when half of HIV-infected persons develop AIDS – some will develop AIDS within a few years, others may take more than a decade, but half will develop AIDS within 7–8 years.

identify the peak rate and peak number of new HIV infections (HIV incidence), the peak rate and peak number of persons living with HIV (i.e., HIV prevalence), as well as the peak numbers of AIDS cases and deaths. One of the UN Millennium Development Goals is to "halt and reverse the spread of AIDS by 2015" but it is not clear to me what this means. As I will explain below, based on UNAIDS estimates of decreasing HIV *prevalence rates* in SSA starting about 2001, the annual HIV *incidence rate* had to have peaked in the mid-1990s. Thus, HIV transmission in SSA "turned the corner" about a decade ago and if reversal of HIV transmission can be considered the same as "reverse the spread of AIDS," then this goal was met about a decade ago.

My analysis of global HIV incidence and prevalence trends indicate that HIV incidence of new infections and prevalence of persons living with HIV infection peaked at different times in different HIV epidemics in different global regions. The reasons for these differences include: the time HIV was introduced into a population or area; the time epidemic HIV transmission may have started; and the primary mode of HIV transmission in a specific epidemic. Explosive HIV epidemics have occurred in MSM, IDU and in FSW in large sex or drug networks.[*] In most developed countries annual HIV *incidence* in MSM and IDU epidemics peaked by the mid-1980s; HIV *prevalence* peaked by the late 1980s to the early 1990s; and annual *AIDS cases and deaths* peaked by the mid-1990s. However, HIV prevalence in developed countries has not been decreasing during the past decade primarily because of the advent in the mid-1990s of relatively effective anti-retroviral treatment (ART) that has prolonged the life expectancy of infected persons. In the Caribbean and Latin America, HIV prevalence peaked prior to the mid-1990s and has been stable or level since then. In SSA, epidemic heterosexual HIV transmission within mostly small (usually less than a dozen persons) but overlapping sex networks has spread much more slowly compared to the explosive epidemics in MSM, IDU, and large brothel-based epidemics in several Asian populations. In some SSA countries annual HIV incidence has taken several decades to finally peak.

As described in Chapter 6, EPIMODEL was designed to calculate annual AIDS deaths based on HIV prevalence trends estimated from HIV data. EPIMODEL uses annual progression rates from HIV infection to AIDS to back-calculate the annual number of HIV infections (annual HIV cohorts) and annual AIDS deaths that are needed to "fit" a specific HIV prevalence curve. The HIV scenario I selected for modeling HIV/AIDS in SSA to estimate when HIV incidence and prevalence may have peaked is the scenario I consider the most likely based on the most recent HIV data and trends. This scenario has the HIV prevalence rate in SSA peaking at about 6.5 percent in the 15–49 year old population in the year 2000 and decreasing to 6.15 percent in 2005. The December 2005 UNAIDS estimates of the HIV prevalence rate in SSA had a peak in 2001 at 7.6 percent, declining to 7.2 percent in 2005. As described earlier in this chapter, I believe that UNAIDS overestimated HIV prevalence in SSA by at least 25 percent and that is why I used a prevalence peak of 6.5 percent rather than the December 2005 UNAIDS peak of 7.6 percent in 2001. In mid-2006, UNAIDS further revised its estimate of HIV prevalence in SSA from 7.2 percent in 2005 to

---

[*] Networks in this context refer to risk sharing groups of persons. Networks can be as small as 3–4 persons and as large as thousands.

6.1 percent which is almost exactly what I had estimated the prevalence rate to be in 2005. Figure 7.8 presents the modeled annual HIV incidence rates and numbers, annual AIDS deaths, and HIV prevalence rate and numbers in SSA for the lower HIV scenario (6.5 percent in 2000 and 6.15 percent in 2005) or what I consider the more likely HIV scenario.

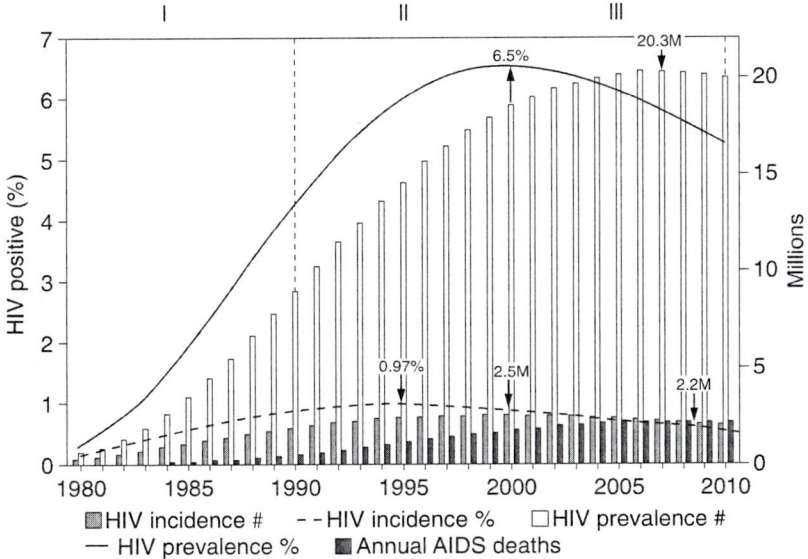

Figure 7.8 The most likely HIV/AIDS scenario in sub-Saharan Africa.

Figure 7.8 is very detailed, but can be readily understood if we focus on this figure by 10 year periods: (I), from 1980 to 1989; (II), from 1990 to 1999; and (III), from 2000 to 2009. The *annual HIV incidence rate* is shown in the lower part of the figure as a dashed line and the *HIV prevalence rate* is shown as a solid line at the top of the figure. *Annual HIV incident numbers* are the small light shaded bars, *prevalent numbers* of persons living with an HIV infection are the tall bars, and *annual AIDS deaths* are the small dark shaded bars. According to this modeled scenario, epidemic HIV transmission started sometimes around the mid-1970s, and by 1980 there were close to a half million African adults living with HIV (prevalence) but very few (about 4000) AIDS deaths. Remember, from HIV infection to AIDS and then death averages close to a decade. Thus, most of the persons infected from 1975 and after would not be dying from AIDS in any large numbers until about 1985 and after, and this is what is seen in Figure 7.8.

During the 1980s, the annual HIV incidence rates and annual HIV incident numbers are steadily increasing and by 1989, the HIV prevalence rate is close to 4 percent and the number of adults living with an HIV infection (prevalence number) is close to 8 million. During the 1990s, the rate of increase of the annual HIV incidence rate (the lower curve) begins to slow and reaches a peak level (0.97 percent) by 1995. The annual numbers of new HIV infections continued to increase after 1995 and do not reach its peak level (about 2.5 million) until the year 2000. The reason why there is this time difference between the peak annual HIV incidence rate from the peak annual incident number is due to the large annual population growth rate in SSA that averages close to 3 percent.[*] It should be noted that during the 1990s, annual AIDS deaths steadily increased from about a half million in 1990 to close to a million in the year 2000. Also, in the year 2000, the HIV prevalence rate peaked at 6.5 percent (19 million prevalent HIV infections). Although the HIV prevalence rate peaked around the year 2000 at about the same time that annual HIV incidence numbers peaked, the number of persons living with an HIV infection is not projected to peak until 2007 about the time when the annual number of AIDS deaths begin to exceed the annual incidence of HIV infections. The numbers of annual new HIV infections (incidence) and annual AIDS deaths explain why HIV prevalence (the number of persons living with an HIV infection) keeps increasing – until the cumulative number of annual AIDS deaths begin to "catch up" to and exceed the cumulative number of new HIV infections.

It needs to be emphasized that the annual HIV incidence rate in SSA would have had to have peaked in the mid-1990s, even if the December 2005 UNAIDS estimate of HIV prevalence of 7.6 percent in 2001 and 7.2 percent in 2005 were accepted and modeled. Thus, I find it difficult to understand how in its December 2005 report, UNAIDS could project an increasing annual HIV incidence in SSA up through 2020 – from about 2.5 million in 2003 to close to about 3.5 in 2020. This is simply not possible if the HIV prevalence rate in SSA has been decreasing since the new millennium! These observations will be reviewed again at the end of the next chapter when UNAIDS' "baseline" HIV scenario of an ever-increasing annual HIV incidence is used to project the numbers of HIV infections that might be prevented over the next 20 years by more intensive and aggressive prevention and treatment programs.

During the remainder of this decade, anti-HIV drug treatment programs (ART) in SSA are not expected to have a significant impact on keeping large numbers of HIV-infected persons from dying from AIDS, but hopefully by the next decade, the impact of ART programs will have to be taken into account when estimating HIV prevalence in this region. Thus, UNAIDS is correct that, as of 2006, the numbers of persons living with HIV in SSA continue to be increasing to record highs. However, this is very misleading because HIV epidemics in SSA began to "turn the corner" when annual HIV incidence rates peaked in the mid-1990s and began to decrease. The decreasing HIV incidence rate in SSA since 1995 can be considered as the beginning of the reversal of HIV transmission rates. The continued increase in the numbers of persons living with HIV in SSA is due to the annual increase in population growth and to the median 8–9 year interval from HIV infection to the development of AIDS and death.

According to these modeling results, HIV prevalent numbers will peak in SSA within a few years before 2010 – more than a decade after annual HIV incidence rates peaked. Thus, regardless of what the definition of halting and reversing the spread of AIDS by 2015 may be, it seems certain to me that this goal has already been achieved or will be achieved by the end of this decade. UNAIDS will be "riding to glory" on the downslopes of all the HIV/AIDS curves.

---

[*] A one percent annual HIV incidence in a population of 100 000 results in 1000 new HIV infections. If the population growth rate is 3 percent, then next year if HIV incidence had peaked and drops to 0.98 percent, then calculation of annual HIV incidence is 0.98 percent times 103 000 for an annual incidence of 1009, etc., etc.

Does this mean that the AIDS pandemic is over? Absolutely not! The TB pandemic must have peaked in different global regions at different times, but the annual toll of TB has kept this disease among the leading causes of global deaths for centuries. For the AIDS pandemic it does mean that the highest annual global incidence of HIV infections has peaked and the annual number of AIDS deaths will also soon peak. Nevertheless, in Africa and Asia, annual AIDS deaths will continue to be at least a couple of million for several decades. In addition, annual HIV incidence in those populations where significant epidemic HIV transmission has occurred will continue to be unacceptably high. In SSA, at least 1 to 2 million new HIV infections can be expected annually for at least another decade or two.

All UNAIDS press releases and reports, as of late 2005, said that the AIDS pandemic was constantly growing and ever-expanding. In mid-2006, UNAIDS finally acknowledged that global HIV incidence probably peaked during the late 1990s. However, the urgent public health need to prevent millions of new HIV infections that are still occurring annually and the need to provide anti-HIV treatment to millions of HIV-infected persons who become eligible to receive such treatment each year requires that current global support of HIV/AIDS prevention and treatment programs be significantly *increased* rather than *decreased*.

Summary and Conclusions

Estimation and projection of HIV infections and AIDS cases and deaths (HIV/AIDS) can be considered more of an art than a science because of the marked limitations of both available data and methods for estimation and projection. These limitations make it possible for UNAIDS and other AIDS program advocates and activists to issue misleading and inflated estimates and projections. For example, in mid-2005 UNAIDS issued a press release on the status of the AIDS pandemic that declared that there was a "quantum worsening in the [HIV] epidemic's trajectory." However, according to UNAIDS' own prevalence estimates through the year 2005, there is a clear trend of leveling or slightly decreasing HIV prevalence rates in SSA and most other global regions. There is not a marked increase in HIV prevalence except for a few countries where HIV epidemics in IDU populations have continued almost unabated. Even in these latter countries, annual HIV incidence probably peaked several years ago. UNAIDS finally acknowledged in mid-2006 that global HIV incidence probably peaked during the late 1990s.

Because HIV prevalence estimates can have a wide plausible range of values, official estimates can be selected to minimize or maximize HIV numbers. In most developing countries there was initially an almost uniform policy that denied high HIV prevalence. In recent years however, there has been a tendency for some developing countries to uncritically accept high HIV prevalence estimates to facilitate receipt of donor support for their AIDS programs. Many countries in SSA and the Caribbean region have, in recent years, carried out population-based HIV surveys that indicate HIV prevalence has been overestimated on average by about 50 percent. HIV prevalence estimates probably remain too high in those SSA countries where population-based surveys have not been carried out and are also probably too high in most Eastern European and Asian countries.

HIV prevalence estimates made by staff of GPA/WHO from the late 1980s up to about the mid-1990s were intentionally conservative. HIV prevalence estimates made or accepted by UNAIDS since the late 1990s have been overestimated. As of early 2006, many prevalence estimates compiled by UNAIDS/WHO remain on the high side. In mid-2006, UNAIDS reduced its adult HIV prevalence estimate in SSA to a more realistic level. A good general rule to follow regarding estimation of HIV prevalence is to be conservative and to use the lower range of any estimate that can be supported with available data. This is the prudent option for public health programs because of the marked limitations of available data and methods used for HIV or AIDS estimation. Furthermore, if a relatively high estimate is made and surveillance data subsequently collected indicate that the previous estimate was too high, it is difficult and confusing to the public and policy makers to reduce the prevalence estimate significantly as UNAIDS has had to do during the past few years.

However, refusal to acknowledge that a prevalence estimate is too high can lead AIDS programs to continue to increase official HIV prevalence estimates falsely year after year to avoid such embarrassment. This is the situation that several developing countries currently find themselves in. It is far easier to revise official HIV prevalence estimates upwards based on new and additional data than to try to defend a high prevalence estimate that cannot be supported by the available data. It is unfortunate that any reduction of an HIV prevalence estimate, even if it is justified based on available data, is considered an attack on, or denial of, the tremendous severity of the AIDS pandemic.

In recent years, UNAIDS has been providing high and low estimates, with a wide range when there may be less certainty of the data used to derive the estimates. However, both high and low estimates are rarely referred to or used. In fact, many news reports or articles by AIDS program advocates use only the high estimate based on their perception that all official estimates are deliberately made too low. In mid-2006, UNAIDS finally accepted lower HIV prevalence estimates for many SSA and Caribbean countries based on population based serosurveys. Nevertheless, the public and policy makers must realize that at least 1 to 2 million new HIV infections (annual incidence) can be expected in SSA for at least another decade or two or until behavior change programs become more successful in modifying and reducing high risk sex behaviors. Unrealistically high HIV prevalence estimates or projections in countries such as China and India will within a few years be exposed as, at best, naïve efforts of well meaning AIDS program advocates and at worst as the work of AIDS "experts" who ignore or deny the leveling or decreasing global HIV prevalence trends to support their own political, social, economic, or personal agendas.

Chapter 8

HIV/AIDS Prevention

During the latter half of the past century, public health programs played a major role in preventing and controlling most major infectious diseases in developed countries, but have been far less effective in developing countries. Much of this success can be attributed to improved environmental sanitation and standards of living. The advent of antibiotics during the 1940s for prevention and treatment of bacterial infections along with the development of effective vaccines for the prevention of almost all severe childhood infectious diseases during the 1950s and 1960s played major roles in this success. However, the public health track record for prevention and control of diseases primarily attributed to human behaviors, such as sexually transmitted diseases (STD), continues to be poor. Prior to the advent of the AIDS pandemic, public health prevention and control of STD had been directed to secondary and tertiary prevention rather than primary prevention.* This was so because most STD physicians were primarily clinicians who were comfortable and competent in the diagnosis and treatment of STD but had little or no expertise in eliminating or reducing sexual risk behaviors.

As of late-2006, the recognized phase of the AIDS pandemic is about a quarter of a century old. During this time, HIV has spread to every country in the world. Primary HIV prevention programs have been carried out by AIDS programs throughout the world over the past two decades with only limited success. Explosive HIV epidemics in IDU populations continue to occur. Prevention of epidemic sexual HIV transmission has been more successful with the 100 percent condom program for commercial sex. However, little progress has been made in the prevention of transmission from HIV-infected persons (regardless of how they acquired their infection) to their regular sex partners. This latter pattern is now the predominant mode of HIV transmission throughout the world. This chapter describes:

1 primary HIV preventive measures and the major issues associated with these public health interventions and
2 problems of measuring and evaluating the success of HIV/AIDS programs in reducing HIV incidence and prevalence.

Primary HIV Prevention

Preventing HIV transmission requires an awareness of transmission dynamics that were described in Chapter 5 and are summarized in Figure 8.1.

---

* *Primary prevention* is preventing or reducing the risk of infection; *secondary prevention* involves identification and treatment of infected persons who may still be asymptomatic; and *tertiary prevention* involves treatment of infected persons who have severe disease manifestations.

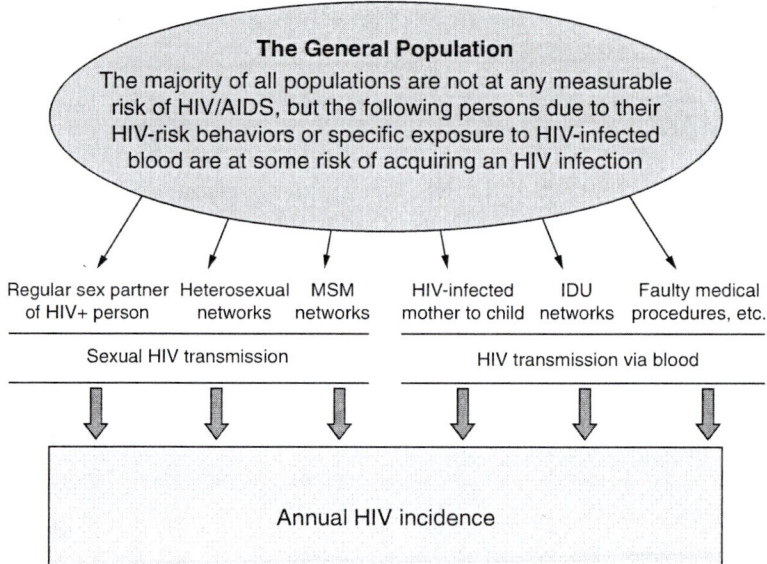

Figure 8.1 HIV transmission.

The patterns and prevalence of each of the above modes of HIV transmission differ between different countries and regions. For example in SSA countries, heterosexual transmission predominates and the numbers of mother to infant transmission and transmission within healthcare settings are the highest in the world. In most developed countries, HIV transmission within MSM and IDU networks[*] predominate and transmission within healthcare settings is rare. However, transmission from an HIV-infected person (regardless of how infection was acquired) to a regular sex partner is, as of late-2006, the predominant mode of HIV transmission in most populations throughout the world. These differences in the patterns and prevalence of these modes of transmission should not be interpreted to imply that specific programs directed to each mode of transmission are not needed in all regions and countries. MSM and IDU networks should be considered to be present in all regions and countries. The specific behavioral patterns and size of these sex and injecting drug networks have not yet been adequately described in most SSA populations primarily because they are overshadowed by the preponderance of heterosexual transmission.

HIV/AIDS programs need to develop specific public health interventions for each of these modes of transmission based on local surveillance data on the patterns and prevalence of these risk factors and risk behaviors. In addition, all HIV/AIDS programs must be aware that nonepidemic sexual transmission (from infected persons to their regular sex partners) will occur regardless of whether or not epidemic transmission has occurred.

The following section provides a more detailed description of primary prevention measures and associated issues for each route of HIV transmission.

---

[*] Networks are groups of persons who share HIV risk with others in their network. A network can be as small as 3 or 4 persons who share sex partners and as large as hundreds or thousands sharing drug injecting equipment.

Mother to Child HIV Transmission

Until the early 1990s, no effective measures were available for prevention of mother to child transmission (MTCT)[*] other than to prevent HIV infections in females. Without public health intervention, about 15–30 percent of infants born to HIV positive women will be infected during pregnancy and delivery and an additional 10–20 percent will be infected through breastfeeding. The use of effective drugs for the prevention of MTCT during the 1990s along with the recommendation that infected mothers avoid breastfeeding have resulted in dramatic reductions and almost elimination of MTCT in most developed countries. However, in most resource-poor countries routine MTCT prevention programs have not been developed, primarily due to lack of funds and trained public health and medical staff. As a result, MTCT remains a major problem in most developing countries, especially in SSA, where as of 2006 at least a half million infants are infected by their mothers annually.

Prevention of MTCT requires:

1 prevention of HIV infection in females of reproductive age
2 prevention of pregnancy in infected females
3 identification of infected pregnant women via routine HIV screening of all ANC attendees
4 provision of anti-HIV drugs to the infected mother prior to delivery and/or to the infant immediately after birth and
5 routine avoidance of breastfeeding by infected mothers.

In developed countries the recommended treatment regimen for preventing MTCT is triple combination therapy that includes AZT: this treatment is effective not only for preventing MTCT but for treating the mother's infection as well. In most resource-poor countries, this recommended treatment is too expensive. Thus MTCT prevention programs have had to resort to short course treatment regimes with inexpensive drugs such as AZT or nevirapine that, although relatively effective, are not as effective as the full prevention regime routinely provided in developed countries. However, until money is no longer an issue for prevention programs in developing countries, even less-than-optimal treatment is better than nothing. Furthermore, until all HIV-infected mothers and fathers in developing countries are routinely provided with triple combination therapy, those infants born to infected mothers who escape infection are doomed to become AIDS orphans. Some progress has been made in the support and development of programs for the prevention of MTCT in developing countries, but MTCT will, much to the shame of international health donors, continue to be a major problem in most SSA countries for the foreseeable future.

HIV Transmission in Healthcare Settings

The initial short doubling time of reported AIDS cases in the early 1980s generated tremendous concern about the potential infectiousness of the causative agent of this emerging disease. Pictures on the front page of newspapers showed

---

[*] It would be more epidemiologically correct to refer to father to mother to child transmission (FMTCT).

healthcare providers in "space-like" suits, helmets and breathing masks to prevent any possible exposure to the unknown but presumed highly infectious agent. We now know that HIV is transmitted via the exchange of blood and sexual secretions such as semen and relatively large amounts of infected blood are usually required for transmission. Studies have shown that transfusion of a pint of infected blood will transmit infection to over 90 percent of recipients while accidental punctures with a needle used on an AIDS patient have resulted in HIV infection in only about 3 of 1000 such accidents.

The first AIDS case related to blood transfusion was reported in late 1982, a little more than a year after the initial report of AIDS in June 1981. It is not clear exactly when most public health agencies and blood banks accepted the fact that the AIDS agent could be efficiently transmitted via blood. But virtually all blood banks throughout the US had accepted that view by 1985. In March 1985 an antibody test for HIV became routinely available in the USA. Prior to that time, prevention of HIV transmission via blood transfusion was accomplished through an inefficient and non-standardized system of voluntary blood donor deferral. Some blood banks instituted strict donor deferral procedures by 1983 or 1984: others not totally convinced that the causative agent of AIDS could be transmitted via blood dragged their feet before instituting a donor deferral system to reduce the number of persons with specific risk behaviors associated with AIDS from donating blood. These latter blood banks paid dearly for delays in instituting strict donor deferral systems. They were sued by blood recipients whose HIV infections were attributed to blood they received. In some developed countries, routine HIV testing of donated blood was not immediately implemented when HIV antibody testing became available by mid 1985 for a variety of reasons. These delays subsequently led to criminal investigations in Canada, France, Germany, Switzerland, and Japan.

As of 2006, over 14 000 persons in the USA have been diagnosed with AIDS after receiving HIV-infected blood or blood products. Almost all of these cases were due to blood transfused before March 1985. This 14 000 is a minimal number of infections since about half of all transfused patients die within 6 months after transfusion from the underlying disease/condition that necessitated the transfusion. Thus, the actual number of HIV infections transmitted via blood transfusion in the USA from about 1980 to 1985 was probably closer to 25 000.

As a result of standardized voluntary deferral of blood donors at risk for HIV infection and routine HIV testing of all blood donations, HIV transmission via blood transfusion has become very rare in the USA. However, infected blood donated by an HIV-infected person who is in the "window period" (the period when the virus is present in blood but HIV antibodies have not yet appeared) continues to be a public health problem. The risk of HIV transmission per unit of blood transfused in the USA in 1995 was about 1 in a half million; by 2003, this risk was reduced to about 1 in 1.5 million due to newer tests that significantly reduced the window period from about 22 days to 11 days.

The success in almost eliminating HIV transmission via blood transfusion in most developed countries stands in marked contrast to the situation in many developing countries. This is especially true in SSA, where blood for transfusion is still not routinely tested for HIV except in major medical facilities in capital cities. As of 2006, transfusions are estimated to account for about 100 000 or more HIV infections annually – with over 90 percent in SSA countries where HIV prevalence in blood donor populations can be as high as 50 percent in many urban areas and HIV testing capabilities remain limited.

In 1987, CDC (Atlanta) issued a set of recommendations for prevention of HIV and other blood-borne agents when providing medical care in or out of medical settings. Under these "universal precautions," blood and certain body fluids of all patients are considered infectious for blood-borne pathogens, including HIV. Universal precautions involve the use of protective barriers – such as gloves, gowns, aprons, masks, or protective eyewear – that can reduce the risk of exposure from potentially infectious materials to the care provider's skin or mucous membranes. In addition, universal precautions recommend that all healthcare providers (teachers in schools and persons giving first aid in any community or home setting) take precautions to prevent injuries caused by needles, or any sharp instruments or objects. Strict adherence to universal precautions has significantly reduced care providers' exposure to HIV and other blood-borne agents in most developed countries. But again, the situation in many developing countries has not been as good. There are no reliable data or estimates on how many HIV infections may be transmitted in healthcare situations in developed versus developing countries. The annual number of such infections in developed countries is probably less than 100 due to low HIV prevalence in the population and good adherence to universal precautions – especially in healthcare facilities. In SSA, if transfusion associated infections are excluded; annual infections among care providers are probably at least several thousand due to the high prevalence of HIV in most SSA populations and to the poorer adherence to universal precautions.

As described in Chapter 5, thousands of hemophilia patients in many countries throughout the world received HIV-infected blood products in the early-to-mid 1980s. This mode of transmission has not been a problem since the mid-to-late 1980s, when manufacturing methods were changed to make these products safe. Extensive transmission associated with HIV contaminated plasma collection equipment was documented in Mexico during the mid-1980s and in China up to about the mid-1990s. It has been estimated that the Mexican problem may have involved hundreds of persons while the Chinese problem was more extensive and may have infected several hundred thousand persons. Hospital or medically acquired HIV infections due to reuse of injection equipment or to administration of small amounts of blood or serum for medical treatment of infants and children have been documented in Russia, Romania and more recently possibly in Libya. These latter problems can be completely eliminated by improved medical education and support to help healthcare providers in developing countries adhere strictly to universal precautions.

HIV Transmission in Injecting Drug Users Who Routinely Share Injecting Equipment

The global war on drugs clearly has not been successful: illicit drug use has been increasing in many populations throughout the world during the past two decades. This increase in drug use, especially in injecting drug use, has coincided with the global spread of HIV. In whatever population HIV may be present and increasing, the potential for HIV to be introduced to injecting drug users and their networks increases. Slow or rapid HIV epidemic spread can be expected after introduction of HIV into any specific IDU network. The rapidity of spread will depend on the extent of sharing injection equipment, size of the sharing IDU networks and the extent of overlap between different IDU networks. As of late-2006, there have been more than 100 documented HIV epidemics in IDU networks throughout the world.

Primary prevention of HIV transmission in IDU populations is conceptually simple and straightforward. If the war on drugs were successful, there would not be ample supplies of illicit drugs for injection. However, such drugs are now cheaper and more available than ever before. During the past decade inflation-adjusted prices for heroin and cocaine in Western Europe were cut by half and global levels of drug abuse have risen persistently. The UN's own report *Global Illicit Drug Trends 2003* reveals that of the 92 countries reporting to the UN in 2001, the vast majority (85 percent) reported that drug abuse had either remained the same or had risen. The stark reality is that injecting drug use is epidemic in many countries. HIV and other blood-borne pathogens are being efficiently transmitted via the sharing of needles and syringes in a varying proportion of IDU. IDU is estimated to account for at least 5 percent of the global total of HIV infections. In some countries – Russia, Indonesia, Malaysia, China, Iran, Nepal, Pakistan and Vietnam – infections in IDU comprise a large percent of total HIV prevalence.

HIV is transmitted among IDU by the sharing of drug injecting equipment and not by the injection of drugs *per se*. Thus, public health programs need to identify and focus harm reduction measures on IDU who routinely share needles and syringes. From the public health perspective, if injecting drug use cannot be stopped, then at least transmission of blood-borne pathogens can and should be prevented by safer injection practices. Harm reduction for IDU means that "clean" injection equipment should always be used rather than sharing potentially contaminated needles and syringes with others. Public health recommendations for harm reduction measures such as not sharing injection equipment, needle exchange programs, etc., have met with resistance from many if not most policy makers, religious leaders, and law enforcement agencies since IDU is unaccepted social behavior and is illegal in virtually all countries. Thus, there has been and continues to be significant tension and opposition to public health harm reduction measures for IDU. Instead of being supportive of harm reduction measures there is usually an emphasis on prohibition and criminalization of IDU in most countries. Until such official opposition to harm reduction measures can be overcome, HIV incidence and prevalence in most IDU populations throughout the world will continue to be unacceptably high.

HIV Transmission in MSM with Multiple and Concurrent Sex Partners

Organized gay* empowerment movements emerged during the 1960s and 1970s in major cities in the USA and Europe. These movements coincided with the heterosexual revolution in most Western countries that were more

---

* Gay is a US term for homosexual males or the more politically correct terminology of MSM (men who have sex with men), and is not commonly used in other parts of the world, such as in Asia.

accepting of greater sexual freedom. However, the sexual revolution and gay empowerment movements also coincided with the introduction of HIV into several gay populations during the 1970s. Thus, along with major increases in the numbers of gay men flocking to cities such as SF, NY, London, etc., there was also a marked increase in sexual risk behaviors among MSM. The development of gay bathhouses where sex contact with many different partners during a single visit was routine created a perfect setting for transmission of sexually transmitted infections (STI). Once HIV was introduced into such a venue, explosive spread occurred. In a cohort of MSM who had blood samples collected because they were enrolled in a hepatitis B vaccine study, HIV prevalence rose from 1 percent in 1980 to 25 percent in 1982 to 65 percent in 1984. With increasing global mobility (jet travel) that became increasingly available during the 1970s, HIV-infected MSM from major cities such as SF, NY, and London rapidly spread HIV to MSM networks in most other major cities throughout the world during the 1980s.

Primary HIV prevention in MSM populations must target those who have multiple and concurrent sex partners since MSM with this pattern of risk behavior have the highest risk of acquiring HIV. HIV incidence in most MSM populations has been reduced from the very high rates present during the initial epidemic phase in the late 1970s and early 1980s to much lower "endemic" levels. Most of the observed decreases in annual HIV incidence by the mid-1980s can be attributed to saturation of infection in those with the highest level of risk behaviors. How much of this decreasing incidence can be attributed to public health prevention programs is not clear and this question will be addressed in the next section of this chapter. However, annual HIV incidence rates in MSM populations are still unacceptably high and currently range from about 1 to 5 percent or higher. Recent studies in the MSM population in San Francisco indicate that annual HIV incidence may now be as low as 1 percent. This decrease in annual incidence may be in part attributable to the new social phenomenon of serosorting, i.e., selecting sex partners based on their known HIV status and the lower viral load of infected persons who are receiving anti-HIV drug treatment (highly active anti-retroviral treatment – HAART). However, even a "low" annual incidence rate of 1 percent (1/100) is still unacceptably high for a severe infectious agent such as HIV.

The MSM community and public health programs will need to work together to reduce annual HIV incidence in MSM populations throughout the world to as low a level as possible. In addition to behavior changes, such as reducing the number of sex partners and consistent use of condoms for penetrative sexual intercourse, much more can and should be done, to reduce the amount of blood or semen that is exchanged during MSM sex contacts.[*] The primary focus of public health prevention of sexual HIV transmission in MSM populations has been on those MSM with the highest number of sex partner exchanges, i.e., on a daily or weekly basis. However, it should be noted that the general patterns of sex partner exchange in MSM are identical to the patterns of heterosexual HIV transmission that are presented in the following section, but the proportion of MSM at the highest level of risk is much higher than in most heterosexual populations.

---

[*] Alternatives to anal sex for MSM can be found at: http://www.man2manalliance.org/

HIV Transmission in Heterosexual Populations

Primary prevention of heterosexual HIV transmission requires an understanding of the different patterns of sex partner exchange associated with different risks of transmission. These patterns and frequency of sex partner exchanges are summarized in Table 8.1.

Table 8.1 Risk of heterosexual HIV transmission based on number, frequency and pattern of sex partner exchange

Annual Number (Frequency of Exchange)	Pattern of Exchange	Annual Risk of HIV Transmission*	Example(s)
Up to 1000 or more (Daily)	Concurrent	Highest	Large brothel-based FSW
Up to several hundred (Daily to weekly)	Mostly concurrent	High	Direct and indirect FSW in small sex networks
Up to dozens (Weekly to monthly)	Mostly concurrent	Moderate to high	20–40% of adults in some SSA countries
Up to dozens (Monthly to annual)	Mostly serial	Low	Up to 20% of adults in Western countries
1 or none (No partner exchange)	Monogamous or abstinent	Zero or close to zero	Majority or large percent of all heterosexuals
Discordant HIV couples (No partner exchange for the uninfected partner)	**Uninfected partner is faithful**	**Annual risk (<10%) cumulative risk is close to 100%**	**Most regular sex partners of an HIV infected person**

* Risk of sexual HIV transmission is positively correlated with HIV prevalence and prevalence of facilitating factors for sexual transmission in specific sex networks. The prevalence of facilitating factors for sexual HIV transmission is positively correlated with the number of sex partners and frequency of sex partner exchange. Male circumcision is an independent protective factor.

Heterosexuals who have the highest annual risk of HIV are those who have almost daily sex partner exchange within large and open sex networks. FSW and their male clients, in large brothel-type establishments, are prime examples of this invariably epidemic pattern of sexual HIV transmission. Direct freelance sex workers plus indirect sex workers (bars, massage parlors, etc.) have fewer male clients annually but may still have sex partner exchanges daily or at least weekly. These FSW and their male clients are at high risk of infection depending on the prevalence of HIV within their sex network(s).

Heterosexuals who have unprotected sex with multiple and concurrent sex partners within smaller sex groupings or networks with some overlapping of these networks are at moderate to high risk of sexual HIV transmission. A varying proportion of different populations have this pattern of sex partner exchange. From 20 to 40 percent of sexually active adults (both males and females) in many SSA populations have this pattern of sex partner exchange but this pattern usually accounts for only a small percent (generally less than 10 percent) of adults in most other populations. In most general populations outside SSA, up to 20 percent of adolescents and adults have multiple but serial exchange of sex partners during their lifetime. The risk of epidemic sexual HIV transmission in populations with this pattern of sex partner exchange is low. When sex partner exchange is on a monthly or annual basis and the pattern of exchange is serial rather than concurrent, no epidemic HIV transmission can be expected.

Prevention of HIV transmission in heterosexuals, who have multiple sex partners, whether on a serial or concurrent basis, is the same and is conceptually simple and straightforward. There is the moralistic approach that declares such behaviors should be prohibited and further those who engage in such behaviors should be punished. If this moralistic approach (**A**bstain from premarital sex and **B**e faithful to one's marital partner) were successful there would be no need for public health risk reduction programs directed to persons who have multiple sex partners. The objectives of most faith-based organizations are different from HIV/AIDS programs. The primary objective of faith-based organizations is to help and support persons to refrain from sex outside of marriage, whereas the primary objective of public health programs is to prevent HIV transmission. Many faith-based organizations consider the provision of **C**ondoms for HIV prevention as condoning premarital and extramarital sex and so have actively opposed condom use for HIV prevention. Public health groups believe that sex workers must be educated about condoms and other preventive practices to lower the risk of HIV infection, but many faith-based organizations declare working with sex workers "perpetuates an inherently evil practice" by inadvertently supporting sex work.

Most public health organizations believe that HIV/AIDS prevention programs should include an appropriate balance of **A**bstain, **B**e faithful, and **C**ondom interventions (**ABC**). For those persons who routinely have multiple sex partners, the total package of **ABC** is needed. For prevention of transmission to an uninfected spouse only **A** or **C** are applicable. Public health professionals point out that it is not essential for every organization to promote all three elements: each can focus on the part(s) they are most comfortable supporting. While this seems a reasonable position, unfortunately some of the most rigidly righteous faith-based organizations do not support any condom use since they view this as supporting or, at the very least, condoning "sinful" behaviors.

In over a dozen SSA countries, where prevalence has, as of 2006, reached five percent or more of the 15–49 year old population, epidemic heterosexual HIV transmission initially accounted for the majority of infections, but nonepidemic heterosexual HIV transmission (from an HIV-infected person to his or her regular sex partner) has been steadily increasing and may now account for more than half of new HIV infections. Therefore, HIV prevention strategies in SSA countries need to be specifically developed to address both epidemic and nonepidemic sexual transmission. In SSA, both the explosive and non-explosive forms of epidemic (R_0 >1) sexual transmission are present. The non-explosive epidemic pattern in SSA consists of small (as small as 3 to 4 persons) sex networks. Education programs, including sex behavior change programs and provision of condoms to all persons who may engage in casual or commercial sex, especially adolescents and youth, have to be given the highest public health priority in SSA. In these high HIV prevalence countries, the primary prevention focus must be given to 10–19 year olds and a secondary focus on adults with the highest sex partner exchange rates. In addition, increased voluntary HIV testing and counseling (VTC) programs are needed to identify regular sex partners of HIV-infected persons to try to prevent "nonepidemic" sexual HIV transmission. Most faith-based organizations will support, or at least not actively oppose, condom use among HIV-discordant marital partners to prevent transmission. Finally, there are accumulating data to indicate that effective anti-HIV treatment (ART) can significantly reduce transmission in discordant couples because ART has the potential to reduce viral load dramatically. In this epidemiologic situation, ART can be considered a tertiary prevention measure for the infected partner and a primary prevention measure for the uninfected partner.

Countries with low HIV prevalence need to monitor closely all situations that tend to increase sexual risk behaviors. These situations include: commercial sex networks, border areas with extensive population movement, migration and/or travel away from stable social environments such as from rural to urban areas for employment, seasonal workers, migrant workers, military, sailors/merchant seamen, long distance truck drivers, large development or construction projects, etc. Primary HIV prevention programs need to target all of these vulnerable populations wherever they may be. In countries currently with low HIV prevalence, the primary prevention focus must be given to persons with the highest HIV risk behaviors to prevent the start of epidemic transmission. If epidemic transmission does not occur in heterosexuals who have the highest sex partner exchange rates then there is no reason to expect epidemic transmission to occur in heterosexuals with lower sex partner exchange rates. In addition to targeting persons with the highest sexual risk behaviors, increased VTC programs should be aggressively implemented to identify regular sex partners of HIV-infected persons to prevent "nonepidemic" sexual transmission.

In low prevalence countries, general HIV/AIDS education programs that focus on youth should be implemented only after targeted programs for persons with the highest HIV risk behaviors are adequately supported. From the epidemiologic perspective, the prohibition of all "sinful" sex is not required to prevent epidemic sexual HIV transmission. However, from the perspective of faith-based organizations the avoidance of premarital and extramarital sex is as vital in low HIV prevalence populations as it is in high prevalence populations.

Other Primary Prevention Measures

HIV/AIDS programs must consider all available public health or medical measures to reduce the risk of HIV transmission, regardless of whether or not epidemic HIV transmission has occurred. This involves, in addition to the **ABC** measures, the reduction or elimination of major facilitating factors such as other STI, especially ulcerative STI, and provision of male circumcision (MC) services. However, as of late-2006, adequate support for and development of STD treatment programs in most developing countries have not materialized to the extent warranted,[*] and

---

[*] There have been some studies that showed that reduction of STD had no significant effect on HIV transmission, but this might vary depending on whether the HIV epidemic was in its early or late stage.

UNAIDS is still calling for additional research on the pros and cons of MC as a public health intervention to reduce sexual HIV transmission. If routine MC programs had been aggressively developed in SSA a decade ago, it is conceivable that this simple measure could have prevented millions of HIV infections. Apparently, UNAIDS and other AIDS "experts" are awaiting the availability of an effective vaccine that would possibly be as effective as MC but the almost mythical HIV vaccine is constantly about a decade away.[*]

Microbicides, chemicals that can inactivate HIV and can be inserted in the vagina or rectum in the form of gels, creams, foams, or films were not, as of 2006, available. However, many are under active development while several are in late stage field testing and may become available within the next few years. If a microbicide as effective as MC in reducing sexual HIV transmission were to become available, it would provide women with a preventive option more under their control. The combined use of condoms, MC and possibly anti-HIV gels, etc., would be far more effective and less costly than any conceivable HIV vaccine might be. Moreover, even *if* an HIV vaccine were to be developed, all currently available measures for prevention of sexual HIV transmission (i.e., **ABC**, STD treatment, HAART treatment of the infected regular sex partner, MC, and possibly anti-HIV gels), could not and should not be eliminated or reduced. Thus, the program cost for use of an HIV vaccine will be added to the prevention budget and should not displace any of the primary prevention measures currently utilized or that may become available in the future. This is not to say that an HIV/AIDS vaccine should not be developed, but to point out that an effective HIV/AIDS vaccine, *if* and when one may become available, will not be the "magic bullet" that the public and policy makers are hoping for.

Two Different African HIV/AIDS Prevention Stories

The official positions taken on AIDS in Africa by the Presidents of Uganda and South Africa have been as different as the course of the HIV epidemics in these countries and have had significantly different impact on the development of HIV prevention programs.

Uganda

In 1986, President Museveni of Uganda was informed by Cuba's President Castro at a summit meeting of nonaligned countries in Harare, Zimbabwe of a major AIDS problem in the Ugandan military. Uganda had sent 60 soldiers to Cuba for military training and they were tested for HIV by the Cubans who found that 18 of the 60 soldiers (30 percent) were HIV positive. Upon being personally informed by Castro of this situation, President Museveni summoned his top health advisers and immediately had them begin developing a national AIDS prevention program that talked openly about AIDS and educated the public about its spread. The Ugandan program did not avoid talking about sexual risk behaviors – on the contrary it emphasized the need for responsible sexual behavior via their "zero

---

[*] Starting in 1984 when HIV was first isolated anyone who asked the question about when an AIDS vaccine might be available got the answer "In about a decade." The answer in late-2006 is still "In about a decade."

[sex] grazing" slogan. Condoms were also promoted for those who might continue with their risky sexual behaviors. HIV prevalence in Uganda has been reported to have decreased from a national high of 15 percent in the 15–49 year old population in 1992 to about 5 percent in 2005. As described later in this chapter in the Ugandan "success" story, most of this decrease in HIV prevalence has occurred after the forceful and balanced use of all the **ABC** interventions.

South Africa

During the 1990s, as major political and social changes were underway in South Africa, HIV spread steadily and was monitored by antenatal HIV testing. HIV prevalence in ANC attendees increased from 2.4 percent in 1992 to 24.5 percent in 2000. It is now abundantly clear that both former President Mandela and his successor in 1999, President Mbeki, did not give HIV/AIDS the attention and priority that it warranted. Former President Mandela has since acknowledged his mistake and is leading national efforts to develop HIV prevention and treatment programs. President Mbeki on the other hand, at the International AIDS conference in Durban in 2000, said that AIDS is a disease caused by poverty, not HIV. He set up a "scientific" group charged with evaluating the country's AIDS problem. His "scientific" advisors included "HIV/AIDS dissidents" such as Peter Duesberg, who believe that anti-HIV drugs such as AZT actually cause AIDS, and that lifestyle choices such as homosexuality or drug addicion can also cause AIDS. The best that can be said about President Mbeki and his Minister of Health is that they have been extremely unhelpful in developing adequate HIV education and prevention programs: they are now hindering rather than promoting anti-retroviral treatment (ART) programs. WHO, UNAIDS, and well meaning and respected social activists such as Paul Farmer, may have to assume some responsibility for the current abysmal AIDS situation in South Africa since they continue, without any scientific support, to invoke poverty as a major determinant of high HIV prevalence. This just reinforces President Mbeki's belief that AIDS is caused by poverty and has nothing to do with sex or HIV.

Public Health and Behavior Change Programs

When I was responsible for communicable disease control for the State of California in the early 1970s, I was summoned from my office in Berkeley to the Governor's office in Sacramento and chastised by his staff for the explosion of STD throughout the State, especially in adolescents and young adults. My response was that I considered STD control in California as a leaky ship in a stormy sea. If I were given more resources (money and staff), I assured the Governor's office that I would be able to patch the leaky ship (STD control) to keep it afloat, but my staff and I could in no way completely "stop the storm" of sexual behaviors. For my frank answer, the STD unit was transferred to Sacramento so that it could be "better" supervised by these political appointees.* The point I want to make is that traditional public health programs did not and currently do not have the capability or expertise for changing population risk

---

* A few years later, the STD unit was silently transferred back to my Infectious Disease Section.

behaviors. In my opinion, most behavioral scientists have focused more on qualitative descriptive studies and much less on the quantitative population aspects of human health risk behaviors. Especially lacking is any demonstrable expertise and capability for changing risk behaviors. Public health's track record for changing risky behaviors such as smoking and routinely using seat belts has not been very good over the past couple of decades. Smoking continues to be an unacceptably high addiction, especially among adolescents and young adults, and seat belt use is clearly not the social norm in most developing countries. From my perspective, the future of public health prevention programs depends on the development of effective behavior change programs. This will require the training of a new generation of public health workers who hopefully will benefit from all the mistakes made by my generation of public health workers. There is a great need for behavioral scientists to focus on the art and science of changing risky health behaviors and not to just study them.

How Effective Have HIV/AIDS Programs Been in Preventing HIV Transmission?

The effectiveness of primary HIV prevention in healthcare settings, especially in preventing transmission from blood transfusions and blood products in developed countries, was clearly shown by the virtual elimination of such transmission after the advent of HIV testing capabilities and the implementation of "universal precautions." Similarly, the virtual elimination of MTCT in most developed countries can clearly be attributed to MTCT prevention programs that have been developed over the past decade. However, the effectiveness of prevention programs in reducing sexual and IDU HIV transmission continues to be far less clear.

Measurement of annual HIV incidence is difficult since the error in measuring HIV prevalence is usually so high that any change in annual incidence could easily fit within this range of error. In addition, HIV prevalence in any country, especially large countries, is comprised of many separate HIV epidemics, each occurring within different sex or IDU networks at different times. In the USA, HIV epidemics exploded in MSM populations in major cities in California and New York during the same time period. Shortly thereafter, explosive HIV epidemics were documented in IDU populations mainly on the east coast, with less severe IDU epidemics in the rest of the country. We now know that the general pattern and prevalence of MSM risk behaviors in San Francisco and New York City were very similar and the HIV epidemic curves in these two cities were also similar in shape and in the general prevalence levels reached. In contrast, the patterns and prevalence of IDU risk behaviors were quite different on the east coast where "shooting galleries"* were present whereas on the west coast IDU networks were generally much smaller. Thus, the lower HIV prevalence in IDU populations found on the west coast can be attributed to the lower risk of HIV transmission within smaller IDU networks and not necessarily to any better HIV prevention programs on the west coast.

---

* Large IDU networks where large numbers of IDU shared common injection equipment daily.

All infectious disease epidemics have similar stages: an early epidemic stage when R_0 (the reproductive number of the infectious agent) is the highest; a slowing of epidemic spread when R_0 begins to decrease; a peaking or leveling of epidemic transmission; and finally a decreasing phase when R_0 is < 1. The impact of HIV prevention programs on any national prevalence trend is very difficult to measure since there are no valid control populations for comparison. If HIV was truly an infectious disease agent for which all or most persons in the population were at about equal risk, then significant differences in HIV prevalence in one population compared with another might be attributed to differences in prevention programs. If prevention programs are implemented when HIV epidemics are at or near their "natural" peaks, the subsequent decrease in prevalence might be incorrectly attributed to prevention programs. Yet most of the observed decrease might more likely be due to a saturation effect – infection of most of the population with the highest risk behaviors. Thus, only a small proportion of the decrease in HIV prevalence might be due to prevention measures.[*] The following section illustrates these problems in attributing reductions in observed HIV prevalence trends to prevention programs.

Decreasing HIV Incidence in an MSM Cohort

Figure 8.2 presents estimates of HIV prevalence and incidence based on point prevalence data from a cohort of MSM in San Francisco. Blood samples were collected from this MSM cohort because they were enrolled in a hepatitis B vaccine study – HIV prevalence rose from 1 percent in 1980 to 25 percent in 1982 to 65 percent in 1984. EPIMODEL was used to fit a prevalence curve to the three HIV prevalence data points and to calculate the annual HIV incidence needed to generate the "fitted" prevalence curve. According to this modeling of the HIV epidemic in this MSM cohort, annual HIV incidence peaked in 1983 at over 20 percent and then decreased sharply and dropped to about 5 percent by 1985.

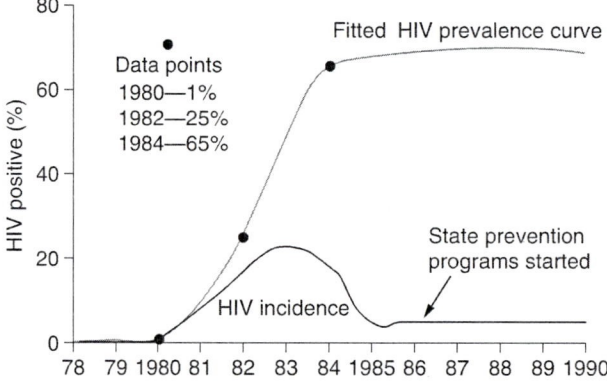

Figure 8.2 Modeling the HIV epidemic in a SF MSM cohort.

---

[*] Dr. Alex Langmuir, the father of the Epidemic Intelligence Service (EIS) program at CDC, Atlanta, referred to this epidemiologic situation as "riding to glory on the down slope of the epidemic curve."

The prevalence curve suggests that by 1983, about half of the MSM cohort, most likely the half with the highest sexual risk behaviors were infected with HIV. After 1983, HIV incidence fell sharply because the remaining half of the cohort probably had less risky behaviors and/or there was some overall reduction in sexual risk behaviors as a result of increasing reports of deaths attributed to this "emerging" disease. It should be noted that funding of State HIV/AIDS prevention programs was not started until after 1985.

The Uganda Success Story

One of the most heralded success stories of a national HIV/AIDS program is that of Uganda. National HIV prevalence in Uganda reportedly peaked during the early 1990s at about 15 percent and then decreased steadily to about 5 percent by 2001. There has been considerable debate as to whether most of the reduction in HIV prevalence can be attributed to changes in sexual behavior such as abstinence and/or being faithful to one's spouse or to the increased use of condoms by those persons with multiple sex partners. However, there is no question that HIV incidence and prevalence rates in Uganda have decreased markedly during the past decade after a government supported HIV/AIDS program that included the whole range of **ABC** interventions was aggressively implemented.

The major epidemiologic question about the Uganda HIV/AIDS numbers is whether the magnitude of the reported decrease in HIV prevalence attributed to prevention efforts might be exaggerated. As pointed out in Chapter 7, there have been marked reductions in the estimated HIV prevalence of many SSA countries since 2001 as a result of population-based DHS HIV serosurveys. In 2001, UNAIDS accepted an HIV estimate of 2.3 million for Kenya and in 2003 the accepted estimate was about half of the 2001 estimate or about 1.2 million. The extent to which Uganda's national HIV prevalence estimate may have been overestimated in the early 1990s compared with its current prevalence estimate is unknown, but overestimates averaging 50 percent have been found consistently in virtually every SSA country where DHS+ or similar population-based HIV serosurveys have been carried out since 2001.

As stated above, there is no question that HIV prevalence in Uganda decreased markedly after 1992, but the decrease recorded in pregnant women in Kampala from 30 percent in 1992 to less than 15 percent by 1996 is simply not possible. Figure 8.3 presents annual HIV prevalence estimates in pregnant women in Kampala based on sentinel HIV surveillance data compared with modeled estimates of HIV prevalence with annual HIV incidence reduced by 25 percent, 75 percent, or 100 percent after 1992. It can be seen that even if all HIV transmission were stopped after 1992, HIV prevalence in these pregnant women would still be just a bit over 15 percent in 1996.* These modeling runs used a median period of 8 years from HIV infection to AIDS death. If a median interval of 10 years is used, an HIV prevalence of 30 percent in 1992 could decrease to only 19 percent by 1992 if all HIV transmission were stopped after 1992.

---

*Sam Okware, initial head of the Uganda AIDS program, showed me the Kampala ANC data when we were together on a World Bank mission in Malawi in 1997. I told Sam then that the decrease from 30 percent in 1992 to less than 15 percent by 1996 was simply not possible and I was sure that the ANC sampling frame was probably changed during this period. He told me he would check it out and get back to me, but I have not received any feed-back.

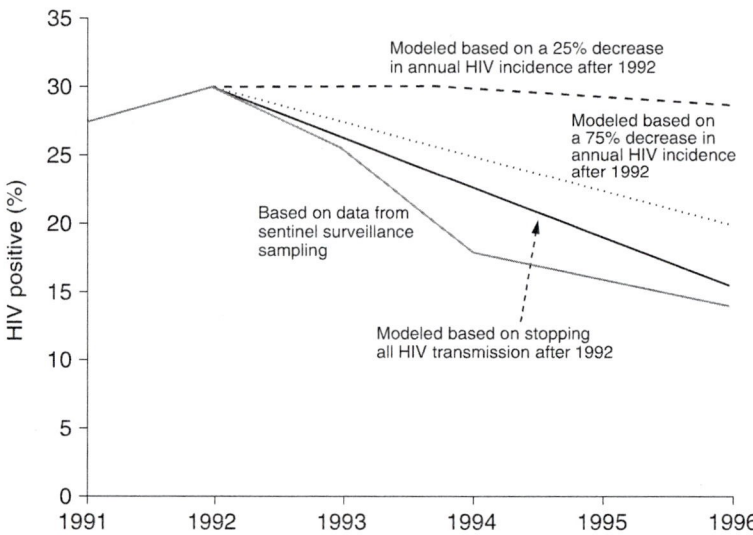

Figure 8.3 Modeled HIV prevalence in antenatal females in Kampala.

I have no doubt that the Uganda HIV/AIDS prevention program was relatively effective and successful, but it could not have stopped all HIV transmission after 1992. The recorded decrease from 30 percent to less than 15 percent is probably, at least partially, due to changes in the sampling of pregnant women in Kampala – either the use of different ANC sites and/or an increase of younger females in the sampling frame after 1992.

Other "Success" Stories

The reduction of HIV prevalence estimates in many SSA countries due primarily to the collection of more representative HIV data from population-based surveys has, in some of these countries, been incorrectly attributed to successful prevention programs. For example, in mid-October 2005, a spokesperson for a faith-based organization in Zambia "...celebrated the very positive progress Zambia has achieved in HIV/AIDS prevention. She quoted the official figure from the Ministry of Health, saying that the HIV/AIDS prevalence rate in the country has reduced from around 20 percent in 2000 to the current 16 percent." Prevention efforts in Zambia may have played some role in reducing or leveling HIV prevalence in Zambia in recent years. However, based on the Zambian studies that looked into the difference between the prevalence estimates derived from sentinel ANC data compared with the estimate from the DHS+, there was no reduction in prevalence, but a higher and lower estimate due to the different methods and data used to calculate national HIV prevalence.

In 1991, I was asked by a high ranking Thai official to project up to 10 million HIV infections in Thailand by the end of the decade if increased prevention efforts were not markedly increased. At that time, I could only project, at most 1 to 2 million infections by the year 2000 since I did not expect any significant HIV spread into the Thai general population. The Thai official still wanted a projection of 10 million or more since he argued that if there would "only" be 1 to 2 million by 2000 the Thai

AIDS program could claim credit for preventing 8 million infections. Such a claim of "success" has been made over a decade later, not from an unrealistically high HIV prevalence projection made in the early 1990s when the Thai 100 percent condom program was started, but from the conclusions of a group of modelers.

In WHO's *2004 World Health Report*, HIV/AIDS success stories about millions of HIV infections prevented in Cambodia and Thailand were featured. These two countries had explosive HIV epidemics in their commercial sex networks and as a result had the highest estimated national HIV prevalence levels in Asia. In both countries, national HIV prevalence in the 15–49 year old population peaked at about 2 to 3 percent. After implementation of the 100 percent condom program for all commercial sex encounters, HIV prevalence has decreased in both countries to less than 2 percent in 2005. There is no dispute that at least some of the prevalence decrease in recent years is the result of the 100 percent condom program. However, WHO has uncritically and with no sound epidemiologic basis accepted a comparison of HIV prevalence levels in Cambodia and Thailand with HIV prevalence levels in high prevalence countries in SSA. Using a curve-fitting and extrapolation model (Asian Epidemic Model), the East-West Center and its collaborators modeled the impacts of HIV prevention efforts. They concluded from their modeling effort that without aggressive prevention programs, both Thailand and Cambodia would now be looking at expanding HIV epidemics with 10 to 15 percent of their adult populations infected, instead of the declining epidemics of 1–2 percent currently seen.

According to these modelers the HIV prevention program started in Thailand in the early 1990s can be credited with preventing several million infections by the year 2000 and over 10 million by 2010 (*see* Figure 8.4). These modelers also projected that about 1 million HIV infections will be prevented in Cambodia by the end of this decade. However, by applying this same naïve comparison method, prevention programs in Myanmar should be credited for keeping prevalence at an estimated 1 to 2 percent. Similarly, there are at least a dozen African countries whose HIV prevalence levels have been less than 5 percent. Should these countries be considered to have better HIV prevention programs compared to African countries that currently have HIV prevalence levels of more than 10 percent? I find the comparison modeling method and conclusions of the East-West Center and their collaborators hard to believe, but apparently UNAIDS and WHO are less critical and more accepting of these modelers' methods and conclusions.

An HIV/AIDS success label has been bestowed on Brazil, but it is unclear what criteria have been used to confer this success label. I agree that Brazil has from the beginning approached HIV prevention with open (transparent) and socially sensitive programs: it is also a model for providing medical care and now ART to persons living with HIV/AIDS. However, estimated HIV prevalence in Brazil and Argentina are both essentially the same at about 0.7 percent of the 15–49 year old population. Does this mean that Argentina has an HIV/AIDS program as successful as Brazil? Using this same naïve reasoning, HIV prevalence in Mexico is estimated to be 0.3 percent and is twice that level (0.6 percent) in the USA. Does this mean that Mexico has an HIV/AIDS prevention program twice as good as prevention programs in the USA – of course not! HIV prevalence can rise only to the level(s) permitted by the existing patterns and prevalence of HIV risk behaviors and the patterns and prevalence of HIV risk behaviors are clearly not the same in all populations.

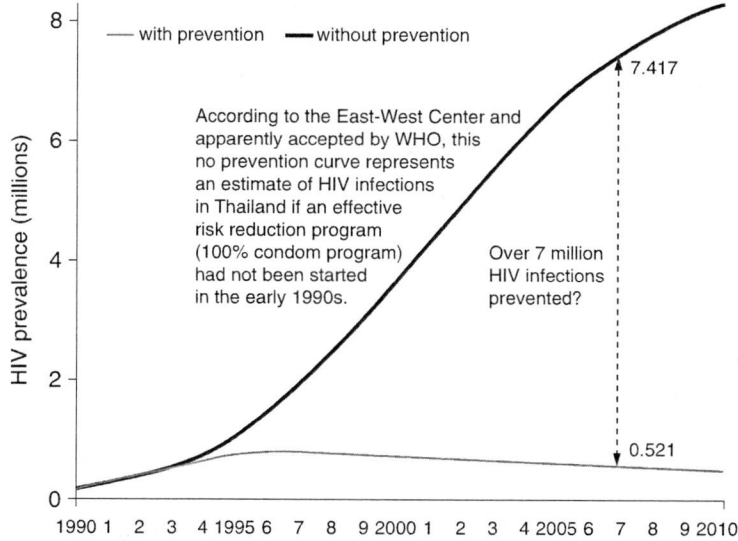

Figure 8.4 Estimation and projection of HIV prevalence in Thailand.

Projecting the Impact of HIV Prevention

As described in the preceding sections, it is difficult to evaluate the past and current "success" of HIV prevention programs because aside from well planned studies with appropriate control populations for comparison, there are no accepted methods that can attribute a low or decreasing HIV prevalence in any population to any specific public health intervention. It is logical to *assume* that in the absence of effective prevention programs HIV prevalence will rise to the level consistent with the existing patterns and prevalence of HIV risk behaviors, but without a good control population for comparison it is uncertain what HIV prevalence level might be reached. It is also logical to *assume* that public health interventions such as risk and harm reduction can reduce HIV transmission, but again, without an appropriate control population it is uncertain how many HIV infections might be prevented. HIV/AIDS models may be helpful to project the relative impact of different prevention and treatment programs on HIV incidence. However, such modeling requires the use of realistic or plausible HIV scenarios since projecting an unrealistically high number of infections will clearly exaggerate the number of infections that might be prevented by different prevention and treatment programs.

UNAIDS in its December 2005 report on the global AIDS epidemic presented the modeled impact of different prevention and treatment programs in reducing annual HIV incidence in SSA.* The HIV scenario selected by these modelers as the "baseline" for comparing future HIV incidence *assumed* that risk behaviors continued at what the modelers believed to be the current levels, and without any major increase in anti-retroviral treatment (ART) programs. This "business as usual" scenario describes what the modelers believe might happen over the next

* Salomon JA, Hogan DR, Stover J, *et al.* (2005) Integrating HIV prevention and treatment: From slogans to impact. *PLoS Med.* **2**(1): e16 [January 11, 2005].

20 years if African and global leaders do not dramatically increase support for HIV prevention and treatment programs. Based on their **assumptions**, the modelers projected a level and unchanging ("stable") prevalence rate in SSA over the duration of the projection – 20 years. In their baseline scenario, annual HIV incidence in 2003 was about 2.5 million and steadily increased to over 3.5 million in 2020. The reason why annual HIV incident numbers increase steadily in this scenario even though annual HIV incidence rates peaked around the mid-1990s is that the modelers *assumed* an unchanging HIV prevalence rate. In order to keep the prevalence rate unchanged, the model has to increase annual incident HIV numbers to compensate for the annual population growth rate of about 3 percent.*

It is not consistent with epidemic theory and HIV transmission dynamics to assume the HIV prevalence rate will peak and then remain unchanged, even if HIV risk behaviors remain the same. These modelers completely ignored the major factor responsible for peaking in all infectious disease epidemics – the phenomena of saturation of infection in persons who are at risk of infection. At the start of any HIV epidemic, virtually all persons with HIV risk behaviors are *at risk* of infection. As the epidemic progresses, fewer susceptible persons *at risk* are present because they have been infected, and the number of secondary infections caused by each infected individual will begin to decrease. When the epidemic peaks, most persons with the highest level of risk behaviors have been infected. There are fewer persons *at risk* to infect and the remaining susceptible persons have lower risk behaviors. Thus, unless HIV risk behaviors begin to increase, HIV incidence will slowly decrease after reaching a peak. There is simply no epidemiologic basis to *assume* that new HIV infections will continue to increase to keep the HIV prevalence rate unchanged even if there is no change in HIV risk behaviors for the next 20 years!

The modeled impact of different HIV prevention and treatment programs in reducing annual HIV incidence from that of the baseline scenario was uncritically accepted by UNAIDS. The modelers projected that a comprehensive prevention and treatment strategy could prevent more than half of the projected total of over 60 million new HIV infections up through 2020. Instead of an annual incidence of 3.7 million infections in 2020, it could be reduced to just about 1 million. Such a reduction would indeed be an impressive public health accomplishment: the extra billions of dollars needed for increasing prevention and treatment programs to the levels recommended would be more than offset by the prevention of close to 30 million new HIV infections. However, is their baseline scenario that has annual HIV incidence steadily increasing up to 2020 possible and plausible? My answer is that perhaps it is possible but not very probable!

At the end of Chapter 7, the most likely HIV scenario for SSA was modeled based on the most recent data on prevalence and trends reported by UNAIDS. The major findings from this modeling exercise were: in order for the HIV prevalence rate in SSA to peak in 2000 or 2001, annual HIV incidence rates had to have peaked around the mid-1990s. Thus, the baseline or "business as usual" HIV scenario developed by these modelers is neither realistic nor plausible! The modelers *assumed* that when the HIV prevalence rate peaked, that it would remain unchanged if HIV risk behaviors remain unchanged. There is simply no epidemiologic basis for such an assumption.

---

* This was described in more detail in the footnote on page 136.

How these modelers and UNAIDS can project an ever increasing annual HIV incidence in SSA for the next 20 years is difficult to understand especially when UNAIDS has reported HIV prevalence rates in SSA to be decreasing and not increasing. UNAIDS' estimate of the HIV prevalence rate in SSA in 2001 was 7.6 percent of the 15–49 year old population and was 7.2 percent in 2005. UNAIDS may well argue that the difference between these estimates is minimal (5.5 percent) and that these estimates are consistent with their contention that HIV prevalence has merely leveled off or stabilized and is not necessarily decreasing. Nevertheless, for the reasons described above, it is difficult to accept their *assumption* that the peak SSA prevalence rate will *persist unchanged for 20 years.*

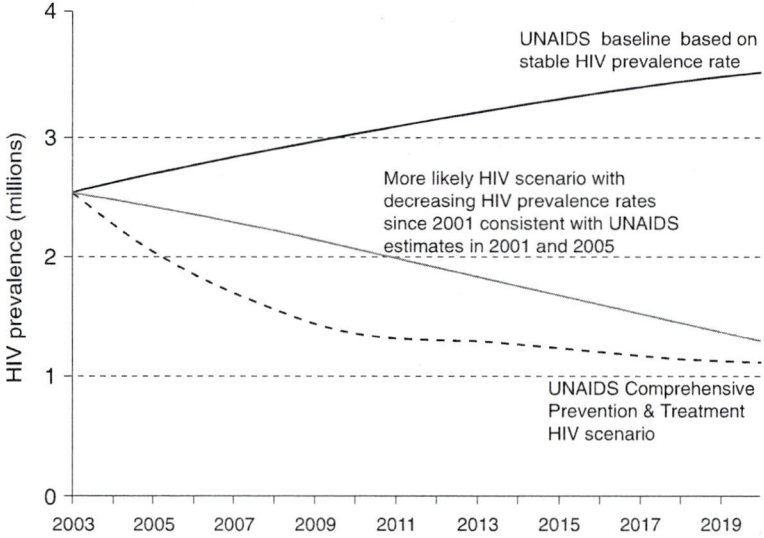

Figure 8.5 Estimated and projected annual HIV incidence in sub-Saharan Africa.

Based on the more likely HIV scenario modeled at the end of Chapter 7, annual HIV incidence in SSA has been decreasing from a peak of about 2.5 million in 2000 and will continue to decrease slowly to a little over 1 million by 2020 (*see* Figure 8.5). How much of this projected decrease in annual HIV incidence might be attributed to public health prevention programs and how much to a natural decrease can and will definitely be the subject for heated debate for the rest of this decade.

A similar modeling study of the impact of comprehensive prevention and treatment programs on annual global HIV incidence was published in early 2006.* Annual global HIV incidence was projected to steadily increase from just less than 5 million in 2005 to close to 6 million in 2015. My comments on this study, that included virtually all of the authors of the paper reviewed above plus several others, is the same as for the first paper. My conclusions, based on HIV prevalence data and trends, are that annual HIV incidence globally peaked by the mid-1990s and has been decreasing since then. These modelers, by ignoring or denying the

---

* Stover J, Bertozzi S, Gutierrez J-P, *et al.* (2006) The global impact of scaling-up HIV/AIDS prevention programs in low- and middle-income countries. *Science Express*, 2 February.

most recent HIV prevalence data and trends, project an ever-increasing HIV incidence over the next couple of decades and then show with their models that increased prevention and treatment programs are capable of reducing HIV incidence during this time period by half or more. My biased opinion is that these "assumption" models, if believed, will enable UNAIDS and AIDS programs to "ride to glory" on the downslopes of HIV epidemic curves!

These modelers have made a "glorious" attempt to develop a strong argument for dramatically increasing support for AIDS prevention and treatment programs. However, they have merely assumed that annual HIV incidence will be constantly increasing over the next couple of decades and that scaled up and comprehensive prevention and treatment programs are capable of cutting their projected numbers in half. As an old infectious disease epidemiologist who has worked with HIV/AIDS modelers for close to 20 years, I'm familiar with how these models work or don't work. I know that if the basic input parameter to the model is that HIV incidence continues to increase, the model will calculate an ever increasing number of infections. If the model is also told that programs x and y will collectively cut HIV incidence in half, the model will do whatever it is programmed to do. It all looks very scientific, but it essentially boils down to whether the basic assumptions and the values for these assumptions, inputted into the model, are credible to begin with.

I clearly do not believe the results and conclusions of these modelers, but regardless of whose estimates and projections are more credible I fully agree that HIV prevention and treatment programs in developed and developing countries all need to be intensified and scaled-up. Although not increasing, HIV incidence and prevalence rates in those populations where HIV epidemics have occurred will continue to be unacceptably high for the foreseeable future. There is a need for AIDS programs to retool future press releases which should abandon the "ever increasing" and "next wave" alarms. Rather they should focus on: preventing the millions of new HIV infections that continue to occur annually; and on the millions of HIV-infected persons who become eligible for ART programs each year.

It should also be fully appreciated that even if AIDS programs could stop all HIV transmission as of 2006, that the moral commitment of the richest countries (G-8) to provide all eligible HIV-infected persons with access to ART by 2010 cannot be met and not just because of insufficient funding. The healthcare infrastructure in most of the severely affected countries needs to be further developed and more medical and technical staff trained. UNAIDS, AIDS program advocates and activists should refrain from making unrealistically high HIV projections in order to maintain and increase the priority that AIDS programs now receive from international donors. Sooner or later, the false alarms and the grossly overestimated and projected HIV/AIDS numbers will be exposed for what they are. There may then be a backlash by donor agencies to the detriment of AIDS programs.

Summary/Conclusions

The major challenges confronting HIV/AIDS prevention programs include the problems of government and official agencies trying to modify or eliminate socially unacceptable and often illegal behaviors with limited authority and resources. Injecting drug use and sexual promiscuity are difficult subjects for government or official agencies to confront. Most AIDS programs are more comfortable trying to cope with the medical and scientific aspects of HIV/AIDS rather than its social and behavioral aspects. There is a preference to treat AIDS primarily as a medical problem: universal support is available from the public and policy makers for the development of effective HIV/AIDS treatments as it is for the development of the scientific "magic bullet" – an HIV vaccine. Similar urgent and universal support for primary prevention and **behavior change programs** has not materialized other than from some faith-based organizations who want to eliminate all sex outside of marital sex.

Interventions for prevention of HIV transmission should be separated into immediate and short-term in contrast to longer-term interventions. Examples of immediate or short-term interventions are those often referred to as "risk reduction" and "harm reduction" – routine and consistent condom use with commercial sex partners and provision of safe drug injecting equipment. These interventions are universally accepted and recommended by virtually all HIV/AIDS programs: they remain controversial because opponents believe that acceptance of these interventions condones these behaviors and/or will tend to promote such behaviors. The primary example of a longer-term intervention is the reduction, modification or elimination of HIV risk behaviors – i.e., having multiple sex partners, especially on a concurrent basis, and/or the recreational use of legal or illegal drugs. These latter measures are also universally accepted. However, it probably takes decades or generations to effect meaningful population change in these behaviors: they remain difficult to achieve because the science or art of changing human behavior (i.e., cigarette smoking, healthy diet and exercise, etc.) is still developing. Ideally, both immediate and longer-term interventions should be fully implemented, but as pointed out above, the immediate risk and/or harm reduction interventions remain controversial or illegal. Faith-based organizations should re-evaluate their active opposition to condom use for casual and commercial sex. If they cannot support public health's need to promote condom use, then at least they should cease their active opposition to condom use.

The following conclusions regarding the effectiveness of HIV prevention programs may be difficult for the public and even many public health workers to understand and accept, but they are nevertheless valid epidemiologic conclusions. These conclusions need to be kept in mind when evaluating the declared "success" of many HIV prevention programs.

1 HIV prevalence is low in most populations not because of effective HIV prevention programs, but because: (a) the vast majority of heterosexuals, even in SSA, do not have multiple and concurrent sex partners; and (b) the infectivity of HIV via vaginal intercourse is very low in the absence of facilitating factors.

2 The effectiveness of HIV prevention programs cannot be measured by low HIV prevalence *per se* since the low prevalence can be more logically attributed to a low risk pattern and prevalence of HIV risk behaviors. However, increasing HIV prevalence can logically be attributed to the lack of effectiveness in preventing HIV transmission.

3 In populations with high HIV prevalence, an increasing prevalence rate does not necessarily indicate that prevention programs are ineffective since it is possible that the prevalence rate might increase even faster without any public health

interventions. Similarly, a decreasing HIV prevalence rate in a population with high prevalence cannot be assumed to be due to public health prevention programs since a decreasing rate will naturally follow after most persons with the highest level of risk behaviors are infected, i.e., when the HIV epidemic has peaked.

Other variables, such as significant changes in specific HIV risk behaviors, are more accurate and reliable indicators of the effectiveness of public health HIV prevention programs.

Regardless of what the future HIV growth potential may be in current low prevalence populations, the most prudent public health strategy is to direct interventions to persons with the highest HIV risk behaviors. Based on observations of past HIV epidemics, it is clear that sustained epidemic heterosexual transmission will occur only in those populations with high risk patterns and high frequency of sex partner exchanges. To assure that epidemic HIV transmission will not occur, public health programs, in close collaboration with relevant NGOs, should implement the 100 percent condom program for all sex encounters in high risk MSM and heterosexual populations (FSW and their male clients). In populations where there are IDU who routinely share needles and syringes, public health programs together with relevant NGOs should implement harm reduction programs for IDU groups to minimize HIV transmission in this very vulnerable population. In the absence of effective public health interventions, HIV prevalence will rise, but only to the levels permitted by the existing patterns and prevalence of HIV risk behaviors.

Effective implementation and evaluation of HIV prevention in any population requires detailed information on the prevailing patterns and distribution of risk behaviors. There is an urgent need for a reliable HIV risk behavior surveillance system in all populations. Findings from such surveillance systems can provide:

1 focus and direction for social outreach programs that provide risk and harm reduction services to those persons with the highest risk; and
2 data to monitor future behavior changes in these populations.

When public health surveillance of HIV/AIDS was initiated in the early 1980s, there were cogent arguments for non-nominal reporting because of the stigma and discrimination to which HIV-infected persons were subjected. A more important reason was the lack of any effective treatment for persons found to be infected. However, current public health as well as personal health implications of not being able to follow up on the infection status of regular sex partners, along with the availability of effective anti-HIV treatment, requires a re-evaluation of the rationale for providing anonymity to HIV-infected persons.

As of late-2006, virtually all countries throughout the world where HIV epidemics have occurred are past the increasing transmission phase and are now at the post peak phase of their epidemics. HIV prevention programs need to re-evaluate prevention strategies to respond more effectively to current patterns of transmission. This means directing primary focus to HIV-discordant couples and/or regular sex partners. All HIV prevention programs need to begin to identify systematically by name infected persons to:

1 provide them with secondary and tertiary prevention services (i.e., ART) as needed and

2 routinely follow-up on all of their regular sex partners to provide them with primary, secondary, or tertiary prevention services, as appropriate. It must be recognized that regular sex partners may be multiple, especially in MSM and many SSA populations where long-term and regular concurrent sex partnerships are common.

The time has come to fully support the more "traditional" public health approach recommended by the New York City Health Department in early 2006 to make HIV antibody testing routine in many clinical settings, with the provision that persons may refuse such tests.

Chapter 9

Dispelling Glorious[*] HIV/AIDS Myths and Misconceptions

As described in Chapters 3 and 4, most of the far out, "flat-earth" type theories of the origin of AIDS and what AIDS is and isn't, were dismissed by mainstream science and public health by the mid-1980s. However, several "glorious" myths and/or misconceptions about HIV epidemiology continue to be accepted and used by UNAIDS and other mainstream AIDS agencies and activists. These myths are needed to support the UNAIDS paradigm that without aggressive HIV/AIDS prevention programs – especially directed to youth – it is just a matter of time before heterosexual HIV epidemics erupt in current low HIV prevalence populations. The studies and observations described in Chapter 5 on HIV epidemiology and transmission dynamics and the global HIV/AIDS patterns and prevalence described in Chapter 7 have led me to far different conclusions about the potential for epidemic HIV transmission in most heterosexual populations. My conclusions are:

1 HIV prevalence can rise only to those levels permitted by the prevailing patterns and prevalence of HIV risk behaviors and the prevalence of facilitating and protective factors and
2 in most heterosexual populations, the patterns and frequency of sex partner exchange[†] are not sufficient to sustain epidemic sexual HIV transmission.

UNAIDS and most AIDS activists believe that these conclusions, especially my second conclusion, are not socially and politically correct and will lead to complacency by the public and policy makers regarding the potential course and severity of the AIDS pandemic.

UNAIDS, other mainstream AIDS agencies, and many social activists believe – without epidemiologic support – that the major determinants of high HIV infection rates are poverty, discrimination and lack of access to healthcare. Without aggressive prevention programs directed to the general public, especially youth, they believe that it is only a matter of time before heterosexual HIV epidemics erupt in almost all developing countries where HIV infection rates are currently low. Some mainstream AIDS "experts" assert that there are insufficient data to support my conclusions or paradigm. My response is that there are *no data* to support their concern that HIV can and will spread into general populations or "ordinary" people if aggressive prevention programs directed to the general public, especially youth, are not implemented. In this chapter, I will provide my evaluation of the glorious myths and misconceptions about HIV epidemiology and transmission dynamics used to support and perpetuate the prevailing

---

[*] Glorious myths are those used for a good cause, i.e., *splendide mendax* (splendidly or gloriously false).
[†] Commonly referred to as sexual promiscuity.

UNAIDS paradigm. I will also describe when and why I began to swim upstream against the orthodox beliefs of mainstream AIDS agencies, but first it would be helpful to review what I understand to be the major determinants of epidemic (i.e., R_0^* >1) HIV transmission.

Major Determinants of Epidemic HIV Transmission

I need to stress that my understanding of HIV transmission dynamics is not very different from most mainstream epidemiologists.[†] The problem in accepting my conclusions and paradigm is that most AIDS activists do not want to acknowledge that epidemic HIV transmission requires the highest risk patterns and prevalence of HIV risk behaviors. These activists do not want to further stigmatize persons or population groups (MSM, IDU, FSW, etc.) who have such high levels of HIV risk behaviors and who are already marginalized. First and foremost, we have to be aware that, as described in Chapter 5, all published sex partner studies show the risk of HIV transmission from any single coital act is very low – about 1 per 1000 or less. By contrast, a pandemic influenza virus would be capable of *generalized* spread in any population because virtually all infants, children, and adults, young or old would be at moderate to high risk of infection to such an agent. However, HIV transmission requires the exchange of a significant amount of blood or sexual fluids. Thus, only a small percent of most general populations or "ordinary" persons would be at moderate to high risk of exposure to and infection with HIV.

There is no question among infectious disease epidemiologists that the primary determinants of epidemic (R_0 >1) HIV transmission are risk behaviors that include having unprotected sex with *multiple* and *concurrent* sex partners and/or routinely sharing drug injecting equipment with other IDU. Epidemic HIV transmission has been documented only where the *highest levels* of such risk behaviors are present. Thus, it is only logical to conclude that in the absence of high HIV risk behaviors, epidemic (R_0 >1) transmission will not occur. What has been essentially ignored is the more important and relevant question: what are the major determinants of HIV risk behaviors? Most social activists do not hesitate to say that poverty and discrimination are the root causes of HIV risk behaviors. However, I don't know of a clear and simple answer to this question, since I consider it more likely that cultural, social, religious, and many other factors, including economic factors, all collectively play some role as determinants of sexual and IDU risk behaviors. Because there is no clear answer to what are the major determinants of HIV risk behaviors, many worthy social agendas have been hitched onto the AIDS program wagon. These social issues, such as poverty, discrimination, gender inequity, and lack of access to healthcare, are major problems that clearly hinder effective HIV prevention and treatment programs, but they are not the major determinants of epidemic HIV transmission!

---

[*] R_0 is the reproductive number of an infectious agent. It is described in detail on page 60, Chapter 5.

[†] I was the principal author of the HIV/AIDS chapter in the 17th edition (2000) of the Control of Communicable Diseases Manual (CCDM), published by the American Public Health Association (APHA).

Glorious Myths or Misconceptions of HIV Transmission Dynamics

Below are what I consider to be the major myths or misconceptions about HIV epidemiology and transmission dynamics that continue to be used by UNAIDS and mainstream AIDS agencies to support the prevailing socially and politically correct, but epidemiologically incorrect, UNAIDS paradigm: *in the absence of aggressive prevention programs directed to the general population, especially youth, it is only a matter of time before epidemic heterosexual HIV transmission will break out in populations where HIV prevalence is low.*

- **Virtually everyone is at almost equal risk of infection with HIV**

The origin of this glorious myth derives from the initial short doubling times for reported AIDS cases in the early 1980s that led to the false conclusion that AIDS was caused by a highly infectious agent. Observations that HIV risk behaviors (sexual promiscuity in homosexual and heterosexual populations and routine sharing of injecting drug equipment) are present in virtually all countries throughout the world also led to the belief that HIV epidemics would eventually occur in all populations. However, it does not follow logically that the potential for extensive HIV epidemics in MSM, IDU, FSW and their clients is equally present in all populations and countries. Further, it is simply not possible for HIV to jump into any "general" population from these high risk groups to spread in epidemic fashion in "ordinary" people. There are no credible STD experts who are concerned that syphilis – which is caused by a bacterial agent that is hundreds of times more infectious per coital contact than HIV – has the potential to sweep through general populations "like a hot knife through cold butter!"

The major characteristic of HIV as an infectious disease agent is that its risk of transmission is, in the absence of facilitating factors, very low for any single sex encounter. This characteristic of HIV is not something that AIDS programs or agencies usually include in their educational messages about HIV transmission. Both Jon Mann and Mike Merson specifically instructed me not to distribute a table I had prepared on the risk of HIV transmission by type of exposure since this table indicated that, in the absence of facilitating factors, the risk of HIV transmission per single coital act was about 1 per 1000 or lower. They were both aware that my table was accurate, but both believed that distributing this information to the public would be sending the public a mixed message about the risk of HIV transmission via unprotected sexual intercourse.

Aside from the low infectivity of HIV, the pattern and prevalence of HIV risk behaviors differ markedly from country to country. As described in detail in Chapter 5, the WHO/GPA surveys of sexual knowledge, attitudes, behaviors, and practices (KABP) carried out in the late 1980s found that:

1 the pattern of sex partner exchange in SSA populations is mainly on a concurrent basis whereas in most developed countries, sex partner exchange is mainly serial, not concurrent and
2 a relatively large percent (up to 40 percent) of females in some SSA countries have sex outside of marriage, whereas less than 1 to 2 percent of Asian females report such behavior.

These findings, as well as the observation that the prevalence of multiple facilitating factors, that can greatly increase the risk of sexual HIV transmission, are more than 10 times higher in SSA populations compared with most other populations, help explain why epidemic heterosexual HIV transmission has occurred in most SSA countries but not in most other populations. In the few Asian countries where epidemic heterosexual HIV transmission has been documented in FSW and their clients, this can be attributed to the large commercial sex networks that were present.

UNAIDS and most AIDS activists have either intentionally or out of honest ignorance ignored the fact that HIV is very difficult to transmit sexually. By refusing to accept the fact that HIV is very difficult to transmit sexually without the highest levels of sexual risk behaviors, AIDS programs have avoided labeling some populations as being more promiscuous than others. It is a much more socially and politically correct public health message to say that sexual promiscuity exists in all populations and thus the risk of epidemic heterosexual HIV transmission to the "general" public, or to "ordinary" people can be prevented only by aggressive **ABC** programs directed at the general population, and especially to youth.

A parallel pandemic of AIDS "experts," most without any epidemiologic training, have used a variety of epidemic models to project large heterosexual epidemics in countries where HIV prevalence rates in the general population are still very low. These "experts" sound alarms that the "next waves" of HIV epidemics are imminent, or HIV is "on the brink" of jumping into the general population from existing foci in MSM and IDU populations. The "next waves" of HIV epidemics predicted for the general heterosexual populations in developed countries during the 1980s have never materialized. Most of these AIDS "experts" have given up sounding alarms about heterosexual HIV epidemics in developed countries and have turned their attention to large populous countries in Asia. For countries such as India and China they project severe heterosexual HIV epidemics, if any sex outside of marital sex is permitted to occur, and education of the general public, especially youth, on how HIV is transmitted, are not aggressively implemented.

- **HIV "bridge" populations will invariably ignite heterosexual HIV epidemics**

Another major misconception about HIV transmission dynamics is that infected bisexual males or infected IDU (male or female) serve as the "bridge" population for HIV entry into the general heterosexual population. What has been virtually ignored over the past two decades is that such "bridging" has and continues to occur from what is described in Chapter 5 as nonepidemic transmission between HIV-discordant couples, i.e., HIV transmission from an infected person (regardless of how infection was acquired) to his/her regular sex partner or partners. This is currently the predominant mode of HIV transmission throughout the world, but these are usually "bridges to nowhere." This is because epidemic heterosexual HIV transmission has not and cannot occur in any population without the presence of a very high risk pattern and frequency of sex partner exchange. In the absence of these latter factors there will not be significant spread within the general population. This is exactly what has happened following the hundreds of HIV epidemics that have been documented in MSM and IDU populations throughout the world since the early 1980s. This also happened with the many HIV-infected persons who traveled out of Africa during the 1960s and 1970s: there were probably hundreds or thousands of such "sparks" that introduced HIV into many populations but they did not start significant epidemic spread until such a "spark" was introduced into a gay bathhouse or an IDU "shooting gallery."

It should be noted that in SSA, where heterosexual HIV transmission has been so extensive, the majority of "general" populations, even in SSA countries with the highest HIV prevalence rates, are at low to no risk of acquiring HIV via sexual intercourse because they are monogamous or faithful to their spouses.

These aspects of HIV transmission dynamics were not fully understood during the late 1980s and early 1990s. In the USA and in most developed countries, where explosive HIV epidemics in MSM and IDU populations occurred during the early 1980s, the anticipated "next wave" of HIV epidemics did not materialize in any "general" heterosexual population. Michael Fumento accurately and in great detail documented this situation in his book *The Myth of Heterosexual AIDS*. However, he also seriously questioned the large and well documented heterosexual HIV epidemics in SSA and Thailand during this same time period.

Mainstream science and public health did not question these large heterosexual HIV epidemics but during this time period were at a loss to explain why epidemic heterosexual HIV transmission was so rampant in SSA and to a lesser extent in a few populations in the Caribbean and Asia and almost nonexistent in developed countries and most developing countries. Some of the initial theories were that: anal intercourse was more prevalent in African and Asian populations than was then believed and/or that poverty was a major determinant of high HIV prevalence. These myths or misconceptions about heterosexual HIV transmission continue to have staunch supporters. There has and continues to be some sort of fixation about anal intercourse that is also not warranted. There is nothing exceptional or mysterious about anal intercourse compared with vaginal intercourse with regard to the risk of HIV transmission. Anal intercourse results in a higher risk simply because of the greater likelihood of tissue trauma and thus more lesions in the fragile rectal epithelium compared to vaginal epithelium. However, there are multiple facilitating factors that can increase the amount of blood or sexual fluids that may be exchanged during vaginal intercourse and as described in Chapter 5, these facilitating factors are highly prevalent in SSA populations compared to most other populations.

- **All high HIV risk behaviors will result in HIV epidemics**

Until the mid-1990s, it was not fully realized that there are major differences in the pattern and size of commercial sex networks. It was believed, almost as a matter of faith, that once HIV was introduced into any commercial sex network, epidemic HIV transmission would inevitably ensue. I don't want to minimize the public health risk that epidemic HIV transmission can occur in virtually all commercial sex networks, but it should be realized that this risk can range from very low to very high. Fortunately, the risk has been very low in those networks where partner exchange rates are not the highest. AIDS denialists such as Duesberg and his followers, who believe that sexual transmission of HIV is a myth, point to the many studies of female prostitutes in developed countries and in many developing countries that show either no HIV infections or only a few to support their theories.

Calculation of the annual probability of a FSW acquiring an HIV infection in a low HIV prevalence country indicates that large annual increases in HIV incidence and prevalence cannot be expected (*see* Appendix 1 to Chapter 5). According to these calculations, if there were several hundred thousand FSW in the Philippines,* less than 100 might acquire an HIV infection each year because of sex work. These infected FSW can be expected to infect several male clients during an arbitrary work span of 10 years as a FSW. However, these numbers will be largely offset by the hundreds of AIDS deaths that can be expected annually from the thousands of prevalent infections in this very low HIV prevalence country. Since the early 1990s, sentinel surveillance in the Philippines has consistently found annual HIV prevalence in registered FSW to be about 1 per 1000. This low prevalence can be attributed to several factors:

1 a very low HIV prevalence in male clients of FSW – less than 1 per 1000
2 most males in the Philippines are circumcised at about the age of puberty
3 most FSW average less than one client a day and
4 reported condom use with FSW in the Philippines is more than 50 percent.

In countries where explosive HIV epidemics have occurred in IDU populations, a major public health concern is that some HIV-infected female IDU will become a FSW in order to support their drug use. Such an increase in HIV-infected FSW has been found in almost all HIV epidemics in IDU populations. These FSW can transmit infection to some of their clients, but as described above such increased transmission in low HIV prevalence countries does not lead to very large increases in annual national HIV incidence and prevalence. The factors needed for sustained epidemic heterosexual HIV transmission include:

1 large open or overlapping sex networks
2 high numbers of daily sex partner exchanges
3 a low percentage of male circumcision
4 low condom usage rates and
5 a high prevalence of multiple facilitating factors.

Thus, the probability of epidemic heterosexual HIV transmission in a low HIV prevalence country like the Philippines, even in the highest risk population (FSW and their clients), is low. The highest public health priority in low HIV prevalence populations is to assure that HIV prevalence in persons with the highest levels of heterosexual risk behaviors (FSW and their male clients) remain as low as possible. This can be accomplished by continuous preaching of **A**bstinence and **B**e faithful, but most likely, for persons with these sexual risk behaviors, promotion of **C** (consistent condom use) for all commercial sex will be the more effective measure for keeping HIV prevalence low in such populations. Aggressive implementation of all **ABC** measures in the general population with a focus on youth is epidemiologically not essential and will have little impact on potential HIV transmission in FSW and their male clients.

In any country, some pockets of very high sex partner exchange rates exist and they include: border areas with extensive population movement; extensive

---

* In the most recent (2005) HIV prevalence estimation exercise in the Philippines, the number of FSW was estimated to be less than 200 000 compared to previous estimates of up to a million or more!

migration and/or travel away from stable social environments such as from rural to urban areas for employment; seasonal workers; migrant workers; military, sailors/merchant seamen; long distance truck drivers; large development or construction projects; etc. Primary HIV prevention programs need to be targeted to these vulnerable populations wherever they may be, regardless of whether the potential for epidemic heterosexual HIV transmission is considered low or high.

- **Poverty, discrimination, and lack of access to healthcare are major determinants of high HIV prevalence**

This litany used by UNAIDS and most AIDS programs includes most of the socially and politically correct myths about major determinants of HIV transmission, but there is no epidemiologic support for these myths and misconceptions. Poverty is a socially and politically attractive hypothesis to account for high HIV prevalence, but available data suggest the opposite. As described in Chapter 5, persons in the top 20 percent for income in Kenya and Tanzania have HIV infection rates 2 to 3 times higher compared to persons in the lowest 20 percent – probably because the wealthiest persons, both males and females, have a greater number of sex partners. Some of the richest countries in SSA have the highest HIV prevalence rates and most of the poorest countries in the world have the lowest rates. Poverty as a major determinant of HIV transmission is a glorious myth that is not easily dispelled even though there are no epidemiologic data to support this myth. I have challenged all students who have taken my class since the new millennium to provide me with data to support this myth and they have yet to come up with any.

In 1987, Jon Mann appropriately declared that the quest for effective treatment and a possible cure for AIDS was an inherent basic human right of all persons living with HIV. However, he went on to say: "…Being excluded from the mainstream of society, or being discriminated against on grounds of race/ethnicity, national origin, religion, gender, or sexual preference, led [leads] to an increase of HIV infection." From my perspective, discrimination clearly raises barriers to HIV/AIDS prevention and treatment programs, but discrimination is not a determinant of HIV risk behaviors and, thus, not a determinant of epidemic HIV transmission. This glorious myth was quickly and uncritically accepted by AIDS activists, and is the centerpiece of UNAIDS' litany that poverty, discrimination, and lack of access to healthcare are major determinants of high HIV prevalence. Personally, I am 100 plus percent against poverty, discrimination, and lack of access to healthcare, but I also believe that even if "we" were able to eliminate these social and public health problems, we would not make much of an impact on the high HIV prevalence rates that are present in MSM, IDU and many SSA populations.

- **HIV prevalence is increasing to record highs. In 2005 there were more than 40 million persons living with HIV and there were 5 million new HIV infections**

These HIV/AIDS numbers are much too high: they cannot be supported by the available data or by recent HIV prevalence trends reported by UNAIDS for most global regions. Also as described in detail in Chapter 7, I believe that virtually all of the UNAIDS estimates in 2001 and 2003 were overestimated, especially for SSA and Asia. In mid-2006, UNAIDS significantly reduced many HIV prevalence estimates in SSA and the Caribbean to more realistic levels. However, I believe that they will need to reduce their lowered estimate for Haiti even more when the population-based HIV serosurveys (DHS+) are completed in Haiti* sometime in 2006. Similar reductions will also need to be made for Eastern Europe and Central Asia (Russia and Ukraine)[†], South and SE Asia (India), and East Asia and the Pacific (China).[‡] I haven't seen any regional estimate that I consider to be an underestimate and I'm convinced that even with the reductions made in the mid-2006 report, UNAIDS will be forced to revise most of their regional estimates further downwards in their next global report on the AIDS pandemic. Global estimates that are more consistent with current data and prevalence trends are about 30 million persons (15–49) living with HIV and closer to 3 million annual new adult HIV infections. Continual denial by UNAIDS of the reality of lower HIV prevalence numbers and continual alarms about HIV being "on the brink" of jumping into general populations will eventually lead to a backlash against AIDS programs for continually crying wolf when there is no epidemiologic basis for such alarms.

UNAIDS considers itself primarily an advocacy agency. Thus, it does not approach the estimation of HIV/AIDS statistics as an objective technical or scientific agency. I recall an exchange I had with the Minister of Health in the Philippines in the early 1990s when I cautioned him about the very high estimate he made by multiplying the 50 reported HIV/AIDS cases by a factor of a thousand to arrive at a national prevalence estimate of 50 000. He told me: "...accuracy is not needed for advocacy!" This unfortunately is how UNAIDS continues to approach the estimation of HIV/AIDS incidence and prevalence. Without all the "doom and gloom" HIV scenarios and without the alarming news releases that warn about constantly increasing HIV infections, AIDS activists fear that the public and policy makers will not continue to give AIDS programs the high priority that it has received up to now. AIDS activists are concerned that the public and policy makers will become complacent about the potential risk of HIV to the general population and will reduce support to AIDS programs if most regional HIV rates are "stable" or decreasing and HIV remains concentrated in MSM, IDU, FSW and their clients, and in most SSA populations.

This is a realistic concern, but as described at the end of Chapter 7:

1 global and regional HIV rates have remained stable or have been decreasing during the past decade
2 HIV has indeed continued to be concentrated in populations with the highest levels of HIV risk behaviors and
3 HIV is incapable of epidemic spread in the vast majority of heterosexual populations.

---

* In the UNAIDS/WHO *2005 AIDS Epidemic Update Report*, the reduction in HIV prevalence for Haiti from about 6 percent to 3 percent was considered as a possible sign that the HIV epidemic in Haiti may have "turned the corner." There was no mention that such a reduction was forced because of low HIV prevalence findings in rural populations.

† There have been large HIV epidemics in IDU populations, but overall HIV prevalence is probably overestimated.

‡ The 2005 report also said that the number of persons in this region living with HIV in 2005 increased by 20 percent compared to 2003. Actually, the official Chinese estimate for 2005 (released in early 2006) showed the opposite. There has been a decrease in HIV prevalence from 840 000 in 2003 to 650 000 in 2005.

Denial of these realities will lead to further erosion of whatever credibility UNAIDS and other mainstream AIDS agencies may still have.

Swimming Upstream Against Mainstream AIDS Agencies

As someone who was in the vanguard of mainstream medical science and public health understanding about the HIV/AIDS pandemic until my resignation from GPA/WHO in early 1992, I fully understand and am sympathetic to the beliefs and positions that AIDS activists have taken and continue to defend. I share the same objectives as my mainstream colleagues; effective prevention and control of HIV/AIDS; and the provision of effective ART for all HIV-infected persons. However, over the past decade, I have come to believe that AIDS programs, especially those developed and supported by international agencies and faith-based organizations, have been politically correct and morally motivated but epidemiologically incorrect.

When AIDS was first recognized in California in 1981, I had already worked as a public health epidemiologist in general communicable disease control for close to two decades. I was rapidly totally immersed in the study of AIDS. In addition to my evaluation of all studies and reports of HIV/AIDS in California as the State Epidemiologist responsible for infectious disease control, I served on a National Academy of Science/Institute of Medicine (NAS/IOM) committee in 1986 that prepared a national report on AIDS.* During the 6-month work period of this committee, I was able to help review and evaluate all of the national and international epidemiologic, clinical, and laboratory studies on HIV/AIDS that were made available to this committee. Thus, when I took early retirement from the California Health Department in 1987 to join Jon Mann at WHO in Geneva, I had been involved almost fulltime in the study of HIV epidemiology for about 6 years.

In retrospect, all of the initial HIV prevalence estimates that I was personally involved with were gross overestimates. I was a member of a small group of epidemiologists who made the first national HIV prevalence estimate for the USA during the 1986 Coolfont Conference in West Virginia. Based on the limited data available to our group we estimated that there were from 1 to 1.5 million HIV-infected persons in the USA. The first HIV estimation meeting that I organized after Jon anointed me to head the Surveillance, Forecasting, and Impact Assessment (SFI) unit at GPA was held in Strbske Pleso, Slovakia in early 1988. In reviewing the HIV prevalence estimates made during this meeting, I now realize that most of these estimates were also gross overestimates: the UK estimate was 40 000 and this estimate was later reduced by almost half; the initial working estimate for France was 200 000 and this estimate was also reduced by more than half after more data became available.

In 1986, Jon Mann estimated that there were from 5 to 10 million HIV-infected persons worldwide; this was the "official" global estimate I inherited when I was appointed Chief of SFI. During the Fourth International AIDS Conference in Stockholm in mid-1988, Bob Biggers, a CDC (Atlanta) epidemiologist who was working in Africa, confronted me in a hallway and challenged the WHO global estimate of 5–10 million. I had been collecting and reviewing all available HIV

---

* *Confronting AIDS: Directions for Public Health Care and Research* (NAS/IOM, 1986).

data from WHO member countries and had to agree with Bob that the estimate of 5–10 million was too high. I brought this situation to Jon's attention and recommended that WHO revise the global estimate to about 5 million since my estimate based on the data I had reviewed could reasonably only support an estimate that was less than 5 million. I even drafted a statement for his consideration for release: "WHO in 1986, based on the limited HIV data available, estimated global HIV prevalence to be 5 to 10 million. However, as of mid-1988, with additional HIV data, the best estimate of global HIV prevalence is closer to the lower range of about 5 million." Jon decided not to issue this statement because he felt sure that at the apparent rate of increase in HIV prevalence in SSA noted in the most recent HIV datasets, that within a year or two at most, global HIV prevalence would be well within the 5–10 million range. Jon proved to be right on the mark and by the early 1990s, global HIV prevalence increased to well within the 5–10 million range.

As I gradually recognized that the HIV estimates described above were gross overestimates, I resolved that any estimate I would be responsible for would be conservative, and further, I would not release an estimate that I could not defend with the available data. After my resignation from WHO in early 1992, I maintained contact with my former staff at SFI and was pleased that HIV prevalence estimates prepared by SFI up to the mid-1990s continued to be conservative and defendable. I was, however, concerned about the urban/rural HIV differential in SSA. Thus, I urged WHO and subsequently UNAIDS staff to devote more effort to measure this differential since the majority of populations in SSA lived in rural areas. This factor has turned out to be the major reason for the 50 percent or more overestimate of HIV prevalence in most SSA and Caribbean countries.

Most AIDS activists were greatly disturbed by any downward revision of official HIV prevalence estimates: they perceived such revisions as a deliberate ploy by public health programs to minimize the severity of HIV/AIDS epidemics. There was and continues to be great distrust of official HIV prevalence estimates by most AIDS activists. During the late 1980s and early 1990s, high and constantly increasing HIV/AIDS estimates were accepted uncritically and assumed to be the unchanging trend of all HIV/AIDS epidemics by AIDS program advocates and activists. Any lowering of an estimate or any projection that HIV or AIDS might be peaking or decreasing was considered to be dangerous to HIV/AIDS programs. It was thought such projections would lead to complacency in implementing prevention and control measures.

Thus, when I predicted in 1991 that "...in developed countries annual AIDS cases were projected to reach a peak before the middle of the decade...," * I incurred the displeasure of Sir Donald Acheson, the Chief Medical Officer in the UK. He apparently was in the audience for my lecture and he immediately dispatched one of his best and brightest medical officers, Dr. Anne Johnson, a very astute medical epidemiologist, to determine if my projection of AIDS cases peaking in developed countries before 1995 could be refuted. Anne Johnson and I had a very cordial and collegial discussion regarding my prediction. As an experienced STD/HIV epidemiologist, she was aware that HIV incidence rates peaked in the USA and the UK before the mid-1980s. Anyone who knew the

---

*State of the Art – Plenary Lecture – Present and Future Dimensions of the HIV/AIDS Pandemic. Seventh International Conference on AIDS, Florence, Italy, June, 1991.

median progression interval from HIV infection to the development of AIDS was estimated to be from 8 to 10 years did not require any complex mathematical model to predict that AIDS cases would peak in these countries before the mid-1990s. Apparently, Anne Johnson was able to adequately explain the epidemiologic basis of my prediction to Sir Donald since I did not hear anymore about this. I had thought my projection regarding the natural decline in AIDS cases that could be expected based on the natural history of HIV infections and on HIV incidence and prevalence trends would be welcomed as "good" news, rather than "bad" news.

Up to the time of my resignation from WHO, I considered myself to be an integral part of mainstream AIDS beliefs. I traveled with Jon Mann and Daniel Tarantola in 1988 to meet with key staff of the WHO Regional Offices in Manila (WPRO) and Delhi (SEARO) to try to kick start some aggressive HIV/AIDS prevention programs in Asia. We exhorted them with the rhetoric that the "window of opportunity" for effective HIV/AIDS prevention in Asia was fast closing. I was convinced by my visits to cities such as Cairo and Manila that it was not a matter of if, but when heterosexual HIV epidemics would break out in these cities. However, by the mid-1990s, when there was no sign of epidemic heterosexual HIV spread, other than in those populations where such epidemic transmission had been documented during the 1980s and early 1990s, seeds of doubt regarding the "gathering storm" of HIV epidemics in Asia began to emerge.

These doubts began to grow but it wasn't until a 6-week USAID mission to evaluate the HIV/AIDS situation in the Philippines in 1995 that I was "converted" to my present understanding of HIV transmission dynamics. I was the epidemiologist and Tony Bennett, who was working for Family Health International (FHI) in their Bangkok office, was the social behavioral expert on this mission. Tony provided me with detailed qualitative and quantitative information on commercial sex networks in Asia. We jogged for close to an hour almost every morning on Roxas Boulevard and pondered why epidemic heterosexual HIV transmission had not erupted in Manila when commercial sex was so visible, especially near all hotels. Tony pointed out that commercial sex for foreigners was readily available and quite visible in virtually all Asian cities but this was not a good gauge of the extent of commercial sex for the indigenous population. It was from these discussions that we both began to realize that the patterns and prevalence of sexual risk behaviors in the Philippines were among the lowest in Asia. Our conclusion has made us *personae non gratae* to the Philippines AIDS program because staff of the national program believes that there is a very high potential for heterosexual HIV epidemic transmission in the Philippines and our conclusion is therefore dangerous and represents "blind optimism."

Tony and I, together with Steve Mills, a social behavioral office colleague of Tony's, prepared a paper that we submitted to *Lancet*. Our paper was rejected on the basis that it was common knowledge that HIV transmission is correlated with sexual risk behaviors and this had been amply documented by many African studies. The basic conclusion of our paper – still not accepted by most mainstream AIDS "experts" – is that countries such as the Philippines and Indonesia will not reach HIV prevalence levels of more than 0.5% (1/200) in their 15–49 year old population because the sex networks and general levels of sexual risk behaviors are insufficient to drive significant heterosexual epidemics. We eventually were able to get our paper published in a special supplemental issue of the journal *AIDS* devoted to AIDS in Asia.[*]

At the 1997 AIDS in Asia Conference in Manila, Peter Piot, in his keynote lecture warned that when HIV epidemics break out in Asian countries, "HIV will cut through Asian populations like a hot knife through cold butter!" Aside from several explosive HIV epidemics in IDU populations, there have not been significant heterosexual HIV epidemics in any Asian country since Peter's dire and colorful prediction. My question to those who believe in the inevitability of HIV epidemics sweeping through general populations in Asian countries is: How many decades do we need to wait before such epidemics might be considered unlikely? Tim Brown told me that, using his HIV/AIDS model, epidemic HIV transmission could occur in FSW in the Philippines within one or two more decades. I told Tim that this would never happen if HIV prevention in the Philippines were to be focused almost totally on populations with the highest risk behaviors (includes IDU, MSM and FSW and their clients) instead of directing a major portion of the prevention budget to educate the general public and youth. My cynical opinion is that pretty soon, AIDS activists will begin to assume full or at least major credit for "successful" HIV prevention programs in Asian and Pacific countries.

After resigning from WHO, I returned to California and became a self-employed[†] independent consultant on HIV/AIDS in developing countries and was able to supplement my retirement incomes with about a half a dozen assignments per year. I was able to evaluate the epidemiology of HIV/AIDS or participate in HIV prevalence estimation meetings in Kenya, Malawi, Albania, Turkey, China, Indonesia, Malaysia, Vietnam, Nepal, Philippines, Hong Kong, Taiwan, South Korea, Laos, India, and Myanmar. In addition, I was asked by several agencies to prepare regional HIV/AIDS reports. Specifically, I was asked to prepare a situation analysis of HIV/AIDS in Asia for the 33rd Annual Conference of the Asian Development Bank (ADB) held in Chiang Mai, Thailand in May 2000. My problem with this report and my subsequent reports was that I tried to be as objective as possible. I kept downplaying the potential for HIV to ever become a "generalized" epidemic in any Asian country. Since such a conclusion was not compatible with the UNAIDS paradigm or with the concerns of AIDS program advocacy organizations such as the International Harm Reduction Association (IHRA), I was considered by mainstream AIDS agencies as not a "team player!"

In spite of my growing reputation as an epidemiologist with unorthodox conclusions about HIV/AIDS, I was asked by the WHO regional offices in Manila (Western Pacific Regional Office – WPRO) and Delhi (South East Asia Regional Office – SEARO) to prepare a report in 2001 on AIDS in Asia and the Pacific regions. I was surprised to be asked and I told my WHO colleagues that I had just finished a similar report for the ADB and I would not be changing much of what I had prepared but I would provide more details and would update the report. This was accepted and I was basically given a blank check during my 3-month assignment to visit any country in the Asia and the Pacific regions to get what updates and details I might need for preparing my report. I finished a draft report for WPRO and SEARO on schedule and was pleasantly surprised

---

[*] Chin J, Bennett A and Mills S (1998) Primary determinants of HIV prevalence in Asian-Pacific countries. *AIDS*. **12**(Suppl B): S87–91.
[†] My wife Anne correctly points out that I was mostly unemployed!

that there were no major changes requested for the final report. The only change I can remember is that the final draft contained the word "promiscuity": I was asked to change it and had no problem changing promiscuity to "a high level of sex partner exchange." To the credit of WPRO and SEARO, they released the 2001 report* in spite of external pressures to stop its printing and distribution. I think that the report was generally well received as an accurate and objective report on AIDS in Asia and the Pacific regions – but that's my personal bias.

Most AIDS "experts" do not understand and don't even want to think about what I have tried to stress constantly in this book. HIV is difficult to transmit sexually and epidemic heterosexual HIV transmission can occur only in the presence of the highest risk pattern and highest prevalence of sexual risk behaviors. Such high levels are not present in most "general" populations. I have found that it is very difficult to change the mind set and beliefs of most "hardcore" AIDS "experts" and activists. Such changes require first and foremost an open mind and in addition it requires a basic understanding of infectious disease epidemiology as well as what I have been referring to as HIV transmission dynamics. Significant heterosexual HIV epidemic transmission has only occurred in populations with the highest risk pattern and prevalence of sexual risk behaviors: mostly in SSA, several countries in the Caribbean, and a few in Asia. In over 100 HIV epidemics in MSM and/or IDU populations in developed and developing countries, no significant heterosexual HIV epidemics have subsequently erupted. This can only be explained by

1 highly effective HIV prevention programs or
2 the fact that in most heterosexual populations, the patterns and prevalence of heterosexual risk behaviors are not sufficient to sustain or fuel epidemic HIV transmission.

I obviously don't think that effective HIV prevention programs can be credited for the low HIV prevalence present in most countries throughout the world!

Over the past few years, virtually all of the graduate students (about half postdoctoral students) who enroll in my class at Berkeley come in with orthodox views and beliefs about HIV epidemiology consistent with the UNAIDS paradigm. I generally find that it takes from 10 to 12 class hours before some begrudging changes start to take hold. The most difficult orthodox myth to dispel is that poverty is a major determinant of high HIV prevalence in developing African and Asian countries. When challenged to provide epidemiologic support for this view, their doubts emerge gradually when they cannot find support for this myth. By contrast, I'm able to show them epidemiologic data that indicate the wealthiest persons in several African studies have the highest HIV infection rates. By the end of the class, I believe that I had converted them to accept my HIV/AIDS paradigm.

I was surprised that I was again asked to prepare a 2003 report on AIDS in Asia and the Pacific regions for WPRO and SEARO. Because of the political sensitivity of my views and conclusions about HIV/AIDS, this second report was probably

---

* This report was available for downloading from WPRO as of August, 2006 www.wpro.who.int/NR/rdonlyres/3E936DD1-BDF6-4669-88F3-854B4D0EA95F/0/ HIV_AIDS_Asia_Pacific_Region2001.pdf

sent to just about everyone working or interested in AIDS in WHO or UNAIDS in Manila, Delhi, Bangkok, and probably Geneva for editorial review. I received such a barrage of comments and suggestions for changes that I finally threw in the towel and told WPRO and SEARO that I agreed to prepare the 2003 report and I would stand by what I had prepared. I was not prepared to rewrite my report based on comments from virtually the total staffs of several offices. Actually, the final 2003 report* eventually released was not very different from what I had initially submitted.

The World Bank also asked me to prepare a detailed report on the prospects for severe HIV epidemics in Asia. I prepared a 50-page report and several months after submitting it I asked about its disposition. I was told that World Bank staff had prepared a detailed situation analysis of HIV/AIDS in the Asia region and my report was "helpful." In the final strategy paper they issued, my report was essentially boiled down to one footnote: "In contrast [to high range projections], low range estimates predict Asia HIV epidemics are constrained by low risk sexual behavior in the general population (Chin, 2003)."

Tony Bennett and I submitted a more detailed paper entitled "The Epidemiologic Basis for Limited Heterosexual HIV Epidemics" to the *American Journal of Epidemiology*. We initially got no response until close to 6 months after submission and then we received a letter of rejection. The reviewers did not believe that we provided sufficient data to support our conclusions. One stated: "…[the] hypothesis discussed in this paper, that heterosexual HIV transmissions is unlikely to reach epidemic proportions in most populations (with the exception of SSA and a few Caribbean and Asian countries) is interesting, and may have merit. However, the data presented and the analyses described are not sufficient to draw conclusions." Our position was and continues to be that there are far less data to support the prevailing paradigm that in the absence of effective HIV prevention, epidemic heterosexual HIV transmission will inevitably occur. I believe that we provided more than ample data to show that extensive sexual HIV epidemics, whether in homosexual or heterosexual populations, have occurred only in those populations with the highest risk patterns of sex partner exchange and that such populations have much higher prevalence (from 1 to 2 orders of magnitude higher) of facilitating factors for sexual HIV transmission compared with populations where no epidemic sexual HIV transmission has occurred. Tony Bennett and I can't figure out what additional data these epidemiologists need or want?

After discussions with my epidemiologic mentor,† he recommended that we submit our conclusions to the *New England Journal of Medicine* for their Sounding Board section which includes brief opinion or editorial type papers. Our submission was rejected on the basis that our paper was not sufficiently noteworthy compared with their waiting list of papers accepted for the Sounding Board section. After this second strike, I persuaded Tony to resubmit our paper that was rejected by the *American Journal of Epidemiology* to the *American Journal of Preventive Medicine*. We redrafted the paper and renamed it: "Heterosexual HIV

---

* This report was available for downloading from a WPRO site as of August, 2006 www.wpro.who.int/NR/rdonlyres/11ED3283-9821-43BE-9B73-B3444A3DADE6/ 0/HIV_AIDS_Asia_Pacific_Region2003.pdf
† Warren Winkelstein, emeritus Professor of Epidemiology, School of Public Health, UC Berkeley.

Transmission Dynamics: Implications for Prevention and Control" and submitted it after I informed the chief editor that we were submitting a paper that had been rejected by another peer review journal.* When we received our third rejection from this journal, both Tony and I agreed that we had struck out – strike 3! It is a bit telling that one of the comments from the reviewer who apparently was the most assertive in rejecting our paper was: "...there is no such thing as nonepidemic heterosexual HIV transmission, since every HIV infection is part of the total AIDS pandemic!" It was quite clear to us that this reviewer did not have a clue as to what we were talking about when we described nonepidemic HIV transmission from an infected person to his or her regular sex partner(s) and the implications this pattern of HIV transmission has for prevention programs.

I realize that I have to walk a very fine line in criticizing the UNAIDS paradigm because I'm acutely aware that the needs of AIDS prevention and treatment programs throughout the world in both developed and developing countries have been and continue to be grossly under funded. HIV/AIDS numbers in SSA, even if cut in half, still constitute one of the largest human disease disasters in modern times! According to what may be the lowest estimate of current adult HIV prevalence in SSA (15 million), about 4000 AIDS deaths can be expected to occur daily! If UNAIDS' prevalence estimate of close to 25 million is accepted, then about 6000 AIDS deaths would occur daily. By comparison, the December 26, 2004 Indian Ocean earthquake and tsunami was estimated to have killed over a quarter of a million persons and the disastrous earthquakes in Pakistan and India in October 2005 may eventually claim up to 100 000 lives. Yet, regardless of which HIV prevalence estimate in SSA may be more accurate, there are now at least 2 million AIDS deaths annually in SSA and this annual number may continue to be this high for at least another decade! Thus, I do not want, in any way, to compromise the international support that has been mobilized for the Global Fund. I believe that even with the lowest possible HIV estimate for SSA, there are insufficient funds to meet the needs of ART programs in SSA and all other resource-poor countries. I do not want the public and policy makers to *throw out the baby* – the severe AIDS problem in SSA and MSM and IDU populations – *with the bath water* – systematic overestimation of HIV prevalence and exaggeration of the potential for epidemic heterosexual HIV transmission in most developing countries outside of SSA.

The following response of a policy person in the WHO Office in Beijing, China after my March 2003 debriefing on the HIV/AIDS situation in China is typical of what I have come to expect from most AIDS program advocates. She said that my conclusions about the low potential for severe heterosexual HIV epidemics in China might well be accurate, but that she could not be certain that it was really an accurate picture of HIV/AIDS in China since UNAIDS paints an entirely different picture. She also said, "What is the harm in keeping the public and policy makers fearful of impending heterosexual HIV epidemics erupting in China if sexual risk behaviors are not reduced or eliminated?"

The basic harm, from my perspective, is that in China HIV prevention efforts are misdirected and essentially wasted on the general public and youth who are

---

* Prior to these rejections, I submitted over 70 papers for publication where I was the sole author (about 50) or was a co-author (about 20), to mostly peer review journals without a single rejection.

at little or no risk of epidemic heterosexual HIV transmission. In China, for the past decade, the primary mode of HIV transmission has been from an HIV-infected person to his/her regular sex partner, i.e., HIV transmission in discordant couples. HIV infection of large numbers of poor farmers via faulty plasma collection procedures probably peaked by the mid-1990s. HIV epidemics in IDU populations have occurred starting in the late 1980s and annual HIV incidence in most of these epidemics peaked or at least leveled off by the late 1990s. For the past decade, there has been great concern that HIV infections from the large pool of infected IDU and the large number of poor infected peasants would "jump" into the general population via infected female prostitutes. Intensified HIV sentinel surveillance was set up in all areas where any HIV epidemic had occurred but as of late-2006, I'm not aware that any significant heterosexual HIV epidemic spread has been detected in China.*

In China and throughout the world, I believe that there has been insufficient attention given to the different patterns of sexual risk behaviors that exist and range from the highest risk (hundreds to thousands of different sex partners annually) to the lowest (a few different sex partners during a lifetime). It is socially and politically correct to assume that, because sexual risk behaviors are present in all populations throughout the world, all populations are, therefore, at almost equal risk of epidemic sexual HIV transmission. There is an occasional disclaimer that perhaps heterosexual HIV epidemics may not ever be quite as severe as those in SSA. As a very old and experienced infectious disease epidemiologist, I fully recognize that any heterosexual epidemic, no matter how "small" in populous countries such as China, India, and Indonesia could quickly total several million or more new HIV infections during this decade. However, I cannot understand the need to have huge numbers of HIV infections to make AIDS a very high priority public health problem. As a global community, "we" would not tolerate a few human mad cow disease cases, yet if a country has "only" a few thousand HIV infections, AIDS activists somehow feel belittled.

I am not preaching public health complacency, but I am preaching that effective prevention of HIV transmission in low prevalence countries must be targeted primarily to the highest HIV risk populations and not to the general public and youth. I am also saying that there has been and continues to be insufficient public health attention and effort directed to the regular sex partners of HIV-infected persons in both developed and developing countries.

Summary and Conclusions

The UNAIDS paradigm is very socially and politically attractive and correct, but there are no data to support the litany that poverty, discrimination, and lack of access to healthcare, are the major determinants of high HIV prevalence in developing countries. To the contrary, all of the available epidemiologic data indicate that having a high risk pattern of sex behaviors (multiple and concurrent sex partners) as well as the highest frequency of sex partner exchanges are the major factors that drive sexual HIV epidemics in MSM or heterosexual populations. My

---

* Aside from published and official HIV data released by China, I have not seen any data that show significant HIV transmission that may be independent of the IDU or plasma collection epidemics.

paradigm, that epidemic sexual HIV epidemics can only occur in populations with the highest risk pattern and highest prevalence of sex partner exchanges, is consistent with all of the current sexual HIV epidemics that have been documented throughout the world. Despite UNAIDS' constant alarms, no epidemic heterosexual epidemics have occurred following hundreds of HIV epidemics in MSM and IDU populations!

Explosive HIV epidemics occurred in MSM and IDU populations in many developed countries during the early to mid 1980s and such epidemic spread peaked (i.e., HIV incidence peaked) by the mid- to late-1980s. Since the new millennium, HIV prevalence has also peaked, but has been decreasing very slowly because:

1 high risk behaviors are still present, albeit perhaps at some lower levels
2 the steady nonepidemic transmission from HIV-infected persons (regardless of how they may have been infected) to their regular sex partners continues to occur
3 effective anti-HIV treatment (ART) programs that became available in most developed countries by the mid-1990s have significantly extended the lifespan of many HIV-infected persons.

These factors explain why HIV prevalence in developed countries are "stable" or may even slightly increase over the next several decades.

In several Asian countries, including several Indian States, explosive heterosexual HIV epidemics occurred within their large and very open commercial sex networks. In addition, several explosive and relatively independent HIV epidemics occurred in IDU populations in many developing countries in Asia and in several countries of the former Soviet Union during the 1990s. The scope of all of these epidemics have been largely exaggerated and the concern that HIV epidemics in IDU populations will inevitably lead to epidemics in the general population or to "ordinary" people continues to have staunch believers. This entrenched myth persists even though there is scant, if any, HIV spread into the general population other than from the infected IDU to his or her regular sex partners. Commercial sex driven epidemics in Asian countries peaked by the mid-1990s and HIV prevalence in countries that had any HIV epidemics have been level or decreasing since the new millennium.

In SSA, heterosexual HIV epidemics have progressed much slower compared to other global regions because the majority of sex networks have been and continue to be relatively small (as small as 3 to 4 in a sex group). According to the most recent UNAIDS estimates, the HIV prevalence rate in SSA peaked around the year 2000, and has been decreasing slowly since then. In order for HIV prevalence in SSA to be decreasing since the new millennium the annual HIV incidence rate in SSA had to have peaked around the mid-1990s. Such decreases in HIV prevalence and incidence are totally inconsistent with UNAIDS' most recent press releases about the ever-expanding and increasing numbers of the AIDS pandemic. UNAIDS and all AIDS activists should be happy to hear that HIV incidence in SSA probably peaked about a decade ago, but they are not willing to even consider this possibility because it would undermine their paradigm.

The vast majority of the public and policy makers have no inkling that the UNAIDS paradigm is inconsistent with established facts about HIV transmission dynamics. This is because they have not had any reason to doubt UNAIDS' information and data. Up to 2006, there has been no criticism or disagreement with the UNAIDS paradigm and its assessment of the AIDS pandemic raised by: any of the major public health and infectious disease agencies (NIH, CDC, APHA, etc); any of the international development agencies (USAID, DFID, etc.); or any of the UN agencies. However, some break from this thundering silence of mainstream AIDS organizations is finally beginning to appear. In late March, 2006, I received a draft of a paper that was submitted to the *Lancet*.* The authors of this paper (technical staff of USAID and the World Bank) reached the same conclusions as I have about the AIDS pandemic peak (end of Chapter 7). Shortly after this article was published, UNAIDS acknowledged in their mid-2006 report to the UN that global HIV incidence probably peaked during the late 1990s. I'm confident that starting in late-2006, UNAIDS will be forced to come up with even more realistic estimates and projections, especially when more mainstream epidemiologists and the news media begin to critically question the epidemiologic basis of the UNAIDS paradigm.†

Regardless of my epidemiologic disagreements with UNAIDS, I totally agree with mainstream AIDS experts who declare that this is not a time to be complacent about the need to strengthen HIV prevention, since annual HIV incidence globally will still be at least 2 to 3 million. However, the glorious myths that are still perpetuated by UNAIDS and AIDS activists, i.e., that the AIDS pandemic is fueled or driven by poverty; the "next waves" of HIV epidemics are inevitable; and the AIDS pandemic is ever-expanding will, sooner or later, all have to be abandoned.

---

* Shelton JD, Halperin DT and Wilson D. Has Global HIV Incidence Peaked? The Lancet.com published online 30 March 2006, DOI:10.10.1016/SO140-6736(06)68436-5.
† Godwin P, O'Farrell N, Fylkesnes K and Misra S (2006) Five myths about the HIV epidemic in Asia. PLoS Med 3(10): e426. DOI: 10.1371/journal. pmed.0030426. Myth number one was: There is a major risk that the epidemic in many Asian countries will have the same disastrous "development impact" as in sub-Saharan Africa, but on a much worse scale, given the huge population sizes of much of Asia.

Chapter 10

The Most Probable Past, Present, and Future of the AIDS Pandemic

The global number of AIDS deaths in 2003 might have been as high as 3 million according to an earlier UNAIDS estimate or as low as about 2 million according to my conservative estimate. Regardless of which estimate may be more accurate, there is no question that AIDS is one of the most severe infectious disease pandemics in the last millennium. This chapter compares the AIDS pandemic with other major infectious disease pandemics to put AIDS in historical perspective. It also compares AIDS deaths with other current leading causes of death to provide a global perspective on the current impact of the AIDS pandemic. I'll conclude by presenting what I believe will be the most likely future regional HIV scenarios.

The AIDS Pandemic in Historical Perspective

How severe is the AIDS pandemic compared with past infectious disease pandemics? From historical records, estimates of the attack rate (i.e., percent of the population infected) and case fatality rate can be used to calculate deaths attributed to each pandemic. Table 10.1 presents these values for plague (The Black Death) in the mid-14th Century, influenza in 1918 ("Spanish flu"), and most recently influenza in 1957 ("Asian flu") and in 1968 ("Hong Kong flu").

Table 10.1 Estimated global deaths in selected major infectious disease pandemics

Pandemic	World pop	Attack Rate	No. of Infections	Case Fatality	No. of Deaths	[Total] Annual Deaths**
Plague (Europe) 1347–1352	*75 million	33 to 66%	25 to 50 million in 5 yrs	1/2	12.5 to 25 million	[1–2 billion] 200 to 400 million
Spanish flu 1918	1.8 billion	40 to 60%	1 billion in <1 yr	3/100	30 million	100 million
Asian flu 1957	2.9 billion	25 to 50%	>1 billion in <1 yr	2/1000	2–3 million	6 million
H Kong flu 1968	3.6 billion	25 to 50%	1–2 billion in <1 yr	1/1000	1–2 million	3 million
HIV/AIDS 1980–2005	6 billion	<1%	70 million in 25 yrs	>9/10	40 million***	[40 million] < 2 million

*Estimated population of Europe only; **Calculated based on 2005 world population; ***The majority of HIV infections acquired after 1995 have not progressed to AIDS and death by the year 2005.

If we assume that the estimated infection and case fatality rates are reasonably accurate,* the deaths caused by each pandemic can be calculated. However, deaths from each pandemic cannot be compared directly because the world's population has increased greatly since the 14th Century and the duration of each pandemic was different. If the attack and case fatality rates for each pandemic are applied to the current global population we get a more valid comparison of their relative severity. Average annual deaths from each pandemic can be obtained by dividing the total deaths by the duration of each pandemic.

The plague pandemic (the Black Death) apparently swept into Europe from Asia in the year 1347 and is believed to have infected from one to two thirds of the total European population (estimated at 75 million). The estimated case fatality rate was about 50 percent and over a 5-year period plague killed up to a third of Europe's population. If these rates are applied to the current world population of about 6 billion we find that 1 to 2 billion plague deaths occurred over a 5-year period for an average of 200 to 400 million deaths per year. The estimated attack or infection rates for the plague and the three influenza pandemics were all high and infected from a quarter to two thirds of the total population. The infection rate for the HIV/AIDS pandemic is about 1 percent of the adult population or about 0.5 percent of the total world population.

These pandemics, except for the AIDS pandemic, can be classified as "generalized" pandemics since virtually the entire global population was at moderate to high risk for acquiring these infections. However, at most, only about 10 to 20 percent of the world's adult population (5 to 10 percent of the total world population) can be considered to have significant HIV risk behaviors and thus be at some measurable risk for epidemic HIV transmission. Epidemiologically, the AIDS pandemic cannot be classified as a "generalized" pandemic. Yet UNAIDS and mainstream AIDS organizations persist in using this designation for AIDS epidemics in SSA countries and in the few countries in the Caribbean and Asia with an estimated adult HIV prevalence rate of over 1 percent.

The case fatality rate for AIDS (> 90 percent) is among the highest for any infectious disease and was also very high for plague in the 14th Century (about 50 percent). Case fatality rates for the influenza pandemics are all much lower but the case-fatality rate for the Spanish flu pandemic was about 30 times greater than for the Asian flu pandemic and 15 times greater than the Hong Kong flu pandemic. If the criterion of severity of an infectious disease is the cumulative number of deaths attributed to that disease, then without question, the most severe human infectious disease, which has been and continues as a major cause of annual deaths, is tuberculosis (TB). During World TB Day 1999 it was reported that an estimated one **billion** persons died of the disease worldwide during the 19th and early 20th Centuries alone.†

---

* Estimates for the plague and the 1918 flu pandemics were derived from several websites on the history of these pandemics: estimates for the 1957 and 1968 flu pandemics were from a CDC (Atlanta) website. I used conservative estimates for each of these pandemics.
† If TB estimators are similar to some AIDS estimators, then a billion may be high, but probably within the ballpark!

Current Global Impact of AIDS

In 1993 the World Bank in collaboration with the World Health Organization and the Harvard School of Public Health sponsored a study to assess the Global Burden of Disease (GBD). This study developed a comprehensive and relatively consistent set of estimates of mortality and morbidity by age, sex and region of the world. The GBD project tried, to the extent possible, to disentangle epidemiology from advocacy in order to produce objective, independent and demographically plausible assessments of the burdens of particular conditions and diseases. Although some of these estimates can be challenged,* overall, they represent the most objective estimates of global diseases and deaths. The following figures were developed from a World Bank groups' analysis of mortality and the burden of disease for 2001. Version 3 revisions of the GBD study[†] were used.

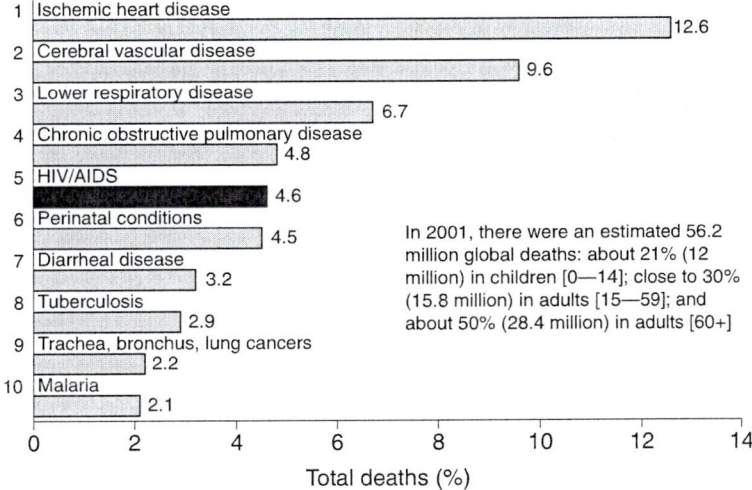

In 2001, there were an estimated 56.2 million global deaths: about 21% (12 million) in children [0—14]; close to 30% (15.8 million) in adults [15—59]; and about 50% (28.4 million) in adults [60+]

Total deaths (%)

Data source: Version 3 revisions of the Global Burden of Disease (GBD) study.

Figure 10.1 Ten leading causes of global death in 2001.

Figure 10.1 presents in rank order the 10 leading causes of global deaths according to the GBD 2001 estimates – AIDS deaths in 2001 were estimated to be about 4.6 percent (about 2.5 million) of the global total of 56.2 million deaths. Version 3 of the GBD study used UNAIDS' revised 2001 estimates of global AIDS deaths (about 2.5 million) because according to the initial 2001 UNAIDS estimate there was a total of 3 million AIDS deaths. Use of the initial 2001 estimate would have raised AIDS deaths to over 5 percent of the global

---

* HIV prevalence and AIDS deaths were probably overestimated by 25 to 50 percent in 2001. Some malaria modelers believe that annual malaria deaths may be at least 3 million or over 5 percent of global deaths!

† Mathers CD *et al.* (2005) Disease Control Priorities Project, Working Paper No. 18, April 2004. *Deaths and Disease Burden by Cause: global burden of disease estimates for 2001 by World Bank Country Groups.* www.dcp2.org/file/33/wp18.pdf

death total in 2001 and raised AIDS deaths to fourth place, ahead of chronic pulmonary obstructive conditions. If my lower estimates of HIV prevalence and AIDS deaths for 2001 are used, AIDS deaths would number about 2 million and this would lower AIDS deaths to sixth place, below perinatal conditions. However, these differences do not change the fact that AIDS is now a leading cause of global deaths. In 1990, AIDS deaths were just starting to increase and by the new millennium they have become one of the leading causes of global deaths.

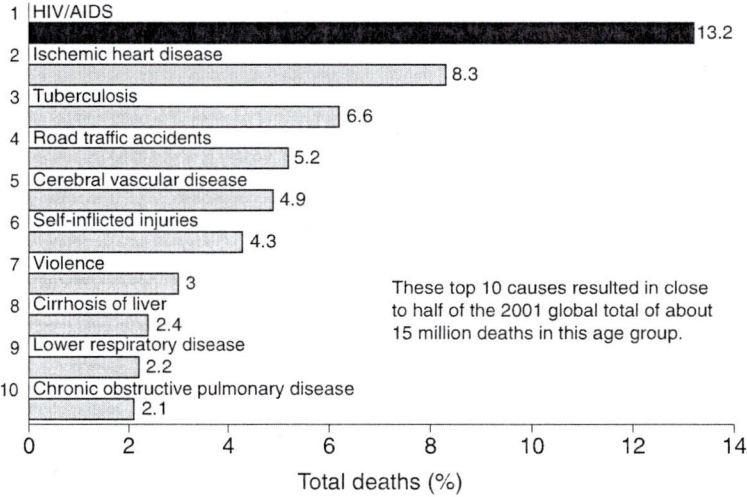

Data source: Version 3 revisions of the Global Burden of Disease (GBD) study.

Figure 10.2 Ten leading causes of death in adults (15–59) in 2001.

The unique characteristic of AIDS deaths is that they occur mostly in young and middle-aged adults who typically have the lowest death rates. The escalation of AIDS deaths during the past decade made it the undisputed leading cause of adult (15–59) deaths by the late 1990s: in 2001 over 13 percent of global adult deaths were attributed to AIDS (*see* Figure 10.2). Even with HIV-related TB deaths attributed to AIDS, TB deaths, independent of HIV, continue to be a major cause (ranked number 3) of adult deaths worldwide. In older adults (age 60 plus), AIDS was not a leading cause of deaths but TB was the 9th leading cause of death in older adults.

On a global basis, it was estimated that less than 0.5 million AIDS deaths occurred in children aged 0–14: the vast majority of these deaths were in SSA. However, as shown in Figure 10.3, diarrheal diseases, malaria, measles, whooping cough, and tetanus, collectively accounted for about a quarter (about 4 million) of child deaths in 2001. Effective and relatively inexpensive preventive measures and/or treatments are available for these infectious diseases. These preventable deaths should give the international health community some cause for soul searching when infectious disease prevention budgets are developed. That these "easily" preventable diseases are still killing millions of children each year is a clear indication that there is a serious flaw in the development of international health priorities.

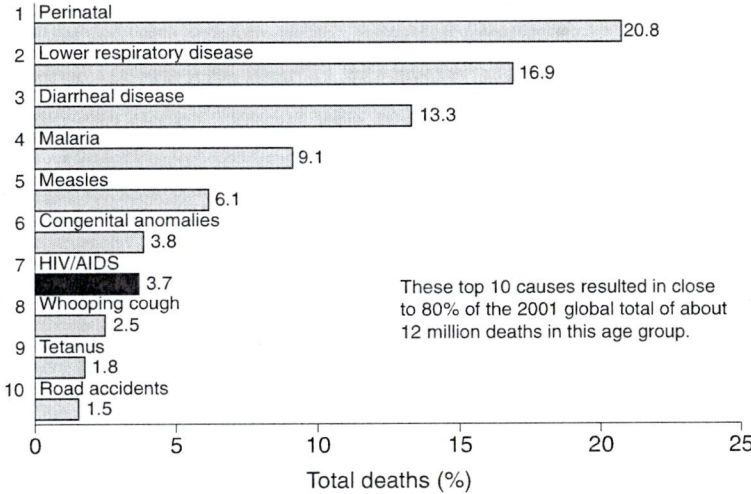

Data source: Version 3 revisions of the Global Burden of Disease (GBD) study.

Figure 10.3 Ten leading causes of death in 0–14 year olds in 2001.

All of the previous GBD estimates were global totals and as shown in Chapter 7, the majority of HIV infections, AIDS cases and deaths are in SSA. Figure 10.4 presents the two leading causes of death in different global regions as defined by the World Bank:

1 high income
2 Europe and Central Asia
3 Latin America and the Caribbean
4 Middle East and North Africa
5 South Asia
6 East Asia and the Pacific
7 SSA

According to these GBD estimates, close to 1 of every 5 deaths in SSA in 2001 was due to AIDS and 1 of every 6 to 7 deaths was due to malaria. AIDS and malaria were estimated to have caused about 30 percent of all deaths in SSA in 2001. Outside of SSA, AIDS deaths were not included in the 10 leading causes of death in any of the regions except for Latin America and the Caribbean where it was the 10th leading cause, and in South Asia where it was the 8th leading cause.

AIDS is by far one of the most devastating human diseases to emerge in modern times, yet the potential for epidemic or sustained HIV transmission in most heterosexual populations is fortunately limited. The extent and severity of heterosexual HIV transmission in SSA is huge compared to any other region and the increasing number of AIDS deaths will have grave impact on all sectors of society in this region. Population growth rates in this region will decline from current growth rates of 2–3 percent down to 1–2 percent over the next few decades. In all other global regions, AIDS will not be a top leading cause of death, but there has been and will continue to be significant focal impact in populations with the highest levels of HIV risk behaviors. The impact may range from up to 50 percent in some MSM and/or IDU populations to "only" a few percent in heterosexuals with the highest sex partner exchange rates.

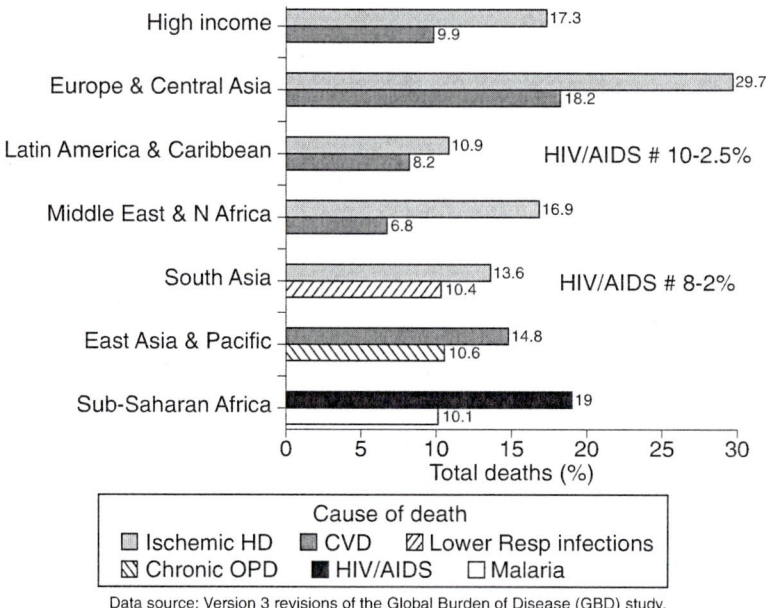

Data source: Version 3 revisions of the Global Burden of Disease (GBD) study.

Figure 10.4 Top two leading causes of death in each global "region" in 2001.

Unrealistic Demographic Projections

The current severity of HIV epidemics in SSA populations will lead to large and measurable impacts on population growth in this region, but it is not clear how severe this impact will be. Demography, the study of human populations, deals with fertility, mortality, and migration – all of which affect the size and composition of populations. Demographers routinely project population growth for 50–100 years. However, estimates and projections of the demographic impact of AIDS deaths for up to several decades or longer requires reliable past and current HIV prevalence estimates as well as reliable projections of future prevalence. The Population Division of the Department of Economic and Social Affairs of the United Nations Secretariat (UNPOP) have prepared official world population estimates and projections since the 1950s. The *2002 Revision* of the official world population estimates and projections tried to measure the impact of AIDS deaths in the most severely affected regions and countries up to 2050. In the *2002 Revision*, UNPOP used HIV prevalence estimates from the UNAIDS Global AIDS report of July 2002. As described in detail in Chapter 7, UNAIDS in its July 2004 Global AIDS report significantly reduced many of the high HIV prevalence estimates in the most severely affected SSA countries by up to half or more.

UNPOP's *2002 Revision* used the UNAIDS initial 2001 prevalence estimates and also accepted the UNAIDS position regarding the continuing increase in HIV prevalence for SSA countries. For projection purposes the following assumptions were used:

1 HIV prevalence and incidence dynamics in the 38 African countries included in the revised AIDS impact projections will remain unchanged until 2010
2 after 2010 HIV prevalence levels will decline according to the UNAIDS model.

Thus, the *2002 Revision* projected a marked worsening of the HIV/AIDS epidemics in these African countries compared with the *2000 Revision* in terms of very much higher morbidity, mortality and population loss. Over the current decade, the number of excess deaths attributed to AIDS in the 53[*] most affected countries is estimated by the *2002 Revision* at 46 million: that figure is projected to increase to 278 million by 2050. Despite these huge HIV/AIDS estimates and projections, the populations of the affected countries are generally expected to be larger by mid-century than today, mainly because most of them maintain high to moderate fertility levels. However, for the seven most affected countries in Southern Africa, where current adult HIV prevalence is estimated at above 20 per cent, these populations are projected by the *2002 Revision* to increase only slightly, from 74 million in 2000 to 78 million in 2050, and outright reductions in population are projected for Botswana, Lesotho, South Africa and Swaziland.

According to the UNAIDS revision of its initial 2001 prevalence estimates and the findings of HIV serosurveys in several SSA countries in 2003, 2004, and 2005, HIV prevalence in this region has probably been overestimated by at least 7 million or more than 35 percent. Instead of about 26 million HIV-infected adults in 2001, the more probable estimate was closer to 19 million. Based on evaluation of the 2001 HIV prevalence estimate and on the leveling and/or decreasing HIV incidence in many SSA countries noted to have started by the mid-to-late 1990s, the demographic impact of AIDS deaths projected to 2050 will likely have to be reduced by at least several folds for the 38 African countries. The demographic impact of AIDS in SSA will be very severe, but not as catastrophic as projected in the 2002 Revision except perhaps for a couple of the highest prevalence countries such as Swaziland and Botswana.

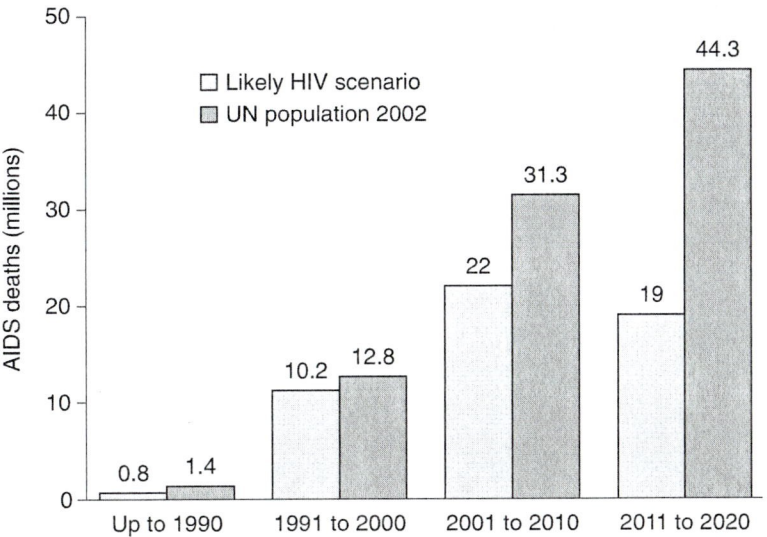

Figure 10.5 Modeling AIDS deaths in sub-Saharan Africa.

---

[*] These 53 countries include 38 African countries, 5 Asian countries, 8 Latin American and Caribbean countries and 2 developed countries.

Projections based on overestimation of HIV prevalence and then compounded by the assumption that prevalence will not begin to decline until after 2010, when many national prevalence rates have leveled off or began to decrease by the new millennium, will result in highly inflated estimates and projections of AIDS deaths as shown in Figure 10.5. During the first decade of the new millennium projected adult AIDS deaths if the 2002 Revision's high HIV/AIDS scenario is used will be 50 percent higher (31.3 million) compared with projected AIDS deaths (22 million) in an HIV/AIDS scenario that is more consistent with the most recent HIV prevalence estimates. During the following decade this difference increases to over 100 percent – 44.3 million adult AIDS deaths projected by the 2002 Revision compared to 19 million using a scenario that is more consistent with the most recent HIV prevalence estimates and trends observed in SSA since the late 1990s.

Another example of the overestimation of AIDS deaths was described for South Africa. South Africa's statistical agency (SA) disputed the *2002 Revision's* forecast that South Africa's population would decline by five million by 2050. According to SA, the UNPOP used a population figure for South Africa that was too low, a total fertility rate that was too low, and an HIV prevalence rate that was too high. SA South Africa estimated: South Africa's total population at 46.6 million, against the UN estimate of 45.2 million; the total fertility rate at 2.77 percent, which is higher than the UN estimate; and HIV prevalence in the 15–49 year old population estimated by the Mandela study at 15.6 percent, which is 6.5 percent lower or 30 percent less than the UNAIDS estimate. While some of these differences appear fairly small, projecting them over 50 years led to the UN forecasting a dramatic population decline, with disastrous effects for the economy, while SA South Africa forecast a population increase. However, even if South Africa's population does not decline by a few million by 2050, the deaths of 10 to 20 percent of the most productive age group over the next few decades will have very large impacts on virtually all major sectors of the country!

Other Examples of Inappropriate Use of HIV/AIDS Models

Mathematical models have been used to develop short and long-range projections of HIV prevalence. However, any mathematical projection model is only as reliable as the assumptions used and the values used for the input parameters. Such models should be used primarily for hypothesis testing and not for making estimates and projections of annual HIV incidence or prevalence for a specific country or population(s). As described in Chapter 6, that was the conclusion of an expert committee that reviewed the HIV/AIDS modeling situation in the UK in 1994. However, many international "experts"[*] and several international and national agencies, including the US National Intelligence Council (NIC), have ignored this sage advice. As a result, some unrealistic HIV prevalence estimates and projections have been inappropriately developed and used in some countries for program and policy decisions.

---

[*] Including yours truly! However, I have learned from bitter experience that one simply should not use an epidemic HIV/AIDS model where an HIV epidemic has not occurred and is unlikely to occur!

It is not only inappropriate but flat out wrong to use an epidemic model (even the improved and updated UNAIDS Asian epidemic model) in populations that have not had significant heterosexual HIV epidemics and where there is no sound epidemiologic basis to expect any heterosexual HIV epidemic to occur. Yet UNAIDS and/or UNPOP have used the new Asian epidemic model to project heterosexual epidemics in China and India. In the five Asian countries included in the *2002 Revision* of the official world population estimates and projections, it was projected that 55 million AIDS deaths would occur in these five countries during the period from 1995 through 2025. This means that there will be a cumulative total of about 100 million HIV infections in these five countries by 2025, with the majority of infections in India and China. Although 100 million HIV infections in an overall adult population of close to 1.5 billion may be possible, it is highly unlikely because the patterns and prevalence of risk behaviors in the vast majority of the heterosexual populations in these countries are incapable of sustaining epidemic heterosexual HIV transmission. The *2002 Revision* would have produced more plausible and useful demographic projections of the potential impact of HIV/AIDS by modeling the most likely HIV/AIDS scenario for the countries selected and not just the worst case scenario that assumes heterosexual HIV epidemics will erupt in these Asian countries. Based on my evaluation of the 2001 and 2003 HIV prevalence estimates and on the leveling and/or decreasing HIV prevalence in SSA and in all of the major Asian countries, I'm convinced that the projection of AIDS deaths in the *2002 Revision* will have to be reduced by at least several-folds.

In addition to the unrealistic HIV projections for SSA and the Asian countries in the *2002 Revision*, the US National Intelligence Council (NIC) developed similar dire projections for India and China in 2002 (*see* Figure 10.6). HIV prevalence will literally have to explode in India and China to get anywhere close to the projections of the NIC or the China Titanic projection. The NIC projected that by the year 2010, HIV infection rates in the adult population of both India and China would increase to about 2–3 percent. This roughly translates to about 20 million HIV-infected adults in China and about 18.5 million in India. The initial China Titanic projection was actually made during the early 1990s and the more than 10 million mark was supposed to have been reached by the year 2000. The Titanic projection was dusted off shortly after the new millennium and the projection pushed forward to 2010. However, there has been no indication of epidemic heterosexual HIV transmission in China and the Chinese and all international "experts" have been looking closely for such transmission in all the HIV epidemic areas in China.

Projections of "generalized" HIV transmission (HIV prevalence of 1 percent or greater in the total 15–49 year old population) in large populous countries such as China and India have been based on the assumption that epidemic heterosexual HIV transmission will occur in these countries. As described in detail in Chapter 5, there is simply no sound epidemiologic basis for this assumption!

The basic problem that HIV/AIDS modelers seem to be oblivious to is: how accurate and representative may any HIV/AIDS dataset be? One can plot a time series of data points – whether they may be of ANC or MSM populations – and use computer programs to calculate the best curve to fit the data points. This is a straightforward mathematical calculation, but can we then assume that the fitted MSM or ANC curve represents the actual HIV prevalence curve for the total MSM population or for all pregnant females, and thus for the total adult

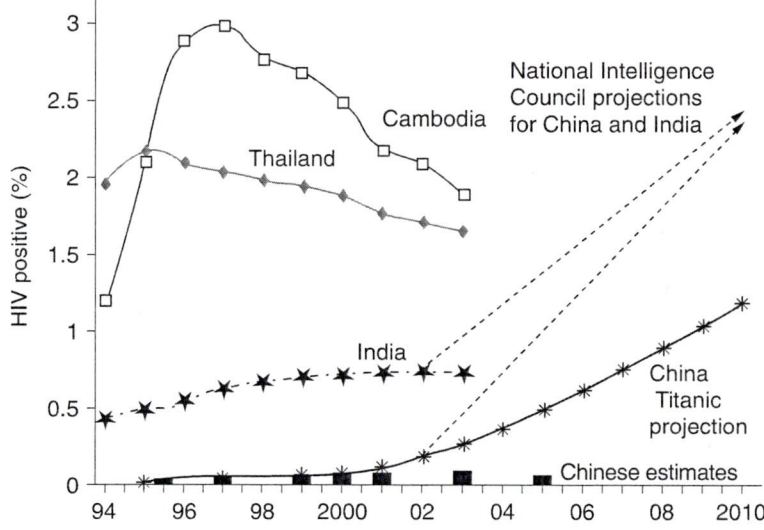

Figure 10.6 Estimated and projected HIV prevalence in selected Asian countries.

population? Even if these curves do represent the national HIV prevalence trend for these populations, how would these curves be able to tell us when prevalence may peak and begin to decrease? The simple and most honest answer is that we do not know and use of virtually any HIV/AIDS epidemic model will produce an HIV epidemic regardless of whether one may occur or not!

The Most Likely Future Regional HIV Scenarios

The AIDS pandemic has been and will continue to be very unevenly distributed globally. This section provides what I consider to be the most likely future HIV scenarios in each of the major global regions.

Sub-Saharan Africa (SSA)

As described in Chapter 7, even though HIV prevalence in SSA was and continues to be overestimated by UNAIDS, this region nevertheless still has by far the highest HIV prevalence of any other global region. By 2001, at least three different prevalence estimates and trends of the HIV prevalence curve for SSA were made (*see* Figures 7.5 and 7.6 in Chapter 7) and from these estimates three different HIV scenarios were developed as shown in Figure 10.7.

The highest scenario that produced the highest prevalence was the UNPOP's 2002 demographic revision for SSA. This scenario that was described earlier in this chapter used the initial 2001 UNAIDS prevalence estimate of 26 million in the 15–49 year old population and also assumed that annual HIV incidence would continue to increase until 2010 and HIV prevalence would increase to about 40 million in 2010. An intermediate scenario used the revised UNAIDS prevalence estimate of 22 million in 2001 and prevalence would increase to about 25 million in 2010. The lowest scenario (the one that I believe is more consistent with recent HIV prevalence estimates for SSA) used a prevalence of

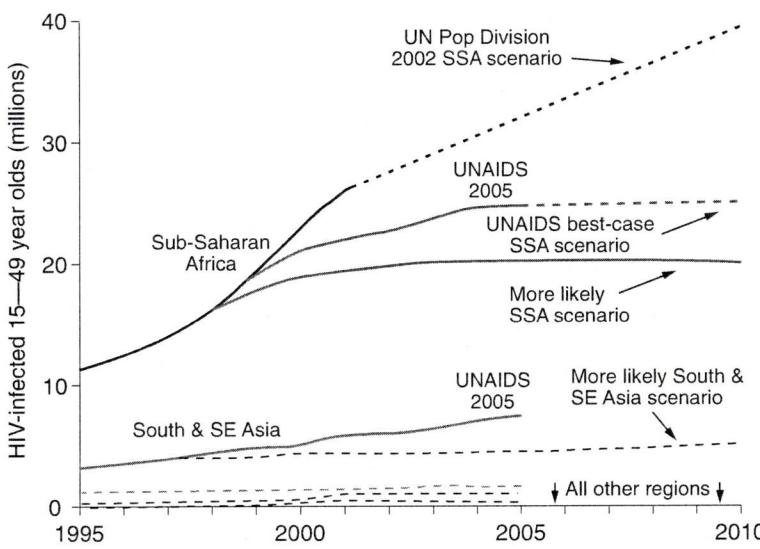

Figure 10.7 Estimated and projected regional HIV prevalence numbers – 1995–2010.

19 million in 2001. In mid-2006, UNAIDS revised their HIV prevalence estimate for SSA to be almost identical to the prevalence estimate used in my HIV scenario for SSA. Even with the lowest HIV scenario, HIV prevalence in the most severely affected SSA countries will still be 10 percent or higher in the adult (15–49) populations for at least another decade or two. Annual HIV incidence in South Africa may have peaked during the late 1990s, but it is unlikely that HIV incidence in this country will decline as dramatically as it did in Uganda. An accelerated decrease in HIV incidence in South Africa cannot be expected until there is full acceptance by policy makers, especially the President, and the general public of the need to significantly reduce sexual risk behaviors. In addition, HIV prevalence will continue to be very high in the SSA region for the next several decades because of the slow but steady nonepidemic sexual transmission in the current millions of HIV-discordant couples. Finally, the slow but steadily developing ART programs in this region will keep many HIV-infected persons living longer.

South and Southeast Asia

This region has the largest population of all global regions – over 2 billion with about half or 1 billion adults aged 15–49. Explosive heterosexual HIV epidemics occurred in Thailand, Cambodia, Myanmar, and several Indian States during the 1980s and early-1990s and all peaked or leveled off by the mid-to-late 1990s. HIV prevalence was initially overestimated in these countries, and all recent national estimates are now less than 2 percent of the 15–49 year old population. HIV epidemics in IDU populations were documented in several other countries in this region, but no significant epidemic heterosexual HIV transmission has, as of mid-2006, been detected in any country in this region except for the first mentioned countries that had explosive epidemic spread in their large commercial sex networks. The overall HIV/AIDS numbers in this region are dominated by India but as of late-2006 it is still not clear whether HIV prevalence in India is closer to

3 million or 6 million. A study of HIV prevalence in young (15–24 year old) ANC attendees in four southern States in India reported that HIV prevalence rates decreased from 1.7 percent in 2001 to 1.1 percent in 2004 for a reduction of about 35 percent.[*] It is extremely unlikely that HIV prevalence in India could increase to over 18 million by 2010 as projected by the US National Intelligence Council. UNAIDS estimated that there were about 7 to 8 million HIV-infected adults (15–49) in this region at the end of 2005. A more likely estimate of prevalent HIV infections in this region as of 2006 is closer to 5 million[†] as shown in Figure 10.7. Over the next few decades, HIV prevalence will be decreasing very slowly in this region because of the slow but steady nonepidemic sexual transmission among discordant sex couples and the increasing development of ART programs that will keep current HIV-infected persons living longer.

Figure 10.8 presents HIV prevalence rate estimates for global regions up through 2005 and the same three HIV scenarios for SSA and a more likely HIV scenario for the Caribbean region up to 2010.

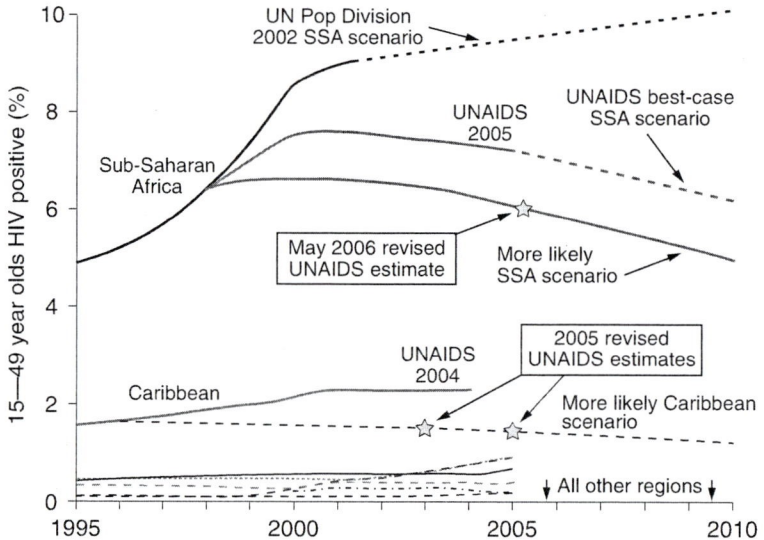

Figure 10.8 Estimated and projected regional HIV prevalence rates – 1995–2010.

Caribbean

In the UNAIDS 2005 report on the global AIDS epidemic, HIV prevalence for this region was reduced from prior estimates of 2.3 percent to 1.6 percent for 2003 and 2005, without any detailed explanation for this reduction. It is clear to me that prior estimates were overestimates and UNAIDS was finally forced to revise

---

[*] Kumar R, Jha P, Arora P. Trends in HIV-1 in young adults in south India from 2000 to 2004: a prevalence study. Lancet 2006; published online March 30. DOI:10.1016/S0140-6736(06)68435-3

[†] This will depend on whether HIV prevalence in India is closer to 3 million as I believe or 6 million. This question should be answered by population-based HIV surveys that are planned in 2006.

the high estimates as a result of an increasing number of population-based HIV serosurveys. HIV prevalence in Haiti was estimated to have been close to 6 percent by the late 1990s, but some recent studies indicate that rural ANC prevalence rates are only about 1 to 2 percent. Since the majority of the Haitian population is rural, this means that the national HIV prevalence in Haiti cannot be more than about 2 to 3 percent or about half of the 260 000 number listed by UNAIDS in their 2003 report. UNAIDS in their May 2006 AIDS epidemic update report reduced the prevalence estimate for Haiti down to 3.8 percent. Prevalence in the Dominican Republic was lowered from about 2.5 percent to close to 1 percent as a result of DHS+ findings. According to my HIV scenario for the Caribbean region, HIV prevalence will not be increasing but will probably not drop much below 1 percent over the next few decades.

Latin America

Aside from a few countries in Central and northern South America (Honduras, Belize, Guyana, and Suriname), most countries in the Latin America region have almost no significant epidemic heterosexual HIV transmission. In most countries in this region HIV prevalence is less than 0.5 percent with a mix of IDU and MSM epidemics. In this region, for the next few decades, I do not expect any major changes from the current HIV patterns and prevalence. ART programs have been well developed in Brazil starting in the late 1990s. As a result, after "Western" countries, this region has the highest percent of HIV-infected persons on ART and I expect that this trend will also continue.

"Western" Countries (North America, Western Europe, and Oceania)

No significant epidemic heterosexual HIV transmission has occurred in this group of high income countries. In the majority of countries in this group HIV prevalence is less than 0.2 percent: most infections are found in MSM and/or IDU populations. Several countries have larger scale IDU epidemics (USA, Spain, Italy, Portugal and Switzerland) and HIV prevalence levels in these countries are close to 0.5 percent or slightly higher. Over the next few decades, I expect these patterns and prevalence levels to remain close to what they are currently. Annual HIV incidence will likely continue to decrease in most MSM and IDU populations, but HIV prevalence will not drop significantly because of slow and steady nonepidemic sexual transmission to the regular sex partners of infected IDU and MSM. HIV prevalence will also be maintained by programs that provide better access to ART programs for the more marginalized persons living with HIV/AIDS.

North Africa and the Middle East

HIV prevalence in this region has been very low. There is no reason to expect significant HIV epidemic spread because sex and IDU networks in countries in this region are all estimated to be relatively small. If southern Sudan was not included in this region, HIV prevalence would be 80 000 in a population of 170 million aged15–49 years. This translates to 0.05 percent or 1 infection per 2000 population aged 15–49. The greatest threat of epidemic HIV transmission in this region will be in IDU groups. But even if some epidemic spread does develop, HIV prevalence in this region would probably rise only to about 0.1 percent at most.

Eastern Europe and Central Asia

Since the mid-1990s, large IDU-driven HIV epidemics have developed in many of the countries of the former Soviet Union and as of 2006 these epidemics appear to be continuing almost unabated. The most severely affected are the Russian Federation, Ukraine, and the Baltic States (Estonia, Latvia, and Lithuania). Also HIV continues to spread in Belarus, Moldova and Kazakhstan, while more recent epidemics have been reported from Kyrgyzstan and Uzbekistan. The current extent of, if any, epidemic heterosexual HIV transmission in this region is unclear and a current estimate of HIV prevalence (over a million as of 2006) may be grossly overestimated. During the next few decades, partly due to saturation of the highest risk IDU networks and partly due to increased and more effective harm reduction programs, HIV prevalence will peak below 1 percent of the 15–49 year old population and then gradually decrease. However, this decrease in HIV prevalence will be very slow because slow but steady transmission from infected IDU to their regular sex partners will continue. In addition, an expected increase in ART program coverage will be keeping HIV-infected persons alive much longer.

East Asia and the Pacific

HIV/AIDS numbers in this region are dominated by China, a country with over 90 percent of the region's population. In 2003, HIV prevalence in China was estimated to be 840 000 (0.12 percent of the 15–49 year old population) and was 0.05 percent for the rest of this region. All of the other countries had an HIV prevalence estimate at or below 0.1 percent except for Papua New Guinea (PNG) where HIV prevalence was 0.6 percent. About 90 percent of HIV infections in China can be attributed to IDU transmission and to faulty plasma collection in paid donors during the early to mid-1990s. I do not envision any extensive epidemic heterosexual HIV transmission in this region with the possible exception of PNG. According to the China "Titanic" projection and the US National Intelligence Council's projection for China, there should have been by 2006 at least several million HIV infections, yet prevalence is still well less than a million. My future scenario for this region consists of slowly decreasing HIV prevalence levels, but the potential for focal IDU epidemics will continue to be high.

All my future scenarios include generally decreasing HIV prevalence with no significant change in regional patterns of HIV transmission that were established during the 1980s and 1990s. In marked contrast to the UNAIDS paradigm, I don't expect or forecast any significant heterosexual HIV epidemics in populations where such epidemics have not occurred. Where epidemic HIV transmission has occurred in MSM, IDU, and/or FSW and their clients, my scenarios project very slow declines in HIV prevalence. I do not expect that high risk behaviors can be eliminated especially since public health interventions for both harm reduction (for IDU transmission) and risk reduction (for sexual transmission) continue to be opposed by some faith-based organizations, particularly by the present US administration. In addition, there will continue to be a high prevalence of nonepidemic sexual transmission, from persons infected as a result of their risk behaviors, to their regular sex partners.

Thus, there will be an unacceptably high "endemic" HIV level in most SSA countries, several Caribbean countries, a few Asian countries, and in most MSM and IDU populations throughout the world. The global patterns and prevalence of HIV have been and will continue to be very similar to those of genital herpes virus (HSV-2), except that HIV prevalence rates have been and will continue to be much lower. The dire projections of: the Titanic scenario for China; the US National Intelligence Council ("next waves" of HIV epidemics for India, China, etc.); the UNPOP Division (*2002 Revision*); and all of the many economic and political "AIDS experts" will all have to be retracted. UNPOP in its 2004 Revision did revise its AIDS death impact scenarios for SSA and Asian countries markedly downwards using UNAIDS revised HIV prevalence estimates. However, my personal and professional bias is that they still have grossly overestimated the numbers of AIDS deaths in these regions. I'm confident that in subsequent revisions that they will eventually have to lower their revised estimates even more!

Summary and Conclusions

The AIDS pandemic is without question one of the most severe infectious disease pandemics in modern times. However, its global impact has been and will continue to be very uneven. AIDS deaths in SSA will continue to be the leading cause of death in this region for at least the next several decades. In addition, in many or most MSM and IDU populations throughout the world, AIDS deaths have been, are, and will continue to be the leading cause of death in these populations for decades to come. In most heterosexual populations throughout the world outside of SSA, there will be minimal to no measurable demographic impact of AIDS deaths.

Although epidemic HIV transmission will not occur in most populations, a major mode of HIV transmission – from an HIV-infected person to his or her regular sex partner – has been occurring virtually ignored by most AIDS programs. As of late-2006, this mode of HIV transmission is probably a major, if not the predominant, mode of HIV transmission worldwide. There seems to be a growing understanding and appreciation of this major mode of HIV transmission and I'm hopeful that routine and systematic follow-up of regular sex partner(s) of persons identified with an HIV infection will become one of the top priorities of AIDS programs throughout the world, as soon as possible.

As a global community, it is clear that "we" would not accept a few human "mad cow disease" cases nor would "we" accept thousands of human rabies cases, yet we are arguing over how many millions of new HIV infections may be occurring each year. In a WHO/FHI workshop in Manila in 2001,[*] I proposed that public health attention be directed away from estimating a specific number of HIV infections in any country, and to switch to classifying countries as having low

---

[*] Intervention strategies and surveillance in countries with low HIV prevalence: A consultation workshop FHI in collaboration with UNAIDS and WHO/WPRO March 29–30, 2001 WHO/WPRO Manila, Philippines.

(having less than 1 HIV infection per 1000 15–49 year olds), moderate (more than 1/1000 and less than 1/100), high (more than 1/100 and less than 1/10), and very high (more than 1/10) HIV prevalence. There was some initial interest in my proposed classification, but the use of specific numbers rather than a range has been so ingrained into the public and policy makers' mind set that "we" will need to continue to play the numbers game to constantly argue over whether the numbers are too high or too low.

What I believe is needed is an objective, evidence-based review of all major disease numbers by a panel of qualified disease experts somewhat along the lines of the GBD study. In the USA, I would propose that the IOM/NAS take on this task for national disease estimates. UNAIDS should provide input to an objective review of HIV/AIDS estimates and projections, but the final decision as to what estimate or projection to accept globally or nationally should not be left in the hands of any primary advocacy organization.

The International* Response to the AIDS Pandemic

This chapter presents my biases and observations on the international response to the AIDS pandemic from the initial efforts of WHO in the early 1980s to the past decade of efforts by UNAIDS and as of 2002, the Global Fund for AIDS, Tuberculosis, and Malaria (ATM). I have relied on a paper† prepared by one of the first WHO staff assigned to help Jon Mann develop a global AIDS program to describe WHO's response to AIDS from its recognition in 1981 until 1987. The description of the international response to AIDS included in this chapter primarily reflects my personal involvement and views and cannot be considered a comprehensive review of the international response to the AIDS pandemic. I will describe the personal politics that I believe prompted Jon Mann to resign from his position as Director of the Global Programme on AIDS (GPA) in 1990, and how after Jon's departure, GPA was converted into a "typical" WHO program by Mike Merson (Jon's successor as Director of GPA). I will conclude by providing a brief overview of the international response to the AIDS pandemic after UNAIDS replaced GPA/WHO in the mid-1990s.

Beginning of the International Response

After the initial report of AIDS in the CDC's MMWR in June 1981, WHO began to gather specialized information on AIDS on a modest scale and subsequently distributed that information in its own Weekly Epidemiological Record (WER). AIDS activity by WHO was restricted to this exchange of information until 1985, when the first International AIDS Conference was held in Atlanta. Participants at the Conference, and in particular the organizer, the United States Centers for Disease Control (CDC), brought heavy pressure to bear on the WHO delegate Dr. Fakhri Assaad, Director of the WHO Communicable Diseases Programme, to persuade the Organization to expand its AIDS activities. On Dr. Assaad's return to Geneva, and at his instigation, WHO convened a meeting of experts and received from them an urgent recommendation to set up an AIDS control program. WHO's reaction was unenthusiastic because funds and staff were lacking and the majority of WHO's Regional Offices (RO), authentic strongholds within the Organization, were reluctant to see their resources reallocated to tackle a problem which seemed to pose no threat to the countries within their area. However, thanks to Dr Assaad's persistence, an international network of some 30 WHO collaborating centers, most of them virus laboratories, was set up; he was then

---

* In recent years, a distinction has been made between *global* versus *international* health. International health focuses on providing aid to countries while global health relates to health issues that transcend national borders. A global approach is needed to respond to the AIDS pandemic, but we have had primarily an international response.

† Tarantola D (1996) The international AIDS control effort in Africa: the big picture and the little details. *Le Journal du SIDA.* **86–87**: 109–16.

able to communicate directly with them from WHO Headquarters (HQ) in Geneva, and thus short-circuited the Organization's bureaucracy. In June 1986, almost one year after the appeal was made to WHO, the Organization set up a small monitoring and information unit with a physician (Jonathan Mann), a secretary (Edith Bernard), and a typewriter.

The Director-General (DG) of WHO, Halfdan Mahler was quite bold to include among global health priorities a problem which was seen, in the mid-1980s, as predominantly affecting minorities in wealthy countries, and in particular homosexuals and drug addicts. He knew that by launching a new program, WHO was running the risk of distracting the attention of Member States and international funding agencies, which had been mobilized with great difficulty in the previous decade, to support Primary Health Care. At the end of 1986, Mahler decided to implement a global program to respond to the pandemic because he had gradually realized the potential seriousness of the situation. At the second International Conference on AIDS, held in Paris in June 1986, alarming news was presented on the spread of HIV/AIDS in several African countries. The problem was again mentioned at Brazzaville in September 1986, at the annual meeting of the Member States of WHO's Africa Region. At the meeting, the Ugandan Minister of Health informed Halfdan Mahler of the worrying AIDS situation in his own country: his concerns were echoed by several other African delegates.

President Museveni of Uganda in a speech at Kampala in December 1995 said that he realized the gravity of the AIDS epidemic in his country somewhat by chance in 1986: "I sent 60 people to Cuba (for military training) and at that time we did not carry out HIV tests because we thought that everybody was all right. When the 60 got there, the Cubans tested them because they are very, very strict. Out of the 60, 18 [close to a third] were found to be HIV positive. When I went to the Non-Aligned summit in Harare that year, Fidel Castro took me aside and said: 'You know there is a big problem in your country,' and he told me the story. I had a meeting with Dr Okware[*] and his group in my office and I did not give them kind words, but out of our quarrel – the quarrel between the political leadership and these doctors – we evolved a program of talking openly about AIDS and educating people about its spread." As a result, President Museveni instructed his ministers to undertake a national and international effort to respond to the epidemic.

GPA/WHO: Early Years

I took early retirement from my position in California and joined WHO in March 1987 as a short-term consultant (STC). When I arrived in Geneva, I was assigned to a small cubicle – perhaps 6' by 10', the standard size for all STC. A few weeks after my arrival in Geneva, Jon asked "...Jim, how are we going to get the AIDS pandemic under control?" My response was – all we have to do is eliminate poverty,[†] prostitution, promiscuity, and drug abuse, and then it will all be downhill! I think Jon then and there decided to assign me to a more technical job – to

---

[*] I worked with Sam Okware on a World Bank mission in Malawi in 1997. He told me that in his initial AIDS unit there were 11 staff persons and in less than a decade eight of his staff had died, all presumably from AIDS.

[†] I remained on the poverty bandwagon until the mid-1990s.

gather and analyze global HIV/AIDS numbers. This was more than OK with me since I had already admitted to having no expertise in being able to "stop the storm" of sexual risk behaviors in California during the 1970s.

I brought along with me a Zenith portable computer that had been "mine" when I was the Head of the Infectious Disease Section of the California State Health Department. The computer was the size and weight of a large piece of luggage or similar to the weight and size of Anne's sewing machine (it had 64k of RAM). It turned out that I was the only person in the Special Programme on AIDS (SPA) who had a computer and it was erroneously assumed that I was a computer expert.* In those days, virtually all offices used Wang machines for word processing and SPA had Wangs but no computers. It turned out that IBM was interested in donating to SPA a total computer system with technical support for a couple of years and this included access and use of the global communication services of IBM's global network at that time. However, petty technical turf problems arose because WHO had just finished wiring the WHO building with a local LAN system that was a generation or two behind what IBM proposed to provide for SPA. The head of the Information Technology (IT) Division at WHO refused to have the IBM system installed just for SPA and as a result, IBM donated only a few desktop computers and printers and walked away.

My initial impressions of SPA, that within a few months was renamed GPA, was that everyone was totally dedicated to his/her work: we were all playing catch-up to get GPA off the ground and into the field so we could help countries evaluate and deal with whatever HIV/AIDS problem might be present. It seemed that all staff worked at least 15 to 16 hour days. I would leave at 7 or 8 pm and still there would be almost half of the staff working away. I would return before 8 am and find more than half of the staff working. This hectic pace was kept up pretty much unchanged until a year or so after Jon resigned and Mike Merson took over as the new director of GPA. I'll discuss this in more

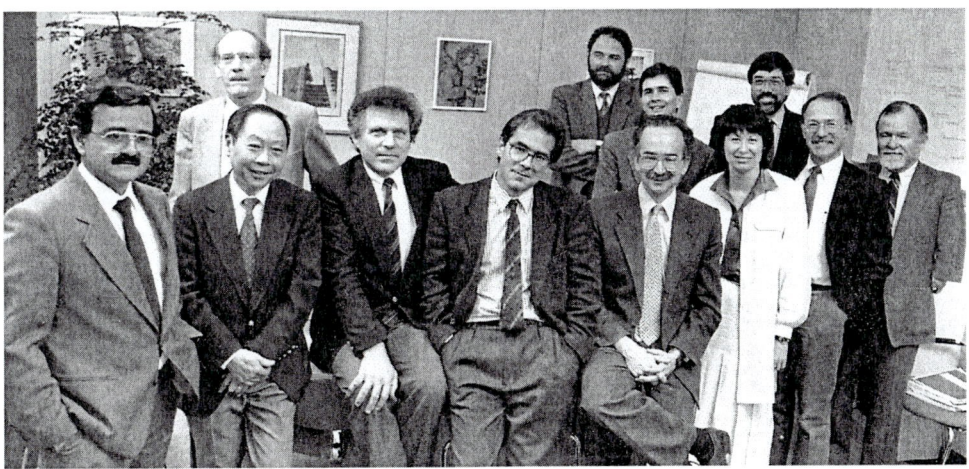

Jon Mann (far right in first row) and senior GPA staff in late 1987. Reprinted by permission of WHO/Erling Mandelmann.

---

*I continue to rely heavily on my number two son (Bennett) for technical assistance for all of my computer needs.

detail later but a year after I resigned from my position at GPA in early 1992, I had an occasion to pass through Geneva on my way to a meeting in Europe. I visited the GPA offices and found the pace of work to be pretty much of an ordinary WHO office – very quiet and not filled until after 9 am and half empty by 4 pm. It was like day versus night – there just wasn't the same *esprit de corps* and vitality of the initial GPA years!

GPA Was Not a Typical WHO Program!

From the beginning, GPA did not function or operate like a typical WHO office. Some of the WHO administrative offices that I had to visit really didn't open much before 9 am, and if you went to most WHO offices after 4 pm you more often than not were likely to find it closed for the day. I have never worked with such dedicated public health professionals. Jon would frequently tell the news media that he had to sail the GPA boat while at the same time he was trying to build it! GPA initially also did not adhere to WHO's bureaucratic rules that required all communications from HQ (Geneva) to be routed through WHO's regional offices[*] and often prepared documents for the Regional Director's (RD) signature. With the hectic pace of program development; the need to communicate rapidly with consultants, national governments and ministries of health; and to schedule and arrange country visits as soon as feasibly possible; GPA had to bypass the Regional Offices (RO). Instead of routing all correspondence through the RO for clearance or approval, which would often take weeks or longer, GPA routinely sent copies of correspondence to the RO to keep them informed but not ask or require their approval.

This was an operational routine that, to say the least, rankled all of the Regional Directors. In addition to correspondence, staff support and/or allocation of program funds from HQ for all WHO programs was to be provided to countries through the RO. Jon had worked for a couple of years in Africa; even though he did not work in a WHO program he knew first hand of the inefficiency and outright corruption in the African Regional Office (AFRO) that was then headquartered in Brazzaville, Congo. He vowed that no GPA staff or country funds/support would be provided through AFRO. My Combating Childhood Communicable Diseases (CCCD) project design team's visit to Geneva and SSA in 1979 included a visit to AFRO, and I was forewarned of the problems in dealing with AFRO. Consequently, our project design team made sure that the CCCD program was not passed through WHO (Geneva) in order to keep our funds out of the potential clutches of AFRO!

The GPA strategy was to get an initial country visit with a small technical program team to help form (if one did not already exist) a national AIDS program office to develop a short-term national AIDS plan. This was to be followed by a longer more in-depth planning mission by a GPA team. The second visit would entail close collaboration with the national AIDS program and other local and/or international experts/partners to develop a medium-term country plan (covering about 5 years) for responding to the nation's AIDS problem. Upon

---

[*] AMRO, also known as PAHO for the Americas, EURO for western European countries, EMRO for countries mostly in the Middle-East and North Africa, SEARO for south and southeast Asian countries, and WPRO for western pacific and east Asian countries.

completion of the medium-term country plan, GPA orchestrated an external donor meeting wherein all interested, potential donors would meet to review and critique the country's medium-term plan. Donors were invited to pledge support for any and all portions of the country plan. This process assured that the country's medium-term AIDS plan would be as comprehensive and complete as possible: Further, it would not require piecemeal development of any part of the plan at the specific behest of a potential donor. This process also tried to minimize or avoid individual donor evaluation meetings. All donors were required to accept a single comprehensive evaluation process in which each donor could participate in, but not dominate.

Thus, GPA inserted itself as the "gatekeeper" for participation of donors or potential donors to national AIDS programs. This requirement, imposed by GPA on all external donors, was received with mixed feelings that ranged from mute agreement with the logic behind this requirement to bitter resentment that an upstart WHO program was precluding independent evaluation missions that were traditional among agencies such as USAID, the World Bank, UNICEF, etc. There were some institutional grumblings, but in the late 1980s, Jon was at the zenith of his power and he had the unfailing support of Halfdan Mahler. All of the UN agencies were "kept in line" and had to acknowledge the primacy of GPA as the "gatekeeper" for all external support for national AIDS programs. A major early GPA concern was that UN agencies would want to be independent of WHO to pursue their own agendas, and this did materialize. In particular, UNICEF wanted to focus their AIDS program support exclusively on the "innocents," i.e. children, thereby virtually ignoring other vulnerable populations characterized by their socially unacceptable behaviors. The administrative mechanism that kept WHO at the center of the UN response to the AIDS pandemic was called the "WHO-UNDP Alliance" and there was a memorandum of understanding setting the respective roles of the two agencies. Among other functions, UNDP was expected to facilitate coordination across the UN and to mobilize resources for support of AIDS programs as well as the transfer of funds by WHO to countries. They operated this financial function quite efficiently.

Jon's Rise and Fall

In retrospect, Jon's triumphs over WHO's bureaucracy and the power and independence of other UN Agencies were to become his eventual downfall. From 1987 to 1990, GPA grew from just Jon and his secretary to a massive global program that had hundreds of staff throughout the world and an annual operating budget of several hundred million dollars. During this period, Jon was adjusting to his "rising star status" and was meeting with the Pope and other global leaders. He was a very articulate and charismatic speaker. His enthusiasm and conviction that persons living with HIV/AIDS had the basic human right to a healthy life propelled Jon's rising star status to that of "superstar." Jon's eloquence in public speaking was maximized in Europe because the French media could not get enough of him! I frequently told Jon that he was just an average epidemiologist, but he would have made a great Rabbi! I'm sure that the preferential treatment Jon received from the Geneva press corps compared with how they treated the new WHO DG, Nakajima, was

a factor in the obvious animosity between the two. I remember clearly scheduled news conferences when Nakajima would open the conference reading in
his stilted and fractured English or French a prepared statement. All of the
reporters would be visiting with each other and there would not be a single
camera or recorder on. When Nakajima was finished, all of the cameras and
lights would go on: the reporters turned their recorders on and were ready to
hear Jon's message – delivered without notes – and then respond to questions
in English or French without pause. I can still see Nakajima smoldering and
fuming in the background.

Why Jon Resigned from GPA

The exact reasons why Jon suddenly resigned as director of GPA in 1990 will
never be fully known. I had expected Jon to provide all the details in a book
describing his professional sojourn with AIDS at WHO, but his unexpected
death in the Swiss Air 111 crash in September 1998 occurred before such a
book could be written. What I have pieced together from my sporadic contacts
with him after his resignation, the basic cause was simple burn-out! On several
occasions after his resignation, I asked Jon why he didn't share any of the
administrative and political problems he had with Nakajima's office with his
senior staff. Jon's answer was that he did not want to get any of us involved
because that would have been the kiss of death for us from the DG's office. Jon
was acutely aware of the battles he would have with Nakajima, who succeeded
Mahler in 1988, about GPA's almost complete independence from the Regional
Offices. During Nakajima's campaign to become Mahler's successor, I'm sure
that he assured his fellow Regional Directors that GPA would be made to
behave as a typical WHO program if he was elected the next DG. Jon, on the
other hand, kept saying that GPA staff and funds would be routed to African
countries through AFRO, "...over my dead body!" Thus, the battle lines were
clearly drawn before Nakajima's arrival. Of course, Jon's upstaging Nakajima at
all international AIDS conferences and press conferences did nothing to endear
Jon to Nakajima.

The apparent straw that broke Jon's back was a personal political game
played by the DG's office in connection with Jon's travel authorization papers
for a high level European AIDS meeting that Jon had organized and at which
he was to be the keynote speaker. Apparently, Nakajima was initially not
invited to this meeting and was rightfully miffed. Jon recognized this oversight
and ensured that Nakajima received an invitation and was also asked to give a
short opening speech. Jon's travel secretary* had sent Jon's travel request for
this meeting to the DG's office for approval a couple of weeks before the meeting, but each time the travel secretary called to ask if the travel request had
been approved, she was told that the DG was traveling or busy and to call back
later. This administrative "dancing" went on up to the last day before the meeting and Jon was convinced that the DG's office was daring him to flaunt WHO
travel authorization requirements. Jon told me that this "cat and mouse" game

---

* Jon had a head secretary, an appointment secretary, a travel secretary and a special occasions secretary as well as Kathleen Kay, his personal executive assistant, and he kept
working them all overtime!

was both personally and professionally wearing: he just plain "snapped" and submitted his resignation without conferring with anyone, not even his administrative superiors at CDC, Atlanta. Immediately afterward, high officials from Washington DC and Atlanta tried to get Jon to reconsider and to withdraw his resignation, but Jon did not change his mind. He was, in my opinion, just "totally burnt out."

After Jon resigned, Nakajima appointed Mike Merson to take over GPA. I was on duty travel when Jon formally turned GPA over to Mike. I was told by several colleagues who were present at this GPA staff meeting that Jon introduced Mike as the lone WHO senior staff who had envied and coveted his position from the beginning. Who furthermore over the years consistently sought to undermine and stab him in the back. With this brief introduction, Jon abruptly left the assembled GPA staff with their new director.

Mike Merson and the Dismantling of GPA

After Mike was made head of GPA, I can say with sincerity and conviction that all of GPA's unit chiefs gave him their full professional support. However, this did not prevent Manuel Carballo and Daniel Tarantola from being targeted for elimination from GPA. One of Mike's first moves was to reorganize GPA to get rid of Manuel Carballo's Social Behavioral Research unit and thereby eliminate Manuel's position. This administrative maneuver was not unexpected because Manuel was the very upfront and visible campaign manager for Nakajima's main rival for the position of DG. The GPA management committee chided Mike for removing such an important research unit, but by then Manuel had moved to another position is Geneva. Several months later, Mike again reorganized GPA to abolish Daniel Tarantola's position. This was also expected since Daniel had worked in the Western Pacific Regional Office (WPRO) when Nakajima was the regional director of that office. Daniel believed that Nakajima considered him to be a disloyal employee since Daniel, as a member of the WPRO staff grievance committee, invariably sided with staff who filed grievances against the RD.[*] Halfdan Mahler was aware of the bad relationship Daniel had with Nakajima: one of his last personnel actions before he turned WHO over to Nakajima was to promote Daniel to a P-6 position. This protected Daniel from being easily dismissed by the DG's office, but could not protect him from being reorganized out from GPA! I did not consider myself in danger of being reorganized out of GPA but I resigned from my position in early 1992.

Why I Resigned from GPA

I resigned abruptly from WHO in early 1992 for a variety of personal and professional reasons. As described above, I was thrilled with my work at GPA for the first few years when Jon was "...trying to sail his boat [GPA] as he was building it." I doubt very much if I would have resigned if Jon had still been director of GPA. My decision to take early retirement from California to join WHO in 1987 took my wife Anne by surprise. It was a difficult situation for her to suddenly,

---

[*] According to Daniel, Nakajima set a WHO record for having the most staff grievances filed against any RD!

without warning, cut her family and personal ties in Berkeley to accompany me to Geneva. We managed to work out a jetsetter arrangement for her to set up a home for us in Geneva while keeping our house in Berkeley for her needed travel back to California for family matters and for her scheduled meetings of the Board of Pensions of the United Methodist Church. Since I joined WHO at the relatively old age of 54 and the mandatory retirement age at WHO was 60, I never considered my move to Geneva as a very long-term venture. After Jon's resignation, Mike's dismantling of senior GPA staff, and conversion of GPA into a "typical" WHO program, my incentive and desire to stay at WHO plummeted. I had just signed a contract extension for two more years in late 1991 when I received, in early 1992, an invitation from Taiwan to participate in an international AIDS conference in Taipei. I immediately took this invitation to the WHO legal office and asked how I might be able to go to Taipei for this conference. I was told that as a WHO employee I could not go to Taiwan. I asked if I could take vacation time to attend the conference and the head of the legal unit said "read my lips – there is no way that you can go to this conference since you are a WHO employee!" I then told him that I'd resign from WHO to go to this conference. He said that since I signed a two year contract I had to give 90 days notice before I could resign. A quick look at the date of the conference indicated that it was exactly 91 days away. I told the legal officer that effective immediately I was tendering my resignation and that I'd go back to my office to draft an official memo of resignation and have it on his desk before the end of the day! That evening, I again surprised Anne by telling her that I just resigned from GPA/WHO and that we would be returning to California.

I did attend the AIDS conference in Taipei and it was necessary that my resignation from WHO adhered to all of the rules. Dr. ST Han, who had succeeded Dr. Nakajima as the Regional Director at WPRO (Manila), somehow got wind of my participation at the Taipei conference. He apparently called WHO (HQ) in Geneva to ask how come Jim Chin, a staff member of GPA/WHO, was attending a meeting in Taipei. He was informed that effective the day of the Conference Dr. Chin was no longer employed by WHO!

Donor Disenchantment with GPA

After the first few "honeymoon" years, bestowed by the major donors to GPA, a combination of donor fatigue and disenchantment of some donors of GPA's operating procedures began to be palpable about the time I resigned from GPA. This disenchantment continued to fester and a couple of years later, in 1994, a group of donors suggested the creation of a joint United Nations program on AIDS. The initial idea was to compel WHO to broaden its partnership with other United Nations agencies and with NGOs. The reasons that donors, and later the developing countries, ratified this decision – which was confirmed by a resolution of the World Health Assembly in May 1994 – include those below.

For the developing countries, assistance from donors was stagnating because of the inability of WHO to provide sustained technical support and adequate funds since the Organization was embroiled in "decentralization" of GPA's implementation. I have no doubt that this decentralization of GPA's operations was simply Nakajima paying his political debt to the WHO Regional Offices, i.e., to make GPA a typical WHO program that would route staff and funds to countries through the

Regional Offices. In the vast Africa region, while AFRO was simultaneously tackling internal management problems and the repercussions of the political instability prevailing in Congo, where its Headquarters were located, decentralization had led to the virtual paralysis of WHO support for national AIDS programs. Donors, for their part, were impatient to see AIDS take its place within the broader framework of social and economic programs with some permanency. Without GPA/WHO as an all powerful gatekeeper, international donors would be able to incorporate funds hitherto allocated to AIDS into complex assistance packages that would conceal the actual decline in the overall amount of funds allocated for AIDS programs. By eliminating GPA/WHO as the gatekeeper, this would also make it difficult if not impossible to directly monitor AIDS funding within the total global development envelope.

Pressure was brought to bear from many angles by the bilateral development agencies, United Nations agencies, beneficiary countries and NGOs for the new program to play a coordinating rather than a direct operational role, especially its gatekeeper role! The underlying motives of the donors and recipient country programs were diverse. In short, the approach around which a consensus emerged made room for a diversity of groups – whether governmental or not – which, during the previous years, had gradually built up their own capacity to intervene.

UNAIDS

UNAIDS was established in 1995 as an advocacy and coordinating agency that almost immediately turned over responsibility for AIDS program funding and technical guidance to other international agencies and donors. However, UNAIDS did not turn over responsibility for the estimation and projection of HIV/AIDS numbers. Since UNAIDS, has declared itself to be primarily an advocacy agency, its objectivity in making or accepting high estimates and projections needs to be questioned. UNAIDS primary mission is to bring coordinated support for HIV/AIDS programs from UN agencies to countries. In this respect, they have not done a great job, largely due to poor UN leadership in countries and territorial fights. My observation of how UNAIDS works in countries is that they establish a theme team of major donors to coordinate all support for country AIDS program activities. I call these "dream" teams since each UN agency or external donor is essentially free to do whatever it wants to do with its support funds or staff. This loose system of "coordination" works well if there is a strong team leader. Usually, however, the group with the largest interest and budget will get to do whatever they believe is best for the country's AIDS program and/or for the donor agency. I often saw what I considered outright chaos with regard to applications for funding to individual donors: arguments over program priorities would be decided by the second golden rule – "Those who have the gold, make the rules!" In addition, a multitude of individual applications for donor support, as well as individual evaluation missions that GPA/WHO had strived to avoid, began to suck up a tremendous amount of country program staff time.

Through the 1990s, most of the UNAIDS country-based staff were, in my opinion, poorly prepared for their task. Most of them, lacking experience, credibility and authority, merely became assistants to the local UN Resident Coordinator. UNAIDS was also expected to lead and coordinate policy development across UN Agencies and other partners. In this respect, they have done a reasonable job where there was a vacuum of interest on the part of UN agencies, but a poorer job when territorial battles impacted on inter/agency collaboration (i.e., UNICEF on children, WHO on care and treatment).

Finally, UNAIDS was supposed to act as an international advocate: in this area, Peter Piot has in the opinion of some, performed well. There has been a plethora of statements, declarations, and resolutions, including those from the UN General Assembly and Security Council for the support of national AIDS programs. This advocacy has helped considerably in the creation of the Global Fund and in limiting instances of HIV-related human rights violations by some governments.

The Global Fund

The concept of a global fund for disease control was apparently first suggested by Bill Foege, a former Director of the CDC (Atlanta), and a former President of the American Public Health Association. I suspect that David Heymann who at the time was Director of Communicable Diseases at WHO presented this proposal to Dr. Gro Brundtland, the WHO Director-General who succeeded Nakajima. She went to the G-8 meeting in Okinawa in July 2000 to present this grand global disease control scheme. The initial idea was to create a global fund and initiative to fight "diseases of the poor." The G-8 did not take up this idea but it was picked up by Japan and a group of countries and eventually became the Global Fund when it was endorsed by the UN Secretary-General Kofi Annan in 2001. However, WHO was not selected as the implementing agency. The primary reasons WHO did not get to manage the Global Fund for AIDS, Tuberculosis, and Malaria (GFATM) were basically the same as those that led to the creation of UNAIDS – to get donor agencies and poor developing countries out from under the dominance of GPA/WHO. UNAIDS was not selected to be the implementing agency of the GFATM for several reasons:

1 UNAIDS declared itself as an advocacy organization and not as a scientific or technical agency
2 UNAIDS did not have much interest in dealing with other, albeit important and major diseases and
3 several of the GFATM founding countries, such as the US, Japan, and Germany, did not want the Fund to be administered by any UN organization. The UK and France were on the opposite side, and developing countries were in the middle, eager to keep their relationship to the UN system while also positioning themselves to access the Fund's money regardless of the implementing agency.

Eventually, WHO was "awarded" the responsibility of providing administrative backing to the Fund (at cost). The World Bank got the honor of safekeeping and channeling funds to countries. WHO was then called upon by countries to help them put together their application to the Fund, always within very short deadlines. The Fund's somewhat naive expectation was that applications would be prepared primarily with the combined efforts of government, private sector, and NGOs. WHO was not paid for this extra effort and staff time, which was a flaw or a bonus in the Fund's design, depending on one's perspectives.[*]

---

[*]Many of the observations and insights about UNAIDS and the Global Fund were provided to me by a former senior WHO official who wants to remain anonymous – his initials are DT.

Development of Global Priorities for Disease Prevention and Treatment

How are national or international health priorities determined for disease prevention and treatment programs? The simple direct answer to this question is that there has not been an objective or consistent method used to determine global health priorities for international disease prevention and treatment. In fact, until the WHO's 3 by 5 ART program, there was a virtual taboo on international support of "routine" treatment programs since this was considered to be a bottomless pit by virtually all international donor agencies. International support for the directly observed treatment strategy (DOTS) program for TB was rationalized on the basis that the DOTS program is primarily a prevention program. Treatment of TB cases renders potentially infectious patients non-infectious and thereby prevents TB transmission to household or close contacts. There have been some scattered attempts to assign priority rankings for major diseases objectively but no method of ranking has been formally accepted by the international health community. The Global Burden of Disease (GBD) ranking of disease and deaths represents the most objective assessment of the relative impact of all major diseases: it may provide the foundation to help international agencies develop a means to rank public health disease prevention and treatment programs. In addition, in 1993 the World Bank published the first edition of "Disease Control Priorities in Developing Countries" (DCPP) with contributions from WHO and public health specialists from both developed and developing countries. This volume examined the priority of 25 conditions based on their public health significance and the cost-effectiveness of preventive and patient management interventions in low- and middle-income developing counties. In 2002, a new DCPP was funded by the Bill & Melinda Gates Foundation. The new DCPP is a joint project of the Fogarty International Center (FIC) of the National Institutes of Health (NIH), the World Health Organization (WHO), and the World Bank. An expanded second edition of DCPP was scheduled to be published in 2005. As of early 2006, the new DCPP has not been released.

No method of ranking causes of disease, disabilities, and death (total disease burden) has, until recently, included risk factors and risk behaviors as the underlying or attributive cause. The WHO's International Classification of Diseases (ICD-10) criteria for assigning causes of death do not include risk factors or risk behaviors. Thus, although there is clear acceptance that tobacco smoking is the primary cause of most lung cancers, ICD-10 coding rules assigns all lung cancer deaths to the disease cancer. This classification of causes of disease and death by conditions is useful for healthcare planning, yet for disease prevention or health promotion a classification of causes of deaths attributable to risk factors or risk behaviors would be more useful. During the past few decades, there has been an increasing awareness of the importance and role that risk factors and behaviors play in disease causation. For example, there is no question that HIV is the etiologic agent responsible for the acquired immune deficiency in all AIDS cases and deaths. However, it is also evident that without HIV risk behaviors epidemic HIV transmission cannot occur. Thus, WHO developed in 2002 a standardized method, designated as counterfactual analysis that estimates different prevalence of a disease by comparative risk assessment.[*] Counterfactual analysis compares diseases and deaths under the prevailing population distribution of a specific risk factor or behavior to a counterfactual exposure distribution. The difference is presumed to be the avoidable or preventable incidence of the disease as a result of changes in the risk factor or behavior. This very simplistic approach is quite logical, but remains to be validated.

My review of the GBD estimated disease burden for 2001 convinced me that prevention of several childhood diseases for which effective vaccines are available – measles, tetanus, and whooping cough[†] – was inadequate. These preventable diseases need to be added to the Global Fund portfolio. The GBD estimates confirm that HIV/AIDS is an almost unparalleled human disaster in SSA. In 2001 almost 20 percent (one out of every five) of all deaths in this region were attributed to AIDS. In contrast, AIDS deaths are not, and will not be, a leading cause of adult deaths in virtually all countries outside SSA. Indisputably in SSA, HIV/AIDS must be given the highest public health priority, but outside SSA, it is more logical to give the highest health priority to the prevention of disease and death attributable to tobacco.

Challenges to International Disease Prevention and Treatment Programs

The basic objectives of HIV/AIDS programs are to prevent HIV infection and provide care and treatment to those infected. With unlimited resources, both objectives might be attained; but with limited resources, a natural tension and competition for resources exists between prevention/control and treatment/care programs. Aside from most developed countries in North America and Western Europe, only a few countries/city states such as Brazil, Australia, New Zealand, Japan, South Korea, Taiwan, Hong Kong, and Singapore, have adequate resources to support both types of programs. In most developing countries, there are insufficient resources to support prevention programs adequately: therefore, the cost of routine anti-HIV drug treatment is completely out of reach. Furthermore, international health agencies have traditionally not funded basic treatment programs in developing countries.

The 3 by 5 program[‡] WHO started in 2003 represented the beginning of international support for HIV treatment programs. The best estimate of HIV-infected persons in developing countries needing ART in 2003–2005 was about 9 million: thus, the target of 3 million on ART by the end of 2005 would have covered only a third of the estimated need. The 3 by 5 target was not met and it is estimated that less than 1.5 million were on ART by the end of 2005. In the ideal world,

---

[*] World Health Report 2002, *Reducing Risks, Promoting Healthy Life*.

[†] I started my international health work in 1979 as the leader of a USAID project design team that developed the Combating Childhood Communicable Diseases (CCCD) program in SSA. It is disheartening now, 35 years later, that these "easily" preventable childhood diseases are still killing millions of children annually in Africa.

[‡] The 3 by 5 target was to distribute anti-retroviral treatment to 3 million people in 50 developing countries by the end of 2005. In late 2005, Dr. Jim Yong Kim, director of WHO's HIV/AIDS department, made a public apology that the WHO had not moved quickly enough to meet its ambitious target.

there would be sufficient support for both prevention and treatment/care programs for all major diseases. However, for most developing countries, the tension and competition between prevention versus treatment/care programs will continue. As a result, risk and harm reduction programs required for effective HIV prevention will continue to be severely under funded.

At the G-8 summit in July 2005, under the presidency of the United Kingdom, the world's most powerful eight nations announced their commitment to "… an AIDS-free generation in Africa, significantly reducing HIV infections, and working with WHO, UNAIDS and other international bodies to develop and implement a package of HIV prevention, treatment and care, with the aim of as close as possible to universal access to treatment for all those who need it by 2010." The G-8 declaration was further enhanced by adoption of the universal access concept by the United Nations General Assembly World Summit in September 2005. The outcome document of the World Summit endorsed "…developing and implementing a package for HIV prevention, treatment and care with the aim of coming as close as possible to the goal of universal access to treatment by 2010 for all those who need it." Whether this moral commitment will be kept is uncertain. Weak health systems, including poor infrastructure and limited trained medical and technical staff, prevent the absorption and effective use of available resources. Although funding has increased considerably during the last three years, it remains insufficient. Sustainable financing mechanisms are still not in place to meet the full costs of implementing HIV prevention, treatment and care programs for all those affected. What is clearly needed is some type of regular and consistent international support, along the line proposed by French President Jacques Chirac in early 2005. His proposal would require a tax on airline tickets to help fund the global fight against HIV/AIDS, tuberculosis and malaria. However, his proposal would raise funds only for treatment and not include support for prevention. The airline tax would be a surcharge on tickets issued to passengers departing from airports in countries participating in the program. President Chirac said the tax would be simple to impose, economically neutral and would take countries' economic status into account. At the end of an AIDS Conference held in Paris in early 2006, 12 countries gave support to a French initiative to impose a surcharge on airline tickets to boost money for developing nations. In addition to France, Brazil, Chile, Cyprus, Congo, Ivory Coast, Jordan, Luxembourg, Madagascar, Mauritius, Nicaragua and Norway agreed to adopt the measure. Britain, while not adopting the tax, said it will divert money from an existing surcharge on air travel for the same purpose: fighting AIDS, tuberculosis and malaria in poor countries, especially in Africa. In July, 2006, France will be the first country to institute the tax, which will add 1–40 euros ($1–$47 US) to each ticket.

Richard Feachem, the Executive Secretary of the Global Fund, has both appealed and challenged the richest countries in the world to meet their moral commitment to adequately support the international efforts to prevent, control and to provide treatment for the most severe and prevalent infectious diseases. Such an international effort would only require a very small fraction of the current global costs for fighting human terrorism. I'm optimistic that global funding for global disease prevention and treatment will eventually be established as a basic international and global responsibility – but the biggest question and problem is when?

AIDS is one of the most severe infectious disease pandemics to occur within the last millennium. However, as I have consistently noted throughout this book, HIV is not and cannot be a "generalized" infectious disease agent. This is because HIV transmission requires a significant exchange of infected blood or sexual fluid. If we exclude HIV transmission in healthcare settings and from infected mothers to their children, only persons with the highest levels of HIV risk behaviors[*] and the regular sex partners of HIV-infected persons are at any measurable risk of infection. The patterns and prevalence of HIV risk behaviors are markedly different in different regions and populations: this accounts for the marked differences in the patterns and prevalence of HIV infection and AIDS cases (HIV/AIDS) currently observed globally.

Summary and Conclusions

The international response to the AIDS pandemic outside of developed countries was hindered by the initial perception that HIV/AIDS was an American disease of homosexual men and injecting drug users. The myths that HIV is not the cause of AIDS and that poverty, not promiscuity, is the driving force of the AIDS problem in poor developing countries have been prominent obstacles to the development of effective behavior change programs in many SSA populations.

The international response to the AIDS pandemic in developing countries formally started in the late 1980s when WHO created the Global Programme on AIDS (GPA). Initial international support for GPA was unprecedented and within a couple of years, GPA grew from Jon Mann and a single secretary to a staff of several hundred with a budget of several hundred million dollars. However, international "turf" problems and petty personal jealousies within WHO doomed GPA's ability to maintain its primary role as the "gatekeeper" to prevent international agencies and donors from pushing their way into a country to pursue their own agendas and priorities.

The AIDS pandemic has exposed the major problems and inequities of international health programs. Prior to the AIDS pandemic, no international agency or donor provided support for "routine" treatment for any disease as part of its international health commitment. Effective, but expensive anti-retroviral drugs that are needed on a daily to weekly schedule have significantly extended the lifespan of HIV-infected persons. These drugs are now provided to virtually all HIV-infected persons who need them in most developed countries. The WHO's 3 by 5 program established an international health precedent by setting a target for the provision of anti-retroviral treatment (ART) to HIV-infected persons in poor developing countries. The responsibility for further development of international support for ART in developing countries has been assumed by the Global Fund. As of late 2006, it is not clear if the moral commitment made in mid-2005 by the world's richest countries to assure universal access to ART in resource-poor countries by 2010 will or will not be met.

I believe there will be significant shortfalls in keeping this commitment over the next decade. However, I'm also "blindly optimistic" that as the concept of global health takes firmer root, there will be a comprehensive and equitable

---

[*] These include unprotected sex with multiple and concurrent partners and routine sharing of drug injecting equipment.

international commitment to support prevention and treatment programs for all of the major human diseases. This will not be accomplished in my life time, and for this failure, shame on my generation! This is a commitment that I believe that my grandchildren's generation can and will accomplish – if not, shame on them!

How will historians in future centuries look upon the international response to the AIDS pandemic? I don't think that they will look too kindly at the inequity of the international response, especially at the initial lack of meaningful support for HIV treatment programs. Historians will, I hope, look back to the AIDS pandemic as the beginning of true global health programs.

Index